AIDS and Representation

Queering Portraiture during the AIDS Crisis in America

Fiona Johnstone

BLOOMSBURY VISUAL ARTS
LONDON • NEW YORK • OXFORD • NEW DELHI • SYDNEY

BLOOMSBURY VISUAL ARTS
Bloomsbury Publishing Plc
50 Bedford Square, London, WC1B 3DP, UK
1385 Broadway, New York, NY 10018, USA
29 Earlsfort Terrace, Dublin 2, Ireland

BLOOMSBURY, BLOOMSBURY VISUAL ARTS and the Diana logo are trademarks of Bloomsbury Publishing Plc

First published in Great Britain 2023

For legal purposes the Acknowledgements on p. x constitute an extension of this copyright page.

Cover design: Tjaša Krivec
Cover image: Mark Morrisroe, Untitled, *c.*1988. Colourized gelatin silver print, photogram of X-ray, 50.5 × 40.3 cm. ©The Estate of Mark Morrisroe (Ringier Collection) at Fotomuseum Winterthur.

A catalogue record for this book is available from the British Library.

Library of Congress Cataloging-in-Publication Data
Names: Johnstone, Fiona, author.
Title: AIDS and representation : queering portraiture during the AIDS crisis in America / Fiona Johnstone.
Description: London: Bloomsbury Visual Arts, 2023. | Includes bibliographical references and index. | Contents: A Crisis of Representation: Constructing an Epidemic – Putting a Face to AIDS: Critiquing Documentary Photography – Mark Morrisroe: A Grandiose Aesthetic Encounter – Robert Blanchon: Abjection, 'Absence' and Autobiography – Felix Gonzalez-Torres: Falling out of Time – Epilogue: In/Visible: Picturing HIV in Endemic Time.
Identifiers: LCCN 2022048173 (print) | LCCN 2022048174 (ebook) | ISBN 9781788311885 (hardback) | ISBN 9781350375031 (paperback) | ISBN 9781350201194 (pdf) | ISBN 9781350201200 (epub) | ISBN 9781350201217
Subjects: LCSH: AIDS (Disease) in art. | AIDS (Disease) and art–United States. | AIDS (Disease)–Patients–United States–Portraits. | Portraits, American–20th century. | Self-portraits, American–20th century.
Classification: LCC N8217.A5 J64 2023 (print) | LCC N8217.A5 (ebook) | DDC 700/.453561–dc23/eng/20230112
LC record available at https://lccn.loc.gov/2022048173
LC ebook record available at https://lccn.loc.gov/2022048174

ISBN: HB: 978-1-7883-1188-5
ePDF: 978-1-3502-0119-4
eBook: 978-1-3502-0120-0

Typeset by Deanta Global Publishing Services, Chennai, India
Printed and bound in Great Britain

For Paul

Contents

List of figures

Acknowledgements

No book is ever truly the work of a single author, and this one is no exception. I am indebted to all the individuals, organizations and funding bodies whose assistance helped to bring this book into being. Special thanks are due to: the staff at Visual AIDS, particularly Nelson Santos and Amy Sadao, who supported my early research there, and Kyle Croft, who helped with obtaining images and permissions in this book's final stages; Teresa Gruber, formerly of the Mark Morrisroe Estate, for sharing Morrisroe's work with me; and the staff at the Downtown Collection, Fales Library, New York University. Ted Kerr gave generous feedback and offered several insightful suggestions for improvements at peer-review stage (any mistakes of course remain my own). Thank you to the following for granting me permission to reproduce images of artworks: Vincent Chevalier, Stuart Marshall and LUX, Nan Goldin and the Marion Goodman Gallery, the Mark Morrisroe Estate, Mary Ellen Caroll and the Estate of Robert Blanchon, the Felix Gonzalez-Torres Foundation, and Kia LaBeija. The AHRC funded the initial research for this volume; part of the writing period was supported by a Birkbeck/Wellcome Trust Institutional Strategic Support Fellowship. Birkbeck School of Arts and Durham University's Institute for Medical Humanities provided me with intellectual community at the beginning and end of this project. Suzannah Biernoff, Jo Winning, Monica Pearl, Mechthild Fend, Patrizia Di Bello, Harriet Cooper, Sophie Jones, Natalie Joelle and Kirstie Imber provided helpful feedback on various drafts of this manuscript and often friendship and encouragement along the way. My deepest debt of thanks is, as always, to Paul Marks, who has supported this project from beginning to end. Without him, this book would not have been written.

Introduction

This book explores how selected artists have used portraiture – particularly self-portraiture – to address individual and collective experiences of HIV and AIDS. Primarily addressing the first two decades of HIV and AIDS in North America, before the use of effective antiretroviral drugs became widespread, it argues that the self-representational practices of artists with AIDS constitute a richly imaginative response to the limitations of early AIDS imagery. While the right to self-representation was a central tenet of the critical discourse informing AIDS activism, in the mid-1980s the options for identification available to a person with AIDS initially appeared to be restricted to the binary visual tropes of helpless victim or activist hero. The challenge for an artist seeking to express their own experience of HIV/AIDS was to develop a more nuanced visual language that could adequately communicate something of the complicated task of living with – and dying from causes related to – the then little-understood and highly stigmatized condition known as AIDS.

This book argues that AIDS changed the very nature of visual representation and artistic practice, necessitating a radical new approach to conceptualizing and visualizing the human body. Its central chapters explore the practice of three artists working in the United States, with a focus on the period between 1987 and 1996: Mark Morrisroe (1959–89), Robert Blanchon (1965–98) and Felix Gonzalez-Torres (1957–96). Working predominantly in the registers of the photographic and the conceptual, their self-representational practices rethink – or, as I shall presently suggest, *queer* – the genre of portraiture while raising important questions about the personal and political complexities of representing their own experiences of AIDS. All three produced works that explicitly challenge earlier iconographies of AIDS, frequently rejecting straightforward pictorial depiction and instead self-referencing through processes of suggestion, substitution and metaphor. The physical body is often rendered elusive and intangible, paradoxically at its most eloquent in the gaps left by its absence. This complex gesture evokes the physical wasting of the body while simultaneously striving to develop a visual vocabulary that might represent the AIDS experience in broader terms than a collection of visible symptoms; it also suggested a strategic approach to increasingly stringent prohibitions on the representation of gay identities or same-sex desire. This book makes a persuasive case for AIDS to be understood as a powerful stimulus for innovative and enduring new forms of art-making.[1] In 1987, six years after initial reports of a rare and mysterious cancer appeared in the English language press, the art historian-turned-AIDS activist Simon Watney described AIDS as not simply a medical crisis but also a crisis of representation.[2] In his book *Policing Desire*, Watney carefully deconstructed the apparent 'truth' of AIDS, as represented in the scientific and popular media of the day, to reveal a number of pre-existing collective social prejudices, including homophobia, xenophobia and an intense anxiety about the sexual potential of the human body. In the same year, academics/activists Douglas Crimp and Paula Treichler advanced similar theses, with Crimp asserting that 'AIDS does not exist apart from the practices that conceptualize it, represent it, and respond to it' and Treichler referring to an 'epidemic of signification'.[3] Essays by all three writers were published in the winter of 1987 in a special AIDS-themed issue of the radical art journal *October*, edited by Crimp. This significant publication contained a total of fifteen articles situating the semiotics and iconography of AIDS in the context of queer identity politics and activism, thus cementing a critical and theoretical framework for thinking about AIDS that has only recently begun to be challenged.

The contributors to *October*'s 1987 AIDS special issue understood cultural production as an active agent responsible for shaping the lived realities of people with HIV/AIDS, not only determining individual perceptions of the condition but also influencing larger policy decisions regarding medical research, public programming and the distribution of government funding. From the mid-1980s onwards, pictures of people with AIDS were omnipresent in the mainstream media. This 'regime of massively overdetermined images' of emaciated and lesion-marked AIDS 'victims' produced AIDS as a punitive spectacle for consumption by a normatively healthy spectator;[4] such pictures offered little in the way of positive identification for individuals and communities actually living with AIDS. Concurrently, activist groups such as the People with AIDS (PWA) Coalition began to create and disseminate their own imagery: a selection of photographs published in the 1987 special issue of *October* was intended to give 'an impression of the self-representation of PWAs'.[5] These intra-community depictions rejected the victim label and offered instead positive pictures of people with HIV and AIDS living full and active lives. Yet these optimistic images could also be experienced as disaffecting, particularly by those whose illness had reached a more debilitating stage. Questions concerning how people with

AIDS should ideally be portrayed, of who had the right to produce and circulate such depictions, in what spaces, under what conditions and for what kinds of intended audiences, were central to discussions about AIDS and representation in the late 1980s and early 1990s and remain deeply relevant to current debates about past and present cultural responses to the ongoing epidemic.

The period covered in this book corresponds with the height of organized AIDS activism in North America, exemplified by the founding of ACT UP (the AIDS Coalition to Unleash Power) in 1987, followed by a gradual decline in activity towards the middle of the 1990s. Previous art-historical accounts of this period have tended to focus on aesthetic responses to AIDS made in an overtly activist mode, such as the politically charged posters and other forms of agitprop employed by ACT UP; on collective visual expressions of mourning, such as the AIDS Quilt Project; or on the graphic materials used to promote public health campaigns.[6] Moving image works have also benefited from sustained scholarship.[7] Portraiture and self-portraiture, however, have received less attention.

Crimp's ambition for the *October* 1987 AIDS special issue was to draw attention to 'a critical, theoretical, activist alternative to the personal, elegiac expressions that appeared to dominate the art world response to AIDS'.[8] In his highly polemical introduction to the issue, Crimp uses a series of rhetorical manoeuvres to establish a near-total binary separation between socially and politically engaged activist aesthetic practices on the one hand and individual artistic production on the other. The former is understood as an essentially collective endeavour, with its proper milieu being not the museum or gallery but the streets and subways; the latter is dismissed as the apparatuses of an 'idealist' conception of art as a conduit for universal truths about human experience. Writing two years later, in the introduction to the catalogue for the exhibition *AIDS: The Artists' Response* held at Ohio State University in 1989, Jan Zita Grover made a similar division, classifying artists' responses to AIDS into two chronological phases.[9] The initial phase, Grover postulated, 'bears witness' to AIDS with descriptive works that memorialize individuals lost to the epidemic; many of these works are portraits, often in traditional media including painting and photography. The second phase emerges from 1987 onwards after the political implications of AIDS become apparent and consists of work carried out by activist groups such as ACT UP or artists' collectives such as Gran Fury, General Idea and Group Material.

This compulsive categorization of artworks as either 'personal' or 'political' – engaged in the work of either mourning or militancy[10] – may have provided an initial strategy for grasping the cultural production of the epidemic during its early years, but no longer holds up to sustained analysis. David Deitcher has rightly pointed out that not all 'second-generation' artists' responses were collectively produced or overtly political, nor were they always encountered outside the margins of the art world.[11] Writing for *Frieze* in 1996, Deitcher offers two examples of well-known artists, David Wojnarowicz and Felix Gonzalez-Torres, whose work is simultaneously deeply personal and politically engaged.[12] More recently, Jonathan David Katz has used these two artists to provide a framework for considering what he refers to as 'the problem of portraiture and AIDS', an implicit reference to the long-standing binary tension that has been set up between personal and political approaches.[13] In a short video presentation made to accompany the exhibition *Hide/Seek: Difference and Desire in American Portraiture*, which he curated for the National Portrait Gallery at the Smithsonian Institution in 2010, Katz discusses two major modes of response. The first is represented by a black-and-white photographic self-portrait taken by David Wojnarowicz in 1990, in which he depicts his face almost buried under a mound of dry earth, his eyes and nose just visible enough to make him recognizable. For Katz, Wojnarowicz's usual modality is 'rage and horror' and 'aggressive in your face activist art' that aims to shock the viewer out of their complacency. The second type of response is exemplified by one of Felix Gonzalez-Torres' piles of wrapped sweets: Katz describes this approach as 'softer, more indirect', not necessarily less political but less obviously so. A new kind of political art work is forged at this moment, as in-your-face activism gives way to camouflaged critique.[14]

The activist and writer Ted Kerr has developed the term 'Second Silence' to describe a period of quietude around AIDS from 1996 onwards (echoing the First Silence during the early years of the epidemic when President Regan refused to acknowledge AIDS as an urgent social and political issue).[15] The first generation of effective drug therapies emerged in 1995 or 1996, leading to a shift in the popular perception of AIDS as no longer a death sentence but instead a chronic yet manageable disease; statistical evidence of a declining mortality rate led to hyperbolic headlines pronouncing the 'ends of AIDS'. The election of Bill Clinton to the White House in 1992, following a campaign that included several gay-friendly pledges, gave the sense that the rampant homophobia of the Regan era was coming to an end. Over the course of the 1990s, the activist practices of the previous decade had declined, in part due to exhaustion and burnout among the survivors, and the visibility of AIDS in the arts had diminished.[16] While this relative quiet was by no means absolute – important cultural references to HIV in this period include the television series *Queer as Folk* (2000–2005), the HBO television film *Angels in America* (2003) and Alan Hollinghust's Man Booker Prize-winning novel *The Line of Beauty* (2004)[17] – the sense of energy and purposeful anger that had characterized the first two decades of the epidemic had largely dissipated.

A turning point occurred in late 2010 when David Wojnarowicz's video montage *Fire in My Belly* (1986–7) – which contains an eleven-second clip of a crucifix swarming with ants – was removed by the Smithsonian Institution from the exhibition *Hide/Seek* following complaints from conservative political leaders and religious groups.[18] This act of censorship was widely understood as a silencing of Wojnarowicz by the American right, a suppression mirroring the one that had taken place almost twenty years previously in the context of the culture wars of the late 1980s and early 1990s.[19] Artists, activists and arts organizations around the world responded with protests and screenings; the artist AA Bronson requested that his own work, *Felix, June 5th, 1994,* also be withdrawn from the exhibition as a gesture of solidarity. The effect of these protests was to galvanize both old and new generations of activists, artists and scholars to readdress the cultural history of the epidemic and to ask pressing questions about the significance of cultural practices in responding to HIV today.

Since 2010 there has been a striking revitalization of cultural production in relation to HIV and AIDS, with a particular focus on addressing the period from the early 1980s to the mid-1990s: activist and writer Ted Kerr has christened this phenomenon 'the AIDS Crisis Re-visitation'.[20] This new wave of creative interest in the histories of HIV and AIDS occurs across a range of media. Films include the documentaries *We Were Here* (David Weissman and Bill Weber, 2011), *How to Survive a Plague* (David France, 2012), *United in Anger* (Jim Hubbard and Sarah Schulman, 2012) and the dramas *Dallas Buyers' Club* (Jean-Marc Vallee, 2013) and *1985* (2018), and *120 BPM* (Robin Campillo, 2018), which splices a semi-autobiographical storyline with archival footage of ACT UP meetings and actions. Larry Kramer's controversial play *The Normal Heart* (1984) was revived for Broadway in 2011 (and subsequently directed by Ryan Murphy for film in 2014),[21] and a new staging of *Angels in America*, directed by Marianne Elliott for London's National Theatre, transferred to Broadway in 2018.[22] Significant museum exhibitions have included histories of activism, such as *AIDS in New York – the First Five Years* (New York Historical Society, 2013) and *Why We Fight: Remembering AIDS Activism* (New York Public Library, 2013); retrospectives of collectives General Idea and Gran Fury; solo shows of individual artists associated with the epidemic; and the pioneering group exhibition *Art AIDS*

America (2015). This revival has been both warmly welcomed and forcefully critiqued. Specifically, its critics have argued that a memorializing approach risks canonizing the epidemic, marginalizing certain AIDS histories – particularly those of women and people of colour – while privileging others; furthermore, by constructing AIDS as a predominantly historical phenomenon, the profusion of recent cultural production frequently fails to engage with the reality of the ongoing crisis in the present moment.

Vincent Chevalier and Ian Bradley-Perrin's poster *Your Nostalgia Is Killing Me* (Figure 1), produced for the Toronto community-based organization AIDS Action Now's *PosterVirus* project in 2013, offers a witty pictorial critique of the hazards of memorialization in the digital age. Employing a deliberately retro 1990s glitchy aesthetic, the computer-generated scene depicts a teenager's bedroom bedecked with cut-and-paste images of canonical AIDS-related visual culture. One wall is plastered with General Idea's AIDS wallpaper and the other with Keith Haring's instantly recognizable cartoon figures; AIDS posters including *Silence=Death* and *AIDSGATE* are hung next to a mock window framing a photograph of an ACT UP die-in; Therese Frare's portrait of David Kirby (used for Benetton's infamous advertising campaign in 1992) is displayed above an artwork by Felix Gonzalez-Torres and a photograph of pop star Justin Bieber attending the 2011 CTM Music Awards wearing an ACT UP T-shirt; on the bed

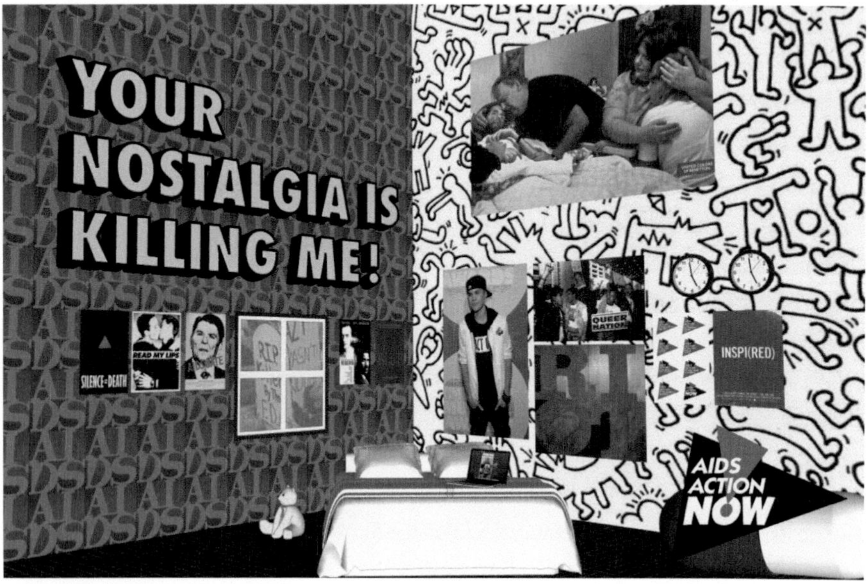

Figure 1 Vincent Chevalier and Ian Bradley-Perrin, *Your Nostalgia Is Killing Me*, 2013. Vincent Chevalier.

an open laptop displays a Tumblr post about Gaetan Dugas (the mythological 'Patient Zero').[23] This assemblage of often asynchronous visual references vividly stages contemporary capitalism's inexorable drive to romanticize and commodify an instantly recognizable version of AIDS history. Nostalgia for this period – exemplified by the reification of ACT UP as representative of a golden age of social activism – is exacerbated by the flattening effects of the internet, where images circulate severed from their original historical, social and political contexts. In a statement released on their Tmblr page, the artists clarified that 'it is not the remembering and it is neither the history, nor the material culture nor the valorization of the battles won and lost that impedes our movement forwards, but rather the unpinning of our past from the circumstances from which the fight was born'.[24] As Chevalier and Bradley-Perrin and their interlocutors make clear, the relentless aestheticizing of the past often goes hand-in-hand with an unwillingness to adequately contextualize (historically, socially and politically) the cultural production of the epidemic or to acknowledge the necessity of (re) activating the very strategies that are being memorialized in order to confront the struggles of people living with HIV and AIDS today.

When the Whitney Museum of American Art mounted the major retrospective *David Wojnarowicz: History Keeps Me Awake at Night* in 2018, contemporary HIV/AIDS activists were dismayed by the exhibition's failure to make the connection between Wojnarowicz's own radical political engagement and the enduring efforts of present-day HIV/AIDS organizations. Declaring that 'The AIDS crisis did not die with David Wojnarowicz', members of ACT UP New York staged an action inside the gallery.[25] Standing quietly next to specific artworks, each protester held up a framed recent news article about the epidemic, formatted to look like museum plaques.[26] Calling on all arts institutions to keep HIV firmly in the present,[27] they explained that 'historicization reinforces distance, a sense of "This is history; this doesn't affect me"', and therefore does a disservice to present activism.[28]

The significant challenges of (re)constructing a complex set of histories while acknowledging the contemporary realities of HIV/AIDS are vividly illustrated by the reception of the exhibition *Art AIDS America.* This groundbreaking show opened at the Tacoma Art Museum in October 2015, having previously been turned down by almost 100 museums – a damning indication of the ongoing unwillingness of major institutions to address HIV and AIDS (and indeed queer culture more broadly). The result of over ten years of careful research and planning on the part of its curators, Jonathan David Katz and Rock Hushka, the show brought together 107 artists working from the early 1980s to the present, with the aim of 'implicitly and explicitly [taking] the museum world to task for its shameful inattention to the greatest art world cataclysm of our time'.[29] Hailed as 'important and necessary', and 'epic' and a 'messy masterpiece',[30] an initially triumphant reception was quickly eclipsed by a storm of protests and public debates accusing the show of whitewashing AIDS history. A local group called the Tacoma Action Collective (TAM) staged a die-in in the museum, displaying posters and stickers with the words 'stop erasing Black people'. The action protested the discrepancy between data from the Center for Disease Control, which shows that Black Americans are disproportionately affected by HIV/AIDS, and an art-world representation of the epidemic, which almost entirely excluded Black artists: 'while HIV prevalence decreases in nearly every US demographic, it continues to increase among Black Americans due to lack of access to medical care'. 'Black Americans represent over 40% of the death toll (nearly 270,000 AIDS related deaths since the 1980s) but only 4 out of 107 contributors to the exhibition are Black.'[31] The protesters demanded more Black staff at all levels of leadership with Tacoma Art Museum, staff training in undoing institutional racism and that the roster of the exhibition be changed to include a greater representation of Black artists before the show toured nationally.

The museum declared themselves open to discussion: the curators explained that they had sought to make a show that challenged the art-historical narrative about AIDS, not to make a show about the crisis itself. This distinction was rejected by the Tacoma Action Collective, as by a number of critics, who argued that 'to make a show that does not reflect the current complex lived reality is irresponsible and untrue'.[32] Further lines of curatorial defence, particularly the claim that they had wanted to focus on 'canonical' works, revealed the entrenched institutional biases of the art world and raised the important question of why so few works by Black artists were considered significant enough to warrant this description. When the show went out on tour – to the Zuckerman Museum, Georgia, Atlanta; the Bronx Museum of the Arts, NYC; and the Alphawood Gallery, Chicago – it became possible to respond curatorially to these criticisms. New works were added, programmes of contextual events were commissioned and a second supplementary catalogue was produced; by the exhibition's final iteration, the original roster had been augmented by an additional fifty-seven works, approximately half of which were by artists of colour.[33]

Writing in the second of the two exhibition catalogues, Katz not only acknowledges the absolute necessity of the critical intervention but also expresses his frustration that 'a show that was already progressive and diverse was targeted for critique while hordes of mainstream museum exhibitions that had never included any African American or for that matter female artists passed by without a word of protest'.[34] Certainly, the criticisms of *Art AIDS America* point to wider inequalities within the art world, as well as changing ideas about the remit of museums, which can no longer continue to operate as if they are separate from the inequalities that exist within the publics that they aim to engage, but have a responsibility to construct their narratives out of direct engagement with the community.[35] Within the museum sector and beyond, reactions to the exhibition demonstrate the necessity of recognizing that the HIV/AIDS epidemic entails multiple histories that are diverse, mutually entangled and enmeshed in an open-ended process of unfolding, telling and retelling that has material effects in the present day.

As the troubled reception of *Art AIDS America* shows, the task of revisiting the crisis is an important and necessary one, yet often seems freighted with the risk of criticism and censure. Given this, it seems important to continue to find new ways to address the epidemic. In his own visual cultural history of the epidemic, *After Silence,* Avram Finkelstein – artist, activist and member of the collective Gran Fury – acknowledges the anxiety commonly experienced by many people over saying 'the right thing about HIV/AIDS, the definitive thing, the final thing'. He concludes that 'everything we have to say about it is the right thing. Saying nothing is the only "wrong" thing'.[36]

This book: Queering portraiture

This book does not aim to deliver a comprehensive art history of the HIV/AIDS epidemic: this history is complex and multifaceted and could not be adequately addressed within a single text. This book's focus is on portraiture and self-portraiture; rather than writing a survey, I wanted to develop a sustained critical engagement with the work of a small number of artists, chosen because their practices reveal something interesting about the possibilities of portraiture for comprehending and responding to the epidemic. Thomas Yingling has suggested that the early years of the epidemic were consumed by a problem of meaning: What did it mean to be a person with AIDS? Cultural production during these early years was based on trying 'to secure a subjectivity for the person with AIDS that was not simply an erasure of his or her previous subjectivity, that did not simply read the illness as the end of meaning'.[37] The practices of the three artists that I focus on in this volume – Mark Morrisroe, Robert Blanchon and Felix Gonzalez-Torres – are richly multidimensional articulations of subjectivity, both individual and collective. In addition to interrogating the question of what it means to be a person with AIDS, their work raises and responds to a more specific query: What does it mean to be an *artist* with AIDS?

There are potential difficulties in interpreting works by artists with HIV/AIDS as self-portraits, especially if, as is the case with a number of examples explored here, those works seem to resist or challenge the normative conventions of portraiture (e.g. by refusing direct representation of the sitter). The problem is particularly acute when an artist's work is framed with the romanticizing narrative of creative genius cut short by an early death. In many cases, reading an artist's practice as an expression of their experiences of illness might be seen as reductive. Robert Blanchon and Felix Gonzalez-Torres were both acutely aware of this and both feared that AIDS would overshadow present and future interpretations of their work; indeed, a number of their pieces addressed in this book actively stage and explore this dilemma.

In each chapter, I situate work that engages directly with HIV/AIDS in the context of the artist's earlier work: in all three cases, the work stimulated by HIV/AIDS represents a consistent development of the artist's earlier practice, rather than a sharp break with it. The fantasy of a 'before' and 'after' is not borne out by these case studies; what we witness instead is artists mobilizing a visual language already developed through their existing practice to address questions raised by their diagnosis and/or illness in an innovative way. Mark Morrisroe extends his established practice of nude self-portraiture and formal studies of the textures of flesh to produce erotic deathbed Polaroid self-portraits and brilliantly hued photograms crafted from medical images. Robert Blanchon's early work interrogates the expectations placed upon portraiture and playfully explores likeness and selfhood as profoundly unstable concepts ill-suited to communication through the single image. Blanchon's conceptual approach to the visual construction of subjectivity is later utilized to underpin a series of meditations on the creative challenges of representing his experience of HIV/AIDS. Felix Gonzalez-Torres' post-minimalist practice has a similarly complex relationship to self-portraiture; his oblique approach allowed the artist to articulate his experience of HIV/AIDS in a codified format that could be displayed by mainstream arts institutions without risk of censorship. These artworks all express a personal and political experience of illness, sometimes implied and sometimes overt; through the necessity of articulating this experience, these artists are motivated to continue to explore and expand the very possibilities of portraiture.

The subtitle of this book, *Queering Portraiture*, signifies in two ways. I deploy the term 'queer' as a heuristic for thinking about systems of normalization and power (including, but not limited to, what Foucault described as the deployment of sexuality and gender).[38] Used as a verb, 'queering' here suggests resistance to, or subversion of, the normative standards of portraiture. Many (although not all) of the self-portraits addressed in this volume explicitly intersect with a category that I have elsewhere described as 'anti-portraiture': that is, portraits that refuse or disrupt the received art-historical conventions of their genre.[39] While portraiture is admittedly 'an unstable, de-stabilizing and potentially subversive art'[40] and is therefore difficult to make generalizations about, standard textbook definitions of portraiture have tended to emphasize the centrality of visual or psychological 'likeness' in the portrayal of individual identity.[41] I argue that an expanded approach to portraiture allowed artists to respond to a range of representational challenges created by the epidemic and its social, cultural and political reception, including the need to avoid the visual stereotype of the AIDS 'victim' and to circumvent potential censorship, as well as to articulate the experiences of a community (rather than privileging the particularized identity of a singular person).[42]

Queering portraiture is also a direct reference to what Cindy Patton has described as the 'queer paradigm' of AIDS.[43] Early in the epidemic, Patton observed that epidemiological literature and public health campaigns were effectively bifurcating target audiences into 'deviant' risk groups and a non-deviant 'general public'. The capacity to acquire HIV became a signifier of social deviance, meaning that 'any category of people deemed epidemiologically significant' and 'all persons with AIDS, regardless of actual sexual orientation', could be 'recategorized as nominal queers'.[44] For Patton, the discursive structures governing the identification and management of HIV rendered AIDS *in itself* categorically queer. While this book focusses its enquiry on the work of three queer men – Morrisroe, Blanchon and Gonzalez-Torres – this is not to imply that queer men are, or have ever been, the only (or even the primary) demographic to be or have been affected by HIV and AIDS or to have made art about the ongoing epidemic. Art has also been produced by women, straight people, trans and non-binary people; the stakes around whose artworks and whose narratives have typically been centralized in art-historical accounts of AIDS are addressed in some depth in the epilogue to this book, through attention to a series of photographic works by the contemporary artist Kia LaBeija.

My methodology combines the close reading of selected artworks with contextual analysis, situating the work socially, culturally, politically and art-historically. (Politics and aesthetics are always intertwined, as Gonzalez-Torres astutely noted.)[45] I have found the concept of 'visual autopathography', a term coined by Tamar Tembeck to describe 'a critical image-language that transforms sickness into a site of aesthetic, political, and even metaphysical inquiry', to be particularly useful.[46] Autopathography is a sub-genre of autobiography that emerged in the second half of the twentieth century; in an autopathography, the narrative focus is on a personal experience of illness, treatment and sometimes death.[47] In contrast to the popular media representations of people with AIDS that I examine in Chapter 2, for example, works by Morrisroe, Blanchon and Gonzalez-Torres can be considered as profoundly autopathographic in that they place personal experience centre stage, paying attention to social and political contexts as well as foregrounding aesthetic considerations such as form. The literary scholar Susanna Egan has pointed out how disability and illness pose challenges to the conventions of life writing, leading to experimentation and 'instability in perspective, narration, medium or authority'.[48] Similarly, the artworks explored here are formally innovative, redefining any entrenched notions about what a visual (self) representation of illness might entail.

A significant body of scholarship on autopathographic texts about HIV and AIDS – novels, memoirs and diaries – emerged in the late 1990s. Ross Chambers' book-length study *Facing It: AIDS Diaries and the Death of the Author* offers useful theoretical frameworks models for thinking about self-representation in relation to AIDS. Chambers argues that in AIDS diaries, the author's literal death transmits a responsibility to the reader to complete the work. Chambers further argues that AIDS diaries distinctly challenge the traditional parameters of the genre of autobiography, which is usually read in the register of memory; rather than being orientated retrospectively, AIDS diaries look forward 'to a future in which they will be read'.[49] The two principal 'death of the author' scenarios in AIDS writing identified by Chambers offer a suggestive framework for considering the three principal case studies addressed in this book. The first, which emphasizes the 'readability' of the work and its subsequent survival in the body of the reader, provides a useful model for theorizing the works of Robert Blanchon and Felix Gonzalez-Torres, examined in Chapters 4 and 5. The second, 'not a survival beyond death but of death itself as a kind of grandiose apocalypse [. . .] a "flamboyance" like that of the setting sun', brilliantly evokes Mark Morrisroe's deathbed strategy of photographic self-inscription, considered in Chapter 3.[50] By borrowing selected elements from the well-established fields of autobiography and life-writing studies, this book is able to develop an enhanced art-historical understanding of the self-representational strategies of artists with

HIV and AIDS as well as a rich theoretical framework for discussing visual self-representations of illness in a wider sense.

In addition to scholarship in literary studies, I have been influenced by an emerging body of research on the visual culture of illness, including writing by Tamar Tembeck, Alan Radley, Lisa Diedrich and Stella Bolaki. Prior to the pioneering work of these scholars, much of the art-historical literature on (self-)portraiture and illness has typically focussed on monographic readings of well-known individual artists. Often, such monographic literature situates an experience of illness almost entirely in the realm of the personal, with little attention paid to the cultural context of the work.[51] The romantic stereotype of the tragic artist dead before their time is remarkably persistent: to take just one example, writing on early twentieth-century artist Egon Schiele's pathographic self-portraits, Gemma Blackshaw observes that Schiele's 'personal history [. . .] has driven a cult of the anguished *Wunderkund* which negates the influence of cultural contexts'.[52] Resisting this entrenched tendency towards monographic interpretation, Tembeck sites the genre of visual autopathography within a 'network of cultural practices that surround the field of medicine', including 'the various social representations of disease that circulate beyond the medical field, and into artists' environments'.[53] As the writings of Crimp, Treichler, Watney and others have shown, HIV and AIDS can only be understood as part of a wider network of practices: a contextual approach is crucial when addressing artworks produced in response to the epidemic.[54]

Art which takes personal illness as its subject has historically been subject to denigration, disparaged as 'victim art' and 'a self-indulgent mining of personal experience'.[55] In a now-infamous article published in 1994, the dance critic for *The New Yorker* Arlene Croce attempted to justify her refusal to review the work *Still/Here* by the openly HIV-positive choreographer Bill T. Jones on the grounds that it included video footage of sick and dying people. Drawing parallels between *Still/Here* and Robert Mapplethorpe's iconic 1988 self-portrait with a skull-topped walking cane, she described Jones and Mapplethorpe as 'victim artists' who, by referring to their illness in their work, have effectively placed it beyond criticism. Such 'pathological' work, Croce claimed, cannot be seriously engaged with as 'art' (in her narrow understanding of the term); referring only to the partisan interests of minority groups, it has no 'spiritual dimension' and lacks the 'power of transcendence'.[56]

For Alan Radley, writing in *Works of Illness*, Croce's approach demonstrates how 'at a superficial level there is a sense that art and illness do not mix, that the values of art . . . cannot serve the needs of ill people'.[57] Countering this,

Radley cautions against approaching art about illness as a transparent window into another person's experience. Images of illness are always (re)presentations, shaped by aesthetic decisions: the essential task, Radley argues, is to ask why people choose to give particular shape and form to their experiences of illness and to understand how such 'works of illness' do their job, both in formally presenting an experience and in eliciting a response from other people. As 'works of illness', the artworks explored in this book are resolutely aesthetic objects: made by artists, they frequently engage with the aesthetic practices and theories of an earlier generation of artists and were predominantly intended for display within art-world institutions, from not-for-profit spaces to museums and commercial galleries.

The period covered by this book constitutes a turning point for the complex intersections of illness, aesthetics and the politics of representation. Until relatively recently, visual representations of illness outside the medical realm were associated with stigma, anxiety and otherness: Sander Gilman has argued that historically, depictions of sickness have typically referred to criminal or foreign bodies.[58] For Gilman, images of illness are images of difference: the aestheticization of illness through art and visual culture offers a way of socially codifying and containing a feared 'other'.[59] Although useful for understanding the construction of AIDS in popular culture, Gilman's arguments are challenged by the self-representational practices examined in this volume: through these works, the artists are less interested in gaining control over an essentially disaffecting encounter with illness and more concerned with exploring and understanding the social and psychical processes through which their experience of HIV/AIDS has been constructed.

Today, the visual representation of illness is no longer laden with the same stigma as it carried previously. Among the many reasons for this shift, we might consider the efforts, during the late twentieth century, of various forms of health activism – including the anti-psychiatry movement, the women's health movement, AIDS activism and disability activism – to remove the shame previously attached to a range of conditions, including mental illness, cancer, HIV and AIDS, and diverse physical impairments. We might also consider the emergence of the figure of the politicized patient and the rise of critical and clinical interest in the patient's own voice as a counternarrative to a medicalized understanding of the experience of illness; Lisa Diedrich has located this emergence around 1980, citing Susan Sontag's *Illness as Metaphor* (1978) and Audre Lorde's *The Cancer Journals* (1980) as significant texts.[60] More recently, web-based technologies such as smart phones and image sharing platforms have allowed self-authored images of illness to gain unprecedented public exposure; Tembeck has described how the resulting phenomena of the 'autopathographic selfie' offers 'a politicized dramaturgy of the lived body'.[61]

Writing on the pre-AIDS histories of health activism, Diedrich has recognized that 'we cannot apprehend an experience and event of illness – like HIV and AIDS, but not only – through discrete disciplines and categories'.[62] Diedrich situates her work in relation to critical health studies and medical humanities, a hybrid field of scholarship and practice that names 'a series of intersections, exchanges and entanglements between the biomedical sciences, the arts and humanities, and the social sciences'.[63] The notion of narrative has been central to the formation of this field: in his foundational text *The Illness Narratives* (1989) the physician Arthur Kleinman differentiated between the terms 'illness' and 'disease', arguing that while disease was predominantly a biomedical concept, illness should be understood more holistically to refer to a wide range of phenomena including 'how the sick person and . . . the wider social network perceive, live with, and respond to symptoms and disability'.[64] Since this point, illness stories have been seen as giving expression to an individual's subjective experience of a particular condition as opposed to a biomedical understanding of disease used by clinicians.[65] Recent interventions in this field have challenged the centrality of narrative for understanding experiences of illness. For Angela Woods, an emphasis on narrative as the normative mode of human expression promotes ideas about a particular kind of self; Woods writes that 'narrative returns us again and again to structure, unity and coherence . . . what place is there for formlessness, for meaninglessness, for silence?'[66] Building on Woods' work, Stella Bolaki has argued in favour of expanding the concept of illness narrative beyond the predominantly textual, and linking it to different media and artistic forms, including fine art practice.[67] Situating her own research on artists' books in relation to the critical medical humanities, Bolaki has argued that to do justice to the complexity of such works, a new set of tools needs to be actively fashioned through a constructive process drawing on different disciplines.[68]

This book participates in the fashioning of those tools. Accordingly, it traverses multiple territories: its subject and its methodological approach are rooted in the discipline of art history, but it shares a set of thematic concerns with medical humanities in its focus on the relationship between aesthetic form and the expression of personal and collective experiences of ill health. Throughout, it demonstrates how medical humanities scholarship can benefit from a slow, attentive and detailed engagement with visual arts practices. Cultural responses to the first decades of the HIV/AIDS epidemic were significant in establishing and extending paradigms that are now central to the medical humanities: in particular, the autobiographical texts that emerged in response to HIV and AIDS helped to cement the status of narrative medicine as both literary theory and clinical practice. While literary treatments of personal and collective HIV/AIDS experiences have received significant scholarly attention and are regularly included on the syllabi for taught medical humanities courses, visual arts practices have received rather less attention in this context. Accordingly, this book calls attention to the complexity of the visual arts practices that emerged in the 1980s and 1990s in response to HIV and AIDS, reading these practices as multifaceted entanglements of personal and collective lived experience with historically and geographically specific art-historical and aesthetic influence and social and political circumstance.

Structure of this book

The first two chapters of this book lay the historical and theoretical groundwork for the three focussed case studies that follow. Chapter 1 establishes an art-historical and art-theoretical context for the book, exploring the intersections between creative practices and theoretically informed written responses to the epidemic in the mid- to- late 1980s. It reads early creative responses to AIDS – including the SILENCE=DEATH logo; the installation *Let the Record Show*, displayed at the New Museum in 1987; and work by artist collectives Gran Fury, General Idea and Group Material – in dialogue with significant texts on AIDS and representation by Simon Watney and Douglas Crimp, including Crimp's introductory essay to *October*'s 1987 AIDS special issue. The chapter also addresses the exhibition *Witnesses: Against Our Vanishing*, curated by Nan Goldin at Artists Space in 1989, which acts as a counterpoint to the unambiguously activist practices listed earlier. While many of the artworks included in *Witnesses* can be characterized as visual expressions of personal grief, the catalogue, which contained an inflammatory essay by David Wojnarowicz, placed the exhibition at the centre of a politicized national debate about the use of public monies to fund 'obscene' art. Throughout, the chapter situates these creative practices and texts in relation to the dominant intellectual currents of the time, with a particular attention paid to the significant influence of the writing of Michel Foucault. Overall, the chapter offers a framework for understanding the art of this period, tracing a shift in focus – in both Crimp's writing and the visual culture that he addresses – from a predominant interest in publicly orientated activist art, to an acknowledgement of the equal significance of highly personal artworks motivated by individual experiences of loss and mourning.

Chapter 2 examines the development of AIDS portraiture as a recognizable genre in both the popular press and fine art photographic practice during the 1980s. It revisits critical responses to photographer Nicholas Nixon's *Tom Moran* series, exhibited as part of his solo show *Pictures of People* at New York's Museum of Modern Art in late 1988, and Rosalind Solomon's *Portraits in the Time of AIDS*, exhibited at New York University's Grey Art Gallery in the summer of that year, and considers these bodies of work in relation to earlier representations of people with AIDS in both the mainstream media and in activist literature. Nixon and Solomon's work – as well as that of Nan Goldin, whose images are also addressed here – sits within the wider genre of social documentary photography; this chapter situates the criticism of Nixon and Solomon's images – and the praise subsequently heaped upon Goldin's – in relation to a specific intellectual heritage exemplified by the writings of Susan Sontag and Roland Barthes and the writings and photographic practices of Allan Sekula and Martha Rosler.

Chapter 3 is focussed on the work of the artist Mark Morrisroe, best known for his highly theatrical practice of self-presentation and for his elaborate manipulations of the photographic negative. His early work includes a large number of self-portraits, frequently nude and all exuding a playful sense of youthful eroticism. Morrisroe was diagnosed with AIDS in 1986 or 1987 and continued to work until his death in early 1989. Black-and-white Polaroid pictures capture a dramatic decline in health, but despite his critical physical condition, these late images convey a similar sensual quality to his earlier nudes. Understood as a continuum, his practice generates a provocative tension between the supposed 'authenticity' of the sick body and the performative quality of self-representation. This chapter is divided into three parts. The first section addresses nudes and self-portraits produced between approximately 1980 and 1986 and explores how the symbolic associations between film and skin are made explicit by the erotic content and erotogenic structure of Morrisroe's early work.[69] Barthes famously described photography as 'a carnal medium'[70] and often used corporeal similes to convey the indexical properties of the photograph; Barthes' metaphor of photograph-as-flesh is mobilized to draw attention to the simultaneously indexical and performative functions of Morrisroe's printed nudes. The second section focusses on Morrisroe's X-ray photograms of 1987 and 1988, which are read through the cultural and historical associations of the X-ray with eroticism and death, and the similarities of the X-ray to another intimate form of figurative representation, the nude. Building on art-historical precedents of the X-ray as a self-portrait and considering its emblematic status as a signifier of medical knowledge, Morrisroe's X-ray photograms are interpreted as complex convergences of clinical 'evidence' and sexualized self-representation. The third section reconsiders Morrisroe's black-and-white Polaroid prints, recasting the dialectic of performativity/indexicality in terms of the erotic/ill subject. Sander Gilman has suggested that AIDS 'wrestled with the discourse of the ugly, un-erotic body and soul from the very identification of the disease': it is telling that Gilman suggests that the one field that resists this discourse is art photography.[71] Comparing Morrisroe's late self-portraits to selected images by Robert Mapplethorpe and paying particular attention to the theatrical quality of both, this chapter shows how both artists employ a visual language inspired by sadomasochistic sexual practices in order to negotiate a flexible subject position that can accommodate both activity and passivity, self-possession and erotic objectification in order to articulate both men's experiences as photographers with advanced AIDS. The chapter concludes by considering Morrisroe's practice in relation to Georges Bataille's definition of eroticism as 'assenting to life even in death'.[72]

Chapter 4 examines the work of the conceptual artist Robert Blanchon, whose theoretically informed, minimalist practice offers a powerful counterpoint to the flamboyant performative presence articulated by Morrisroe's work. The chapter takes its starting point from Sasha Archibald's assertion that Blanchon's practice is 'an archive of absence'.[73] Examining 'absence' in relation to the artist's early works, it offers an overview of Blanchon's strategies of self-portrayal, which challenge the historical associations of portraiture with the bounded individual and recast the subject in terms of fragmentation, incoherence and contingency upon others (including the viewer). Works such as *Untitled (Death Valley Self-Portrait)* (1995) and *Untitled (Death Valley Horizon)* (1997) suggest the artist's fascination with the prospect of his own death and disappearance: reading these in dialogue with other works, including *Untitled (Self-Portrait)* (1991), which interrogates the assumed solidity of the portrait subject, this chapter argues that this fascination should not be understood merely as an effect of the artist's HIV-positive diagnosis but must be recognized as a deliberate artistic strategy to undermine outmoded assumptions about the stability of the subject. The chapter extends these insights to consider the installation *Protection* or *Carcharodon Carcharias (Jaws)* (1992–5) and imagined public art project *4 opportunistic infections for public viewing and consumption* (*c.* 1992), both of which activate an autobiographical voice while deliberately producing an 'I' that is equivocal and unclear. Given the text-based nature of much of Blanchon's work, the chapter draws on scholarship in life-writing studies, focussing particularly on the distinctions between traditional autobiography and other forms of life writing, such as confessional texts, memoirs and diaries, which typically imply a productive relation with a reader. The second part of the chapter focusses on the exhibition *gum, waste, indentations, stains + envelopes*, shown in 1996 at the Randolph Street Gallery, Chicago, and widely interpreted in the press as an autobiographical show by an HIV-positive artist. Drawing on the confessional form, the exhibition maps the body topographically as a series of visual enigmas, oscillating between the individual and the collective, and forcing the viewer to reconsider the portrait as a form that articulates the interplay between personal and group experience; accordingly, this chapter reads the exhibition through selected literature on confessional practice, focussing particularly on the role of the interlocutor/viewer. The thematic of absence identified and explored in the first part of the chapter is here theorized through Simon Watney's ground-breaking essay on the 'impossible object' constituted by the homosexual body, a phantasmatic entity that is only permitted to enter public visibility in a blemished and abject form.[74] Applying the insights of Watney and others, the chapter argues that Blanchon's installation plays on cultural stereotypes of queer abjection to critique a dominant discourse about the social consequences of the AIDS epidemic, particularly in relation to the hyper-visibility/invisibility of the gay male body.

The work of Felix Gonzalez-Torres, examined in Chapter 5, is the subject of a vast existent critical literature. At the risk of adding to this, it is necessary to address his work in this book because, perhaps more so than any other artist, Gonzalez-Torres has become indelibly associated with the AIDS epidemic. In particular, his work has been formative in shaping Jonathan Katz's curatorial practice and scholarship on the epidemic.[75] However, this association in itself has proved challenging for his estate, the Felix Gonzalez-Torres Foundation, who have repeatedly resisted attempts to tie the work specifically to HIV/AIDS, ultimately resulting in accusations about the commercial art world's erasing or sanitizing of AIDS.[76] This book's engagement with Gonzalez-Torres' work raises the question of to what extent it is appropriate to contextualize an artist's practice in relation to their serostatus. More broadly, it asks what is at stake in deciding whether a biographical reading of an artwork is appropriate or not. Reading Gonzalez-Torres' work provocatively through the lens of portraiture and self-portraiture, as both personal and community illness narratives, the chapter uses the concept of queer temporality to trace the changing critical reception of the work over time. It addresses a range of classic works, including the paired clocks of *"Untitled" (Perfect Lovers)* (1987–90); the series of hand-painted 'bloodwork' charts produced between 1988 and 1994; and the sweet spills and paper stacks (also known as 'giveaway' pieces) produced between 1989 and 1992. The clocks of *"Untitled" (Perfect Lovers)* establish Gonzalez-Torres' practice as one of paired self-portraiture or double autobiography, as acknowledged by Robert Storr and Nicholas Bourriaud, among others.[77] This chapter develops existing understandings of this well-known work by reading the twinned timepieces through selected scholarship on film-making, queer time and cancer survivorship, bringing together issues of illness, eroticism, temporality and somatic experience. The 'bloodwork' charts (hand-painted paper graphs mimicking the medical image of a declining T-cell count) are read in relation to another illness narrative, an extract from *Roland Barthes by Roland Barthes*, in which the author gives a short account of his experience as a young boy inside a tubercular sanatorium. By thinking through these well-known works in relation to other forms of visual or written illness encounter, the chapter aims to recuperate them as 'works of illness' or visual autopathographies (to use terms coined by Alan Radley and Tamar Tembeck, outlined earlier in this introduction).[78] Finally, the sweet spill works, which Nancy Spector has recognized as 'pushing the limits of the [portrait] genre'[79] are also explored through the mutability of queer temporality, here read in terms of repetition, affectivity and touching across time.

An epilogue addresses the ongoing art historicization of the epidemic through a close reading of selected photographic self-portraits by the multimedia artist Kia LaBeija (b.1994), which explore the artist's experience as a born-positive queer woman of colour. LaBeija rose to public prominence after her work was included in the exhibition *Art AIDS America;* she became an articulate commentator on the under-representation of artists of colour in the show, ultimately appearing in several public talks designed to broach the issue. In interviews and panel discussions, LaBeija emphasized her loneliness as the only HIV baby in the room and as the only woman of colour; it is not that other such people do not exist, she argued, but that their existence is not recognized or attended to, especially by institutions of power such as major art organizations.[80] Attending to selected works by LaBeija in relation to the themes of this book – presence and absence, visibility and invisibility – this epilogue addresses emerging debates about the contemporary visual imaginaries of HIV in America today.

1

A crisis of representation

Constructing an epidemic

On 5 June 1981, a short story in the Center for Disease Control's bulletin, *Morbidity and Mortality Weekly Report*, described five deaths in Los Angeles from the rare *pneumocystis* pneumonia. As the editorial explained, 'the occurrence of pneumocystis in these 5 previously healthy individuals without a clinically underlying immunodeficiency is unusual. The fact that these patients were all homosexuals suggests an association between some aspect of a homosexual lifestyle or disease acquired through sexual contact and Pneumocystis in this population'.[1] Less than a month later, on 3 July, the story appeared in the general press in the form of a short piece in *The New York Times* titled 'Rare Cancer Seen in 41 Homosexuals'. While acknowledging that the cause of the outbreak was still unknown, the article postulated a link with 'multiple and frequent sexual encounters with different partners – as many as ten sexual encounters each night up to four times a week' or with the use of drugs such as amyl nitrates or LSD in order to highlight sexual pleasure.[2] This marked the beginning of an unshakeable association between gay male sexual activity and the condition that would eventually be named acquired immunodeficiency syndrome (AIDS), initially known informally as gay-related immune disorder (GRID), although this acronym was never officially adopted.

Over the next few years, further groups were placed on the at-risk list, including intravenous drug users, haemophiliacs and other people who had received blood transfusions, men and women of Haitian origin and (briefly) sex workers, although this category was eventually removed from the CDC's official list.[3] Despite the identification of a range of epidemiological groups 'at risk', AIDS remained conceptualized almost exclusively as a 'gay disease' until at least the mid-1980s, as scientists continued to insist that it posed no threat to heterosexuals. John Langone's article 'AIDS: The Latest Scientific Facts', printed in the December 1985 edition of the science journal *Discover*, is typical in its marshalling of scientific authority in support of the 'gay disease' hypothesis. Langone explains that the virus is only able to enter the bloodstream via the 'fragile' anus and urethra; in contrast, the vagina, designed for rough intercourse and the delivery of children, is too tough a barrier for the virus to penetrate. Thus AIDS, Langone is able to conclude, 'isn't a threat to the vast majority of heterosexuals [. . .] It is now – and likely to remain – largely the fateful price one pays for anal intercourse'.[4] The article is accompanied by three illustrations that demonstrate the relative porosity of the bodily membranes in questions; to drive the point home, these are labelled 'vulnerable anus', 'fragile urethra' and 'rugged vagina'. The double-page spread is titled in capital letters: 'Why AIDS is likely to remain a gay disease'.

In the same year as Langone's article was published, the film star Rock Hudson issued a statement confirming that he had AIDS. This constituted a major turning point in public awareness of the epidemic: the average number of AIDS news stories per month increased by 270 per cent, as mainstream publications were suddenly filled with human interest stories about the victims of this new killer disease.[5] *Newsweek* ran a cover image of a haggard-looking Hudson, captioned with a text describing AIDS as 'the nation's worst health problem [. . .] fears are growing that the AIDS epidemic may spread beyond gays and other high risk groups to threaten the population at large'.[6] Hudson's illness corresponded with increasing anxiety about the possibility that AIDS might affect the 'general population', a group that was implicitly heterosexual, monogamous and white. This was reinforced by the development of a test for HTLV-III, identified as the causative agent for AIDS; if the person with AIDS had initially been visually identifiable by the presence of lesions, now the threat of infection could also be embodied by those who appeared perfectly healthy. A cover story for *Life* magazine warned 'Now No One Is Safe from AIDS', illustrated by three images of atypical AIDS sufferers: a young woman, a blond family of three and a saluting African American soldier in uniform.[7] The media began to distinguish between AIDS patients according to their perceived culpability, with numerous stories devoted to the 'innocent' victims of the epidemic (as opposed to gay men and IV drug users who were frequently framed – implicitly if not explicitly – as responsible for their own situation). Ryan White, a twelve-year-old with haemophilia who had been excluded from school when it became known that he had AIDS, became America's AIDS poster boy, featured in numerous newspapers and magazines and appearing on talk shows, his life eventually providing the story for the 1989 television movie *The Ryan White Show*. Kimberley Bergalis, a photogenic young woman who had contracted HIV after dental surgery, became another celebrity victim. The media debate around Bergalis' illness focussed on her virginity as a symbol of her innocence; in an article in *People* magazine, her own father is actually quoted as saying, 'Her sickness would have been easier to accept if she had been a slut or a drug user. But she had everything right.'[8]

Yet despite widespread media coverage of heterosexual AIDS patients, AIDS continued to retain its image as primarily a gay disease. This presented something of a paradox, as the very community most strongly associated with the illness (and most heavily affected by it), was barely represented in the media. Writing in 1987, Crimp claims that 'not a single piece of government sponsored education about AIDS for young people, in Canada or in the United States, has been targeted at a gay audience, even though governments never tire of emphasizing the statistics showing that the overwhelming numbers of reported cases of AIDS occur in gay and bisexual men'.[9] The enduring association of AIDS with homosexuality (in the United States) is partly due to the way in which the initial epidemiology of the disease was skewed by class and racial bias, meaning that early cases were visible in middle-class gay men with access to healthcare, but not, for example, in IV drug users, who were dying unnoticed throughout the 1970s and early 1980s.[10] It is also partly a consequence of homophobia; Watney has argued that AIDS was effectively used as a pretext to justify calls for the regulation of socially unacceptable groups such as gay men.[11] Finally, it is a result of the fact that the practical response to the epidemic was largely through gay community organizations: in Crimp's words, 'the gay movement is responsible for virtually every positive achievement in the struggle against AIDS during the epidemic's early years'.[12] One of the largest and best known of these organizations, Gay Men's Health Crisis (GMHC), was set up in early 1982, initially with the aim of raising money for research into this mysterious new killer disease.[13] Within a few months, the organization realized that it also needed to disseminate educational information and coordinate volunteers to help those most severely affected. Hotlines were set up, staffed by helpers hurriedly trained in the intricacies of the immune system or in negotiating the bureaucracy involved in obtaining disability and social security benefits.[14] By 1987, GMHC was the largest AIDS service organization in the United States, providing support for both gay men and the wider community.

Yet the gay community's response to AIDS was far from unified, and the well-documented tension between the founding members of GMHC is a case in point. This conflict is dramatized in Randy Shilt's popular novel *And the Band Played On* (1987), a journalistic account of the early years of the epidemic up to Hudson's diagnosis in 1985. One of the heroes of the novel is the filmproducer-turned-activist and playwright Larry Kramer, one of the original members of GMHC. Kramer wants to lobby the government for policy change; his co-founders prefer to remain apolitical. Eventually Kramer resigns from GMHC and writes a well-received play about AIDS, *The Normal Heart*, which accuses the gay political movement of defining itself solely through promiscuity: 'being defined by our cocks is literally killing us' [. . .] 'millions of men [. . .] have singled out promiscuity to be their principal political agenda, the one they'd die for before abandoning' . . . 'why didn't you guys fight for the right to get married instead of the right to legitimize promiscuity?'[15] Kramer's sexually conservative position mirrors Shilts' own: although Shilts is an openly gay journalist and sympathetic to those affected by the crisis, his text is moralistic and judgemental in its lurid descriptions of bathhouse scenes and anonymous sex. The novel attracted criticism from within the gay community: Crimp accuses Shilts of internalized homophobia, of disavowing his own subject position as a gay man in a homophobic society, of writing in 'flagrant disregard' of people with AIDS and of blaming the gay community for the unchecked spread of AIDS.[16] Crimp's attack on Shilts (and by extension on Kramer) highlights the way in which the epidemic drove sex (a supposedly private activity) into the public and political realm, with strongly expressed views on both sides. As a corrective to Kramer's injunction that gay men 'stop thinking with their dicks', Crimp proposes that on the contrary, 'it is our promiscuity that will save us'.[17] The diversity of sexual practices available to gay men paradoxically offers multitudinous opportunities to practice safe sex, as gay people 'have always known that sex is not, in an epidemic or not, limited to penetrative sex'.[18]

While GMHC transformed into an organization delivering care, but with no political agenda, ACT UP – the AIDS Coalition to Unleash Power – was explicitly political in its aims. ACT UP New York formed in March 1987, and other regional groups soon formed across the country. Over the course of its life there were more than eighty ACT UP groups within the United States.[19] ACT UP specialized in confrontational, direct-action activism: their work included demonstrations, disruptions, acts of civil disobedience, street theatre and agitprop, as well as direct meetings with government and other officials.[20] Numerous participants attest to the energizing, even erotic, nature of ACT UP meetings.[21] As the artist and documentary video maker Gregg Bordowitz remembers:

> We were serious, angry, defiant, and proud. We were silly, theatrical, campy, and irreverent. We were sexy. The regular Monday night general meeting was the

> hottest place to be in New York. Over five hundred people crammed into the first floor of the Lesbian and Gay Community Services Center. You had to touch a hundred bodies to cross the room. It was a great place to cruise.[22]

It was his experience of ACT UP that influenced Crimp's production of *October*'s AIDS special issue. Crimp had initially anticipated just a couple of articles – a review of Watney's *Policing Desire*; an essay on Stuart Marshall's video *Bright Eyes*, recently seen by Crimp in an exhibition at the New Museum; and a second essay on a public information video produced by the collective Testing the Limits. As part of his preliminary research, Crimp contacted Bordowitz, a member of Testing the Limits, who suggested that Crimp should attend an ACT UP meeting with him. As Crimp recalls, 'I was hooked . . . [ACT UP] utterly transformed the nature of this special issue that I did, both what I commissioned for it; the size that it grew to; and the kind of balance between, or the juxtaposition of more academic essays and more directly activist work.'[23] Crimp's statement reveals the absolute interconnectedness of intellectual and activist approaches to AIDS. Existing boundaries, real or imagined, between academic theory and 'real-world' practice were dissolved as scholars from a variety of disciplines became involved in the complicated business of caring for friends with AIDS, attending ACT UP meetings and demonstrations, and fighting to end the crisis.

Critical engagements: Historicizing responses to AIDS in theory and practice

The year 1987 was also significant for the publication of two early and important texts on AIDS and representation: Simon Watney's *Policing Desire*, published in the spring, and Crimp's *October* Winter 1987 special AIDS issue. Both *Policing Desire* and many of the essays included in *October* are polemic in style, written with a sense of urgency (*Policing Desire* was completed in just six weeks). Although Watney's book addressed the situation in the United Kingdom rather than the United States, it failed to make an impact in Britain, where it was dismissed as a defence of pornography and 'self-indulgent hot air'.[24] In contrast, it was well received in the United States; it was a significant influence on many of the essays published in *October* and went into its third print run in 1997.

Watney's text and many of the *October* essays are based on an awareness of the reciprocal relationship between representation and lived experience. Representation, be that visual or textual, is understood not simply a passive reflection of the real but as a complex force that actively shapes all aspects of material existence. In Crimp's introductory essay to *October's* AIDS issue, he asserts this in the strongest possible terms, arguing for the political importance of interrogating the cultural constructions of the epidemic:

> AIDS does not exist apart from the practices that conceptualize it, represent it, and respond to it. We know AIDS only in and through these practices. This assertion does not contest the existence of viruses, antibodies, infections or transmission routes. Least of all does it contest the reality of illness, suffering and death. What it does contest is the notion that there is an underlying reality of AIDS, on which are constructed the representations, or the culture, or the politics of AIDS. If we recognize that AIDS exists only in and through these constructions, then the hope is that we can also recognize the imperative to know them, analyse them, and wrest control of them.[25]

In Crimp's analysis, knowledge is power: by understanding the discursive field in which representations of AIDS operate, Crimp hopes to be able to diminish their potency.

Watney and Crimp, like many other AIDS activists, were both strongly influenced by the writings of Michel Foucault, the French philosopher and historian of ideas (who had himself died of causes related to AIDS in 1984); Foucault's work investigates the relationships between knowledge and power, and explores how those relationships manifest through institutions. Gregg Bordowitz has explained how Foucault's texts provided him with the tools to critique the dominant clinical discourses surrounding AIDS: 'Foucault taught us to reject the authoritarian gaze of the medical profession [. . .] we learned from Foucault's methods. When he analysed penal institutions he listened to prisoners, not their jailers [. . .] Following these examples we struggled to give voice to people with AIDS.'[26]

The popularity of Foucault's ideas among activists has been noted in several historical accounts of the epidemic. As Nancy Stoller observes in her chronicle of ACT UP, 'Foucault's radical analysis, as well as his identity as a gay man, has made him and his work objects of sustained attention by gay intellectuals and activists. His theoretical sophistication and attention to the body as a site of political struggle mirror the practice of New York City ACT-UP.'[27] Similarly, David Halperin has noted that Foucault's speculations about power 'seem to have found their most receptive audience among cultural activists, members of political direct-action groups, participants in various social resistance movements with some connection to universities and – most of all – perhaps, lesbian and gay militants.'[28] Halperin asks rhetorically, 'What book do we imagine the more reflexive members of ACT UP to carry about with them in their leather jackets?', and answers *The History of Sexuality, Volume 1*, 'the single most important intellectual source of political inspiration for contemporary AIDS activists'.[29] This text addressed a number of concepts at the heart of the AIDS activist movement, including an emphasis on the body as the locus of power relations and the pathologization of 'deviant' sexualities.

The influence of Foucault to the contributors of the 1987 AIDS special edition of *October* is clear in Crimp's opening assertion that that 'AIDS does not exist apart from the practices that conceptualise it, represent it, and respond to it'. Crimp has elsewhere explicitly acknowledged Foucault as an 'intellectual idol'[30] and had drawn on Foucault's work in his earlier research, applying Foucault's theories to the institution of the museum and the discipline of art history in his essay 'On the Museum's Ruins' (1980) and drawing on Foucault's reading of Velasquez' *Las Meninas* in *The Order of Things* for his essay 'On Painting' (1981).[31] While Crimp does not refer to Foucault's texts directly within his two essays included in *October's* AIDS special issue, his methodology is clearly derived from an understanding of Foucault's writing.

A Foucauldian influence is even more apparent in Simon Watney's book, *Policing Desire*. Watney suggests that AIDS discourse is formed by the re-invigoration of long-standing cultural fantasies about the 'homosexual body' as inherently effeminate, contagious and degenerate.[32] (The term 'homosexual body' is often italicized by Watney to emphasize its status as a powerful fiction rather than a biomedical reality.) For Watney, these dominant representations literally shape reality and are as damaging to gay men's perception of themselves as they are to the acceptance (or lack of it) of homosexuality by the culture as a whole: 'We can only ultimately conceive of ourselves and one another in relation to the circulation of available images in any given society'.[33] While this view may have currency within relatively specialized academic circles, Watney suggests, in the real-world images in newspapers or television broadcasts are still widely assumed to either represent or misrepresent a single, unified 'truth'. Watney's project is thus to demonstrate that there is not a single 'truth' to be told about AIDS, but rather that the virus has been used to articulate a range of social fears than encompass homophobia, xenophobia and a deep-seated anxiety about the sexual potential of all human bodies.

Watney is particularly influenced by Foucault's understanding of the body as shaped by relations of power, quoting at length from *Discipline and Punish*:

> The body is directly involved in a political field; power relations have an immediate hold upon it: they invest it, train it, torture it, force it to carry out

> tasks, to perform ceremonies and to emit signs. The political investment of the body is bound up, in accordance with complex, reciprocal relations, with its economic use; it is largely as a force of production that the body is invested with power and domination; but, on the other hand, its continuation as labour power is possible only if it is caught up in a system of subjection . . . the body becomes a useful force only if it is both a productive body and a subjugated body.[34]

The voluntary subjugation of the body occurs through a wide variety of cultural imperatives: in the name of health, beauty, masculinity, respectability and so forth. Attitudes towards the body and by extension towards sex and homosexuality are, Watney argues, never simply private but are enmeshed in a network of social and national values.

The dominant theoretical response to AIDS, represented here by the collection of essays published in *October*'s special AIDS issue and by Watney's *Policing Desire* (both in 1987), can therefore be historicized in terms of a post-Foucauldian understanding of models of power, knowledge and discourse. Foucault's work laid the intellectual groundwork for the work of Crimp, Watney and others and made it possible to consider AIDS as actively constructed through a range of linguistic, visual and material practices, in diverse discursive fields that include scientific research papers, the printed press, television and political speech. This enabled activists to contest the truth-value of such representations and provided a positive position from which to challenge the relations of power embedded within them. In particular, an emphasis on the historically and socially constructed nature of 'sexuality' was instrumental in delegitimizing pathologizing discourses of homosexuality.

Art is not enough: Activist aesthetic practices in the late 1980s

Among the most powerful creative responses to AIDS of the late 1980s were the politically charged posters and other forms of agitprop aimed at raising awareness of the epidemic, drawing attention to the lack of an adequate official response to the crisis, and combatting the misinformation disseminated by the mainstream media. The graphics needed to be reproduced quickly and inexpensively, and communicate essential information in a straightforward way; hence text was often privileged over image, or combined with simple but striking visual forms.

The SILENCE=DEATH logo is the most enduring example: created in 1987 shortly before the formation of ACT UP, the neon pink triangle and insistent white capitals on a dense black background are now indelibly associated with AIDS activism. The six men who created the logo – Avram Finklestein, Brian Howard, Oliver Johnston, Charles Kreloff, Chris Lione and Jorge Socarrás – had initially gathered together as a personal consciousness-raising group, transforming into a political collective with the aim of creating a poster that would galvanize a community into action while simultaneously suggesting to anyone outside that community that mobilization had already taken place.[35] The men were acutely aware that they were 'selling' activism in a not-yet political moment: to achieve this, the poster needed to *be* advertising. Accordingly, almost every aspect of the production of the SILENCE=DEATH poster was a tactical decision, informed by the creative and commercial backgrounds of the group members (five of the six have attended art school, four were graphic designers and two were art directors).

The image content needed universal appeal. Reacting to William F. Buckley's call for the surveillance tattooing of all HIV-positive people, the group initially considered using a picture of a tattooed body. However, this risked being too exclusionary: how could people of different races and genders be represented through a single image? The pink triangle, with its associations with Nazi concentration camps, felt like an obvious way to connect Buckley' remarks to the concept of genocide; combined with the SILENCE=DEATH tagline, the symbol invited comparisons between the historical and contemporary persecution of gay people, suggesting that speaking up against current forms of oppression might be necessary for future survival. As Finklestein recalls, the inversion of the triangle was accidental, the group discovering this only after the posters had gone to press; the change in orientation, as well as the modification in colour from pale pink to vibrant fuchsia, suggested a reclamation of the historically freighted symbol. The black background allowed the graphics to stand out and offered a meditative space in New York's already saturated visual environment: with associations with fashion, interior design and various music scenes, and well as – more sombrely – death, black was in Finkelstein's words: 'sexy, authoritative [and] to be taken seriously'.[36]

Deciding where to place the posters was also carefully considered. Wanting to give the impression of an organized community, the posters were hung in commercial advertising spaces alongside other advertisements; to maximize visibility within a budget, a professional sniper company was paid to wheat-paste the posters across demographically targeted neighbourhoods. The image was soon adopted by ACT UP for use on portable placards at demonstrations, the repetition of the image giving the impression of highly organized and cohesive group and creating memorable visual impact: ultimately, graphics would become central to ACT UP's success.[37]

The SILENCE=DEATH logo formed the centrepiece of the first major art installation to explicitly address AIDS, a tableau titled *Let the Record Show*, which was displayed at the New Museum in late 1987; the museum's curator described the logo as 'among the most significant works of art that had yet been done which was inspired and produced within the arms of the crisis'.[38] Just over two decades later, the logo would feature prominently in the Harvard Art Museum's 2009 exhibition *ACT UP New York: Activism, Art, and the AIDS Crisis, 1987–1993*, thus completing its transition from street propaganda to institutionally legitimated art object. As the case of the SILENCE=DEATH logo suggests, the distinction between activists' visual materials and more traditional art objects is not always clearly delineated. An involvement in AIDS activism inevitably shaped the individual creative practices of many artists; for example, the artist Simon Leung, who was enrolled in the Whitney Museum's Independent Study Program (ISP) between 1988 and 1989 has recalled how many people in his year were involved in ACT UP: 'At least five or six of us in the program were extremely active in ACT UP. We would go to the Monday night meetings, attend seminars on Tuesdays and Thursdays, and do political/art work simultaneously. A few people in the ISP made no distinction between art and activist work.'[39]

Yet despite this, the dominant narrative of creative responses to AIDS between 1987 and the early 1990s is shaped by the assumption that 'art' and 'activism' are mutually exclusive categories. Often practitioners themselves were at pains to extricate their work from the suspect label of 'art', a term negatively associated with a conservative network of established museums and commercial galleries that showed little interest in exhibiting work concerned with pressing contemporary social issues. In 1988, Gran Fury, a New York-based activist collective that operated as an affinity group to ACT UP, placed a black-and-white advertisement in *The Village Voice*, pairing an image of a placard-carrying protester with the injunction 'Art Is Not Enough. Seize Power through Direct Action'. As the slogan suggests, Gran Fury's tactics were to prioritize impact over aesthetics, public-facing interventions over museum shows and thus, both explicitly and implicitly, 'activism' over traditional 'art'. Their favoured medium was the poster, which frequently consisted simply of text, as in the slogan's subsequent reappearance, 'With 42,000 dead, art is not enough'. Gran Fury's recurrent use of the 'Art Is Not Enough' slogan is echoed in their declared aim to 'get out of Soho, get out of the art world',[40] and in a 2012 panel discussion, former members of the collective (which disbanded in 1994) continued to insist that they had not been making 'art', but rather 'propaganda'.[41]

This overt rejection of the objects and images approved by the established art world finds theoretical support in Crimp's introductory essay to *October*'s AIDS special issue. 'AIDS: Cultural Analysis/Cultural Activism' sets up a series of binaries: activism/art, street/museum, political and social engagement/timeless and transcendent values. Crimp criticizes a traditional 'art world' response to AIDS, the Art against AIDS auction, established in June 1987 with the laudable aim of supporting AIDS research through the sale of donated artworks. In the words of its curator, Robert Rosenblum, the auction comprised 'an anthology of gifts from hundreds of renowned as well as lesser known names'; generous dealers donated works by 'names like Picasso, Giacometti, Pollock, David Smith, artists who lived and died in a world without AIDS', while works contributed by an older generation of living artists – 'de Kooning, Nevelson, Bourgeois' – sat alongside those gifted by a younger cohort – 'a Johns, a Rauschenberg, a Stella, a Lichtenstein, a LeWitt'.[42] In the auction catalogue, Rosenblum describes art as emotionally affirming, but lacking in practical application in the face of a medical crisis:

> By now, in the 1980s, we are all disenchanted enough to know that no work of art, no matter how much it may fortify the spirit or nourish the eye and mind, has the slightest power to save a life. Only science can do that. But we also know that art does not exist in an ivory tower, that it is made and valued by human beings who live and die, and that it can generate a passionate abundance of solidarity, love, intelligence, and most important, money.[43]

For Crimp, Rosenblum's 'traditional idealist conception of art [. . .] entirely divorces art from engagement in lived social life' and implies that the only real-world value of art is as a tradable commodity.[44] In order to recognize that art *does* have the power to save lives, it is necessary to abandon this outdated idealist model of art in favour of 'an engaged, activist aesthetic practice'.[45] Crimp rebuffs the suggestion that art can be consoling or emotionally sustaining with the rousing declaration: 'We don't need a cultural renaissance; we need cultural practices actively participating in the struggle against AIDS. We don't need to transcend the epidemic; we need to end it.'[46]

Crimp's critical position is based not only in a rebuttal of the art market but also in a rejection of modernist cultural practices that he perceives to be exhausted and outmoded. As David Deitcher notes, Crimp had been one of the most forceful advocates of 'critical postmodernism' throughout the early 1980s, long before he became involved in AIDS activism.[47] Crimp and other exponents of critical postmodernism (including Rosalind Krauss, Hal Foster and Craig Owens, all of whom Crimp was associated with through his work at *October*) had sought to shift the debate 'beyond the self-referential concerns of modernist cultural practice to shed light on the ways power is exercised through language and representation'.[48] In an introduction to the edited volume *Postmodern Culture* (1985) – which also contains essays by Krauss, Crimp and Owens – Hal Foster posits the existence of an 'oppositional postmodernism' or a 'postmodernism of resistance' that aims to 'deconstruct modernism' and to 'change the object and its social context'.[49] Crimp's contribution to this collection, 'On the Museum's Ruins', first published in *October* in 1980, draws parallels between an aesthetic break (the displacement of the 'natural' pictorial field of modernist or pre-modernist painting) and an epistemological one (the 'archive' of modern knowledge).[50] The notion of an epistemological rupture is borrowed from Foucault's *The Order of Things*; the methodology informing Crimp's 'critical postmodernism' can thus be seen as directly influenced by Foucault's own 'archaeological' enterprise.

Crimp suggests that the strategies of critical postmodernism undermine 'notions of originality, authenticity and presence, essential to the ordered discourse of the museum';[51] this view anticipates the resistance to established art institutions expressed in his writings on AIDS almost a decade later. Reading Crimp's critique of art-world responses to AIDS in 'Cultural Analysis/Cultural Activism', one might assume that in 1987 museums were entirely opposed to exhibiting socially or politically engaged art. Yet from the late 1970s onwards, the museum was already beginning to reshape itself in response to pressures from a number of directions, including the women's movement, postcolonial discourse and gay and lesbian struggles, and by the late 1980s, selected art institutions were arguably already open to work addressing current social and political issues.[52] This period should therefore best be understood not in terms of an absolute binary between institutionalized blue-chip artworks and Crimp's notion of 'an engaged activist aesthetic practice', but rather in the context of the frequently overlapping boundaries between these two perceived poles of creative activity.

In the winter of 1987, the New Museum of Contemporary Art became the first major art institution to give space to an explicitly political work about AIDS. Situated in lower Manhattan in the slightly shabby environs of the Bowery, the New Museum was at the time known for being more progressive in its curatorial policies than established institutions such as MOMA or the Guggenheim. One of the New Museum curators, Bill Olander, had joined ACT UP after noticing the appearance of the SILENCE=DEATH posters on the subway; Olander was able to offer the group temporary use of the large, street-level window space that faced out onto the main thoroughfare and could thus be seen by casual passers-by as well as by visitors to the museum. Over thirty contributors worked on the installation over a period of several months. Tom Kalin, one of the subsequent members of Gran Fury, described the process as 'additive, like a collage': people would turn up to meeting with cuttings from newspapers, which would then inform the direction the work would take.[53] Others volunteered practical expertise in specific areas: for example, one person would bring the knowledge of how to make a photo mural, while another would facilitate access to an LED.

Titled *Let the Record Show*, the installation at the New Museum (Figure 2) aimed to reproduce the atmosphere of an ACT UP demonstration, where protesters would shout 'shame' at political figureheads who were failing to react to the crisis. Six life-sized black-and-white cardboard cut-outs of well-known people were installed against a photomural of the Nuremberg Trials. Each figure held an engraved mortuary slab: illuminated in turn by a shifting spotlight, their legends revealed a damning response to the epidemic from both government and media:

> The logical outcome of testing is quarantine of those infected. (Senator Jesse Helms)
>
> It is patriotic to have the AIDS test and be negative. (Cory Servaas, Presidential AIDS Commission)
>
> We used to hate faggots on an emotional basis. Now we have a good reason. (anonymous surgeon)
>
> AIDS is God's judgment of a society that does not live by his rules. (Jerry Falwell, televangelist)
>
> Everyone detected with AIDS should be tattooed in the upper forearm, to protect common needle users, and on the buttocks to prevent the victimization of other homosexuals. (William F. Buckley, Columnist)[54]

A sixth and final slab was blank, held by President Reagan to indicate his persistent silence on AIDS. Reagan has been widely criticized for his lack of timely response to AIDS: Crimp and Rolston refer to a 'six-year-long failure to make any statement at all about the nation's number-one health emergency',[55] and many historians have argued that Reagan all but ignored the epidemic.[56]

High above this tableau glowed the neon logo SILENCE=DEATH; the implicit corollary of this slogan is, as Lee Edelman points out in his Derridean

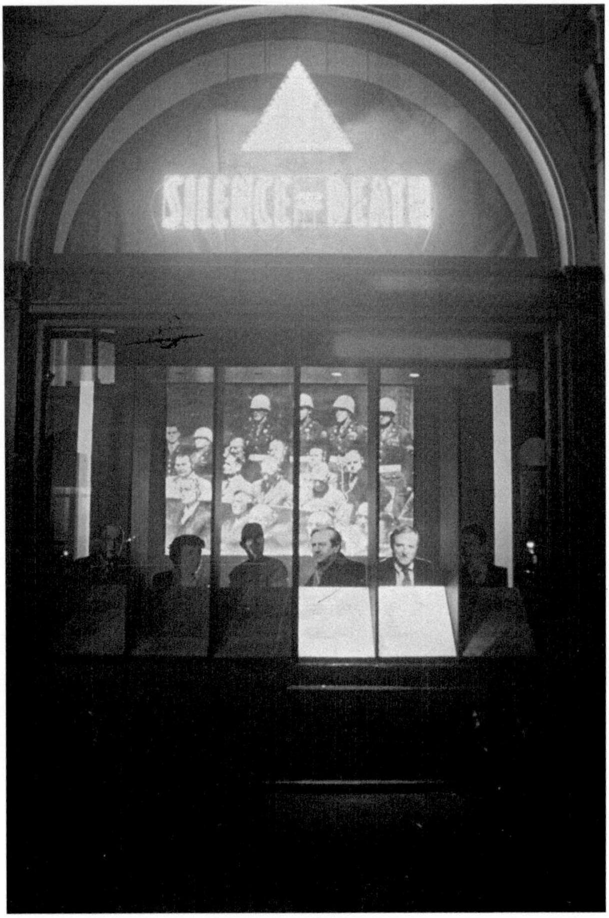

Figure 2 Installation view: '*Let the Record Show . . .*', New Museum, New York, 1987. Photo: Fred Scruton.

deconstruction of the logo, Discourse = Defence.[57] Accordingly, the third aspect of the installation comprised an electronic installation board across which was broadcast ten minutes of running text about the government's failure to address the crisis.

> Let the record show. . . . William F. Buckley deflects criticism of the government's slow response to the epidemic through calculations: 'At the most three years were lost . . . Those three years have killed approximately 15,000 people; if we are talking 50 million dead, then the cost of delay is not heavy . . . '

> Let the record show. . . . The Pentagon spends in one day more than the government spent in the last five years for AIDS research and education . . .

> Let the record show. . . . In June 1986, $47 million was allocated for new drug trials to include people with AIDS. One year later only 1,000 people are currently enrolled. In that time, over 9,000 Americans have died of AIDS.
>
> Let the record show. . . . In 1986, Dr. Cory Servaas, editor of the Saturday Evening Post, announced that after working closely with the National Institutes of Health, she had found a cure for AIDS. At the time, the National Institutes of Health officials said that they had never heard of Dr. Cory Servaas. In 1987, President Reagan appointed Dr. Cory Servass to the Presidential AIDS Commission.[58]

In a short text produced to accompany the installation, Olander anticipates the question 'but is it art?' by providing a defence of its artistic credentials. Olander argues that all historical periods have produced works of art with 'extra-artistic functions', citing Jacques-Louis David's *Death of Marat*; the revolutionary aims of the Russian avant-garde; and the more contemporary example of Hans Haacke's *U.S Isolation Box, Grenada, 1983,* a reproduction of the eight-foot-square, poorly ventilated wooden cubes used by the US military to detail prisoners in Granada.[59]

As Olander acknowledges, art-world precedents for *Let the Record Show* can be found in the conceptual, language-orientated artworks of the preceding decades. A clear influence can be seen in the work of Jenny Holzer, who had begun experimenting with text in the late 1970s: her *Truisms* (1977–9), a series of one-line political, social and sexual slogans, were initially hand typed onto sheets of paper, printed inexpensively and anonymously as posters and hung from buildings around lower Manhattan. In 1982, selected *Truisms* were relayed onto a twenty-by-forty-foot Spectacolor electronic sign installed in Times Square; Holzer found this medium granted a far greater visual impact than the typed texts and allowed her to reach a much larger audience, and from this point on the use of electronic text became a signature feature of her work.[60] For her 1986 show *Under a Rock* at the Barbara Gladstone Gallery in New York, Holzer installed a single strip of electronic running text in front of sombre rows of granite benches, each engraved with a disquieting sentence (e.g. 'It takes a while before you can step over inert bodies and go ahead with what you were trying to do'). The solemn, chapel-like atmosphere, the running electronic text and the engraved, tomb-like slabs, supported by the date and location of the installation, make it tempting to hypothesize *Under a Rock* as a likely inspiration for *Let the Record Show.*

Another potential artistic influence on the activist aesthetic can be found in Barbara Kruger's provocative juxtapositions of text and imagery in collage works that address issues of feminism, power and consumerism. Initially trained as a designer and picture editor, from 1979 onwards Kruger began to appropriate and re-photograph black-and-white pictures from existing sources, layering them with typeset phrases presented in red lacquered frames.[61] Frequently employing a tactic of direct address with phrases such as 'Your gaze hits the side of my face', these collages are often defined by the active confrontation of the spectator. The influence of Kruger's collage techniques can be found in activist graphics such as Gran Fury's posters *Read My Lips* (1988). Used to advertise a same-sex kiss-in protest again homophobic responses to AIDS, these posters matched vintage images of kissing sailors and a pair of lesbian flappers from a Broadway play with the capitalized text 'READ MY LIPS'. As Ann Goldstein has written, Kruger's work 'has consistently positioned itself within the world';[62] displayed both in public areas and within the 'private' space of the museum, Kruger's collages, like Holzer's electronic texts, disrupt the binaries that have commonly been used to underpin discussions of activist art at this particular historical moment.

The *Imagevirus* project, carried out by the Canadian artists' collective General Idea, drew on similar consumer advertising strategies as Kruger, combining these with 'high art' references, and using art-world structures to distribute work that was essentially underpinned by activist objectives. The group had been working with notions of copyright and branding since the 1970s; *Imagevirus* came about 'as a way of creating an image that could travel through the world as easily as Indiana's *LOVE* image had'.[63] The concept was simple: they took the letters of the acronym AIDS and arranged them into a logo, placing the letters 'A' and 'I' on top of the letters 'D' and 'S', to resemble the famous *LOVE* logo made by Robert Indiana in 1966. The design was first created as a six-foot square painting for the fundraising AmFar exhibition of June 1987; a few months later, it was printed onto 4,500 posters and distributed through the New York subway system. Replicated in various formats as prints and posters, stickers and sculptures, the logo was disseminated internationally, appearing on trams in Amsterdam, an electronic billboard in Times Square, as a sculpture in a public square in Hamburg, as wallpaper in art galleries from Frankfurt to San Francisco and on the front cover of the *Journal of the American Medical Association*.

General Idea were strongly influenced by William Burroughs' thoughts about the viral properties of language, a communicable medium that self-transforms and proliferates via a parasitic attachment to organic matter.[64] Accordingly, viral infection is the creative principle behind *Imagevirus*: the rearrangement of the acronym suggests mutation, while its persistent repetition across different mediums evokes both the relentless spread of the 'real' virus and the corresponding infection of the representational field. In turning 'LOVE' into 'AIDS', *Imagevirus* exploits the common associations of the epidemic with sexual activity, highlighting the constructed nature of AIDS as a social as well as biological phenomenon. *Imagevirus* was not universally accepted as a successful 'activist' intervention: some people felt that the equation of LOVE and AIDS was too problematic, while others criticized the project for failing to make any meaningful practical efforts to end the crisis (such as providing safe-sex information or fighting for access to medical treatments).

The impact of conceptual art strategies was arguably as significant in shaping creative activist responses to AIDS as the more prosaic requirements of disseminating information quickly, cheaply and efficiently. By the close of the 1980s, art institutions had become increasingly accustomed to commissioning and exhibiting politically and socially engaged art; while the critical art practices of the previous decades had paved the way for this, such extensive acceptance is unlikely to have ensued were it not for the state of emergency characterized by the AIDS crisis in the late 1980s.[65] Many of Gran Fury's projects were made economically feasible through collaborations with important contemporary arts institutions, including their participation in the Whitney's *Image World* (1988–9), the New Museum's *The Decade Show* (1990) and the Venice Biennale (1990). This doesn't mean that the relationship between art institutions and activism was always a comfortable one: at the Biennale Gran Fury's contribution, a pair of billboards entitled *The Pope and the Penis* – which challenged Catholic doctrine on AIDS education by juxtaposing a photograph of the pope with an image of an erect penis – caused such a scandal that Italian customs officials initially refused to release it at the airport.[66]

While the conceptual art strategies employed by General Idea, Gran Fury and other activist collectives undeniably facilitated a level of rapprochement between fine art institutions and activist practices, the appropriateness of such techniques was occasionally open to debate. Between 1988 and 1989, the New York-based collective Group Material were given a four-part show 'Democracy' at the DIA Art Foundation in New York; the fourth and final part of the show was titled *AIDS and Democracy: A Case Study*. A review by Elizabeth Hess for *The Village Voice* notes that a conceptual approach has replaced the more usual photographic materials common to a museum show about AIDS: gone were the images of ill and emaciated victims, supplanted by didactic information presented on video, in newspaper clippings, pamphlets and other handouts and by artworks displayed on the walls.[67] For Hess, this was the strength of the piece: by juxtaposing 'hot' information with 'cool' art, all artworks, no matter how abstract, begin to take on a particular meaning in relation to AIDS, thus revealing how 'AIDS unavoidably changes the picture of art, which is exactly what all major life and death disruptions do'.[68] In a response piece published a week later, Kim Levin accused the show of failing to directly confront the 'horror of reality'.[69] What Hess calls conceptual, Levin calls non-confrontational: the conceptual strategies of distancing and mediation act as 'psychic shields'.[70] The physical and emotional devastation of AIDS are glossed over, and the show fails to elicit the emotional response that should lead to compassionate action. Citing Gran Fury's poster, Levin concludes, 'Art is not enough'.

The activist collectives discussed thus far – General Idea, Gran Fury and Group Material – had several things in common, including a predominantly conceptual approach to their creative practice; an emphasis on text, either on its own or in conjunction with graphics; and a focus on getting out of the art world (but also using the structures of that art world when necessary). Significantly, they all also shared a focus on collaborative working, rejecting the notion of individual authorship that had traditionally structured the art market and gallery and museum system. The membership of many of the groups waxed and waned: for example, Group Material (1979–96) initially consisted of ten to fifteen members, fell to three in its second year, and thereafter stabilized at between three and four members (Doug Ashford joined Julie Ault, Tim Rollins and Mundy McLaughlin early on; Felix Gonzalez-Torres joined in 1987, when Rollins left).

The theoretical precedent for this rejection of authorship can be traced to the writings of Roland Barthes and Michel Foucault. Barthes' essay 'The Death of the Author' (1967) famously argued that texts should be understood not in terms of a single 'theological' meaning determined by the intentionality of the author but in terms of multidimensional spaces 'in which a variety of writings, none of them original, blend and clash'.[71] Thus, the previously God-like author figure was deposed by the birth of a newly empowered reader. The applications of this theory in the world of visual art are clear to see. Foucault implicitly critiques Barthes' position a few years later in his own essay, 'What Is an Author?' (1969).[72] Foucault's criticism of the 'death of the author' concept is that it doesn't destabilize the privilege of the author, but actually preserves it, via the concepts of 'the work' and 'writing'. The name of the author (or artist) is not simply a proper name but implies a specific function, suggesting ownership of a number of texts or discourses. Most importantly, Foucault suggests that an analysis of the author function can help us 're-examine the privileges of the subject'. By depriving the subject of its role as originator, it becomes possible to analyse the subject as function of discourse. These ideas were immensely influential on artistic practice and will be returned to in this book in relation to works by Robert Blanchon and Felix Gonzalez-Torres. However, this popular critical position, combined with an activist emphasis on collaborative working, seemed to some artists to leave no room for expressive, individually motivated works exploring personal experiences of AIDS. AIDS brought real-life resonance to Barthes' death of the author scenario, while simultaneously challenging it. As Gregg Bordowitz has noted, 'I never rejected Barthes's contention that texts have many authors, including its readers, but AIDS compelled me to recognize the contributions of singular figures.'[73]

By examining a number of activist aesthetic practices, the first part of this chapter has shown how the dominant distinctions between art and activism, far from denoting an absolute binary separation, were in fact breaking down at that moment in time. Nonetheless, the distinction between the two types of work seemed very real to many artists at the time. Bordowitz has commented upon the polarity between art and activism that existed during this period: 'Many of us, particularly the younger artists not yet professionally established, felt we had to make a choice between art and activism. The position of the gallery or museum seemed, to my mind at the time, aligned with the very same institutional apparatus enforcing a rule of silence about the most urgent issue of my life.'[74] From the late 1980s to the early 1990s, many artists felt compelled to make politically engaged work at the expense of their own individual practice. As David Deitcher recalls: 'For gay artists and writers it was difficult not to feel as if continued engagement in independent artistic practices amid the devastation of plague was comparable to Nero fiddling while Rome burned.'[75] This would change over the next decade, as an overtly activist aesthetic was gradually replaced with a more nuanced, individually expressive style of work.

Witnesses: Against Our Vanishing (1989)

The first exhibition dedicated to personally motivated, intimate explorations of AIDS opened in November 1989 at Artists Space, a non-profit gallery in downtown Manhattan that had been established in the early 1970s to promote the work of emerging artists. Evocatively titled *Witnesses: Against Our Vanishing*, the show was guest-curated by the photographer Nan Goldin at the invitation of the gallery's director Susan Wyatt. At the time Goldin was already a successful artist (her well-known work *The Ballad of Sexual Dependency* had been published as a critically acclaimed book in 1986) and had recently emerged from a long period in a rehabilitation clinic, where she had been treated for a drug addiction.[76] On returning to her old life in the East Village, she found a community devastated by AIDS. Many of her friends were sick, and others had already passed away. In the catalogue, Goldin describes how a mounting death toll resulted in a modification of the exhibition's conceptual focus, resulting in a finished show that was not 'issue' orientated, but instead a subjective expression of grief:

> Over the past year four more of my most beloved friends have died of AIDS. Two were artists I had selected for this exhibit. One of the writers for this catalogue has become too sick to write. And so the tone of the exhibition has become less theoretical and more personal, from a show about AIDS as an issue to more of a collective memorial.[77]

Witnesses was, in essence, an intimate tribute to a group of friends and was dedicated to a number of recently deceased artists to whom Goldin was close: Kenny Angelico, Keith Davis, Max diCorcia, Peter Hujar, Mark Morrisroe, Vittorio Scarpati and Bibi Smith are among those named. Later losses include Goldin's muse, the writer and actress Cookie Mueller, who contributed a text to the catalogue and who died less than a week before the exhibition was due to open.

The show included works in a variety of media, from painting, drawing and photography to sculpture and mixed-media assemblage. Portraits and self-portraits dominate, and individuals are often represented through portraits executed by fellow artists as well as by their own work. For example, Vittorio Scarpati (1953–89), the Italian artist who had married Cookie Mueller in 1986 and who had died in the fall of 1989, a few months before *Witnesses* opened, is the subject of both his own cartoon-like sketches and of a black-and-white Ektacolor print taken by Philip-Lorca di Corcia, the photographer who would later become famous for his 'Hustlers' series (1990–2).[78] In a simple pen-and-ink line-drawing (one of many produced in order to pass the time as he lay attached to the machine that ensured the functioning of his pneumonia-ravaged lungs), Scarpati depicts himself resting weakly against a pillow, holding open a sketchbook of images in which his diseased lungs mingle with stars and winged beings, each page rising, wresting loose from its bindings and ascending skywards. The caption reads, 'What happened to my lungs? I do not know. This is it, they turn into a book page & page & page & page.' This simple sketch speaks of the importance of fantasy and imagination in the mundane world of illness and hospitalization. Scarpati's compromised lungs are inscribed on the pages of his notebook as a visual text to be read and diagnosed, but, more importantly, as the sheets of paper fly up into the air like the pack of cards in Tenniel's *Alice in Wonderland*, they also become a fantastical object with a richly imagined existence of their own. Di Corcia's photograph of Scarpati conveys a similar mix of the prosaic and the transcendent, as its subject lies in a hospital bed, his features bleached by an aureole of dazzling white light. Any spiritual or religious connotations are undercut by the faintly comical presence of an IV pole garlanded with a cluster of brightly coloured, slightly deflated balloons, and topped with a straw boater hat. A reviewer for *The New York Times* read di Corcia's image as a testimony to the warmth of the friendships that formed this community, as well as indicating the therapeutic potential of photography to offer a temporary respite from suffering: 'An AIDS patient lies in a hospital. All around him are the marks of festivity. Colored balloons ride the ceiling. A vintage summer straw hat makes a cameo appearance. Focus is everywhere soft and sweet. For the time it takes to activate the camera, pain and despair and indignity are defeated.'[79]

However, the show was not simply a personal expression of grief; it was also at the centre of a national debate about the use of public monies to fund 'obscene' (i.e. sexually graphic and particularly homoerotic) art.[80] In 1986, the Attorney General's Commission on Pornography, led by Edward Meese and informally known as the Meese commission, concluded that pornographic images – including those labelled as 'art' – posed a serious threat to traditional American family values. The commission recommended that government should actively regulate dangerous erotic images by passing laws to curtail their production and circulation. As Carol Vance and Janet Kraynak have pointed out, the report constituted a protracted investigation into the power of visual images; its conclusion is founded on the implicit assumption that to be able to control photographic representation is equivalent to wielding a form of social and political power.[81] Fundamentally reactionary, the Meese commission echoed the principles of religious conservative groups such as the American Family Association (AFA), who had reacted to the liberal gains of the 1960s and 1970s by increasingly zealous calls for a return to 'traditional American moral values'. As Vance evocatively writes: 'To enter a Meese Commission public hearing was to enter a time warp, an inviolable bubble in which the 1950s was magically recreated. Women were virgins, sex was dirty, shame and secrecy were rampant.'[82] The retrogressive moral conservatism exemplified by the Meese Commission would, over the course of the late 1980s and early 1990s, exert an increasingly negative influence on the willingness of arts organizations to exhibit work that might fall foul of the censors.

By the time *Witnesses* took place, the debate about art and obscenity had reached a newly critical level. At the beginning of 1989, Andres Serrano's *Immersion (Piss Christ)* (1987), a sixty-by-forty-inch Ciberchrome print of a photograph of a small plastic crucifixion submerged in a glass of the artist's urine, attracted the ire of the chairman of the American Family Association (AFA), the Reverend Donald Wildmon. In 1986, Serrano had been given a $15,000 fellowship by the Southeastern Center for Contemporary Art in Winston-Salem, North Carolina, who in turn had received monies from the taxpayer-funded organization, the National Endowment for the Arts (NEA).[83] Wildmon was outraged that public money had effectively been used to finance the 'demeaning disrespect and desecration of Christ',[84] and organized a public letter writing campaign that brought *Piss Christ* to the notice of Congress. More than twenty senators were equally scandalized by what they saw as a 'deplorable, despicable display of vulgarity'[85] and wrote to the acting chair of the National Endowment for the Arts calling for a reform of the grand awarding procedure. The senator for North Carolina, Jesse Helms, took up the case of indecency in the arts with particular enthusiasm, and in the summer of 1989, he proposed a law that would outlaw the federal funding of artworks deemed 'obscene', including within the definition of obscenity images depicting 'sadomasochism, homoeroticism, [and] the sexual exploitation of children or other individuals engaged in sex acts', as well as any works 'determined not to possess serious literary, artistic, political or scientific value'.[86] The Helms Amendment, as it became known, thus legally redefined obscenity in the visual arts not only in terms of pictorial content but also as an aesthetic judgement.

The debating of the Helms Amendment in Congress that summer caused considerable anxiety in the art world, especially affecting organizations in receipt of NEA funding. In 1988, the ICA in Philadelphia received a $30,000 grant from the NEA to finance an exhibition of Robert Mapplethorpe's photography, entitled *The Perfect Moment*. The show included works of a potentially pornographic nature, including homoerotic images of nude males, often engaged in sadomasochistic practices (among the best-known of these is a self-portrait of Mapplethorpe with a bull-ship inserted into his anus). The exhibition opened in the fall of 1988 without controversy and then travelled to Chicago in February 1989. It was due to open at the Corcoran Gallery in Washington in June 1989, but the director of the gallery, keen to avoid jeopardizing future funding, chose to act cautiously and cancelled the exhibition in its entirety. His decision led to widespread protest among the art community and a subsequent public apology. *A Perfect Moment* was eventually shown at the Contemporary Art Center in

Cincinnati in 1990 where gallery officials were indicted for pandering obscenity (they were later acquitted).[87]

Goldin was explicit about wanting *Witnesses* to include work that articulated a 'gay aesthetic'; such works include elegant male portrait photographs taken by Peter Hujar; a conceptual work by Allen Frame, which pairs photographs of men taken in the fifties with those taken in the present in order to provide 'evidence of a continuum of gay sensibility'; Clarence Elie-Rivera's photographs of Black and Latino drag queens; and Darrel Ellis' pen-and-ink nude *Self-portrait after Photograph by Robert Mapplethorpe*. A section of the exhibition dedicated to Mark Morrisroe (who had died in the July of that year) includes three graphically erotic nude self-portraits from the early 1980s and a fourth image of two men embracing (the two men in the image are not identified, but it is likely that they are Morrisroe and his lover at the time).[88]

Yet despite this deliberate emphasis on homoerotic imagery, *Witnesses* did not attract the censor's attention for its visual contents, but for a powerful catalogue essay penned by the artist and writer David Wojnarowicz, 'Postcards from America: X-rays from Hell'. Written in the first person, the essay initially foregrounds the personal experiences of Wojnarowicz (who was diagnosed HIV positive in spring 1988)[89] and his circle. After visceral descriptions of friends who had recently undergone blood transfusions, been struck by sudden blindness or lost thirty pounds within a week, Wojnarowicz recounts an acquaintance's apocalyptic observation: 'There are no more people in their 30s. We're all dying out'. He reflects how his own life is 'being unwound and seen through a frame of death'.[90] In the central – and most politically problematic – part of the essay, Wojnarowicz rails against the government's lack of response to the AIDS crisis, effectively accusing politicians of wholesale murder by alluding to the way in which the ban on the representation of homosexuality prevented gay men's health groups from producing and distributing safe-sex information, leading to an increase in the rate of infection and ultimately to a higher death toll. In breathless prose, Wojnarowicz describes Cardinal John O'Connor, a central figure in the blocking of federal funding for safe-sex education, as a 'fat cannibal from the house of walking swastikas' and a 'creep in black skirts' who has 'kept safer-sex education off the local television stations and mass transit advertising spaces for the last eight years of the AIDS epidemic thereby helping thousands and thousands to their unnecessary deaths'.[91]

The director of Artists Space, Susan Wyatt, decided to 'warn' John Frohnmeyer, the chairman of the NEA, of the essay's contents before the catalogue went to press. Frohnmeyer immediately rescinded Artists Space's grant; in response Wyatt met with the Board and publicly issued a one-line letter to Frohnmeyer rejecting the rescindment of the grant. After a significant amount of press coverage, the NEA grant was eventually reinstated, with a disclaimer stating that it had not been used to fund the catalogue (additional monies for this had been provided by the Robert Mapplethorpe Foundation). The furore over the NEA grant generated a significant amount of press coverage, bringing a new audience to Artists Space and transforming the exhibition into a widely recognized success.

On the one hand, *Witnesses* can be understood signalling the start of a turn away from publicly engaged activist aesthetic practices and towards a new preference for individually expressive works. In its emphasis on mourning the deceased, it anticipates the deep sense of melancholy and personal loss that is said to characterize the second wave of artistic responses to AIDS. On the other hand, the controversy generated by Wojnarowicz's essay suggests that it was possible for an exhibition about AIDS to be simultaneously personally expressive and politically significant, implicitly challenging the polemical opposition of art or activism that Crimp had advanced two years previously in 1987.

Mourning or melancholia? Creative responses to AIDS in the 1990s

In 1989, Crimp offered a more nuanced rethinking of his earlier position, in an essay that attempted to reconcile the popular opposition of mourning and political activism. 'Mourning or Militancy?' opens by acknowledging that, for many activists, mourning 'is not respected; it is suspect'; from an activist perspective, public mourning rituals such as candlelit vigils often seem 'indulgent, sentimental, defeatist'.[92] Nonetheless, Crimp insists that we must recognize the psychological necessity of practices of grieving and searches for a way to make activism and mourning compatible. He finds his answer in Freud's 1917 essay 'Mourning and Melancholia'.[93] Initially Freud's text would seem to suggest that mourning and activism are indeed irreconcilable: 'profound mourning', according to Freud, 'involves a *turning away from every active effort* that is not connected with thoughts of the dead'.[94] Crimp admits to some difficulties in using Freud's text for a theory of mourning in relation to AIDS deaths. First, for Freud mourning is a solitary activity, whereas the modes of AIDS mourning that interest Crimp – candlelit marches, memorial services and the AIDS Quilt – are mainly communal.[95] Second, Freud assumes that when the work of mourning is complete, a return to normality will be achieved; Crimp suggests that for gay men, who have been consistently labelled non-normative by medical and psychological discourse, there can be no return to a 'normality' to which they were not admitted in the first place. Crimp points out that AIDS mourning is taboo in many parts of society, citing the opening anecdote from Watney's *Policing Desire*:

> [Bruno's] funeral took place in an ancient Norman church on the outskirts of London. No mention was made of AIDS. Bruno had died, bravely, of an unspecified disease. In the congregation of some forty people there were two other gay men beside myself, both of whom had been his lover. They had been far closer to Bruno than anyone present, except his parents. Yet their grief had to be contained within the confines of manly acceptability. The irony of the difference between the suffocating life of the suburbs where we found ourselves, and the knowledge of the world in which Bruno had actually lived, as a magnificently affirmative and life-enhancing gay man, was all but unbearable.[96]

When gay men are denied the right to grieve *as gay men*, the work of mourning is effectively blocked by 'the violence of silence and omission'.[97] Freud suggests that mourning is a confrontation with reality;[98] for Crimp, a confrontation with the reality of a world where queer mourning goes unrecognized or is marginalized or interdicted must *necessarily* lead to militancy.[99]

In the second half of his essay, Crimp broaches the topic of AIDS melancholia. For Freud, while mourning is a natural process that eventually leads the bereaved back to normality, melancholia is a pathological condition denoting a mourning that has not been completed. Both mourning and melancholia are characterized by 'a profoundly painful dejection, cessation of interest in the outside world, loss of the capacity to love [and] inhibition of all activity', but only melancholy is characterized by 'a lowering of the self-regarding feelings to a degree that finds utterance in self-reproaches and self-revilings and culminates in a delusional expectation of punishment'.[100] This lowering of self-esteem, Freud argues, is 'predominantly moral'; Crimp suggests that the 'moralising self-abasement' characteristic of melancholia is 'only too familiar to us in the response of certain gay men to AIDS'.[101]

Crimp suggests that the media have been only too keen to give voice to this self-abasement, which is characterized by a rejection of sexual activity and a turn towards conservative values such as gay marriage. He is keen to connect this turn towards an increasing sense of exhaustion as the epidemic moves towards the end of its first decade. In a piece of text worth citing in full for its sheer accumulation of exhausting detail, Crimp lists the problems faced by activists and the gay community:

> Most people dying of AIDS are very young, and those of us coping with these deaths, ourselves also young, have confronted great loss entirely unprepared. The numbers of deaths are unthinkable: Lovers, friends, acquaintances, and community members have fallen ill and died. Many have lost upwards of a hundred people. Apart from the deaths, we contend with the gruesome illness itself, acting as caretakers, often for very extended periods, making innumerable hospital visits, providing emotional support, negotiating out wholly inadequate and inhuman health care and social welfare systems, keeping abreast of experimental treatment therapies. Some of us have learned as much or more than most doctors about the complex medicine of AIDS. Added to the caretaking and loss of others is often the need to monitor and make treatment decisions about our own HIV illness, or face anxiety about our own health status.
>
> Through the turmoil imposed by illness and death, the rest of society offers little support or even acknowledgement. On the contrary, we are blamed, belittled, excluded, derided. We are discriminated against, lose our housing and jobs, denied medical and life insurance. Every public agency whose job it is to combat the epidemic has been slow to act, failed entirely, or been deliberately counterproductive. We have therefore had to provide out own centres for support, care, and education and even fund and conduct our own treatment research. We have had to rebuild our devastated community and culture, reconstruct our sexual relationships, reinvent our sexual pleasure. Despite great achievements in so short a time and under such adversity, the dominant media still pictures us only as wasting deathbed victims; we have therefore had to wage a war of representation, too.
>
> Frustration, anger, rage, and outrage, fear, and terror, shame and guilt, sadness and despair – it is not surprising that we feel these things; what is surprising is when we don't. For those who feel only a deadening numbness or constant depression, militant rage may well be unimaginable [. . .][102]

Reflecting back on this essay from the vantage of 1992, Crimp writes:

> Throughout the early 1990s AIDS became increasingly an unbearable and therefore more deeply repressed topic, AIDS activism became virtually invisible, and gay politics moved steadily Rightward. I had begun to see this configuration of repression, trouble among activists, and moralistic politics at the turn of the decade. 'Mourning and Militancy' [. . .] was my first attempt to theorize this turn.[103]

The social turnaway from activism corresponds with a slowing in creative production from activist collectives and a change in the kind of artwork about AIDS that was exhibited by institutions. Activist slogans and interventions began to decline and the 'elegiac' style of work of which Crimp has initially been so dismissive became more prevalent. In 1992, *From Media to Metaphor: Art about AIDS* opened in New York and subsequently toured the United States and Canada for two years. The exhibition covered a wide range of different art practices, from the photographic documentation of activism (Ellen B. Neipris and Diane Neumaier), to photographic portraits of people with AIDS (Nicholas Nixon, Gypsy Ray, Jane Rosett and Rosalind Solomon), to conceptual works (Felix Gonzales-Torres). Roberta Smith, writing for *The New York Times*, suggested that the show revealed how the politically motivated, media-orientated work of the mid-1980s had increasingly given way to a more personal and metaphorical style of art.[104] *Significant Losses: Artists Who Have Died from AIDS*, held at the University of Maryland Art Gallery in 1994, suggested that AIDS was perceived as a less pressing issue than in previous years and that numbers of new artworks being created about AIDS were declining. Actively historicizing the epidemic, *Significant Losses* aimed to consider the effect that AIDS had had on the art world: 'AIDS has changed the way in which art is conceptualised, produced and critiqued. Art will never be the same, ever again.'[105]

Writing in 1996, David Deitcher described the cultural perspective of the late 1990s as 'quietist', lamenting:

> Scare indeed is the rancour – but also the acerbic style and wit – of the AIDS activist graphics that once peppered public space to incite anger about the government's neglect of AIDS. Gone as well is the art that exploited the prestige and public reach of prominent art institutions to memorialize the dead, galvanize the living, and counter the popular media construction of AIDS as the natural – and inevitably fatal – consequence of behaviours that the majority disdains to this day as sinful or antisocial.[106]

Many activist-orientated creative collectives dissolved or disbanded: two key members of General Idea, Felix Partz and George Zontal, have both died in 1994, leaving AA Bronson as the only surviving member. Gran Fury split in that same year, issuing a collective statement suggesting that the original strategies of AIDS activism had become outmoded.[107] Group Material separated in 1996, following the death of Felix Gonzalez-Torres.

The period from 1996 until approximately 2010 is often understood as one of 'quietism', to use Dietcher's term. This is not to say that cultural production addressing AIDS came to a total standstill in this period. Dion Kagan's book *Positive Images* (2018) explores a range of popular visual culture (predominantly film and television) and written literature about AIDS produced during the first fifteen years after 1996, a period that he describes as the 'post-crisis' period.[108] However, a detailed history of fine art practices responding to HIV/AIDS during this period remains unwritten, although it is unfortunately beyond the scope of this present book.

This chapter has outlined the theoretical, artistic and institutional background to cultural production during the first sixteen years of the epidemic, with a particular focus on the perceived tensions between activist and fine art practices. It has examined a range of activist aesthetic practices in the late 1980s, including the installation *Let the Record Show*, selected posters by Gran Fury, the *Imagevirus* project by General Idea, and exhibitions by Group Material. It has compared these practices to the predominantly personal, emotionally expressive works included in the exhibition *Witnesses: Against Our Vanishing*, curated by Nan Goldin at Artists Space in 1989, arguing that this exhibition symbolizes an affective turning point from 'militancy' to 'melancholia' (to use Crimp's terms). The following chapter will consider how this intellectual heritage shaped critical responses to the photographic portraits of people with HIV and AIDS that were circulated and displayed in museums and other fine-art contexts from 1988 onwards.

2

Putting a face to AIDS

Critiquing documentary portrait photography

Nicholas Nixon's *Tom Moran* series, displayed as part of his solo show *Pictures of People* at New York's Museum of Modern Art in late 1988, and Rosalind Solomon's *Portraits in the Time of AIDS*, exhibited at New York University's Grey Art Gallery in the summer of that year, are acknowledged as the first photographic portraits of people with AIDS to be exhibited by mainstream art institutions.[1] While many professional art critics praised Nixon and Solomon's efforts to bring a taboo topic to a wider audience, their projects also attracted intense criticism from members of the communities most affected by AIDS, with Nixon's exhibition occasioning a modest but important demonstration by ACT UP, where protesters complained that his sensationalist images portrayed people with AIDS as silent victims and AIDS as a death sentence. Within a year, two influential essays had added to the criticism of Nixon and (to a lesser extent) Solomon: Douglas Crimp's 'Portraits of People with AIDS', first presented at the conference 'Representing AIDS' in November 1988, and Jan Zita Grover's 'Visible Lesions: Images of the PWA', first published in *Afterimage* in summer 1989.[2] Today, there is emerging recognition for Nixon and Solomon's images as urgent, complex portrayals of people with AIDS made and received at a particular historical moment. This chapter contextualizes the hostile reception of these images by situating Crimp and Grover's responses in relation to a particular intellectual heritage, exemplified by a rich literature of 'anti-photography' photography criticism that emerged in the late 1970s and early 1980s.

Early photographic portraits of people with AIDS

Between 1981 and 1982, AIDS was rarely visible in mainstream visual culture: the microscopic views of biopsy specimens and close-ups of KS lesions that appeared in medical journals were intended only for an expert clinical audience, and in any case were radically abstracted from any recognizable human referent. Early articles in the gay press, the only other medium at that point interested in the epidemic, tended to duplicate these scientific emblems, so that in these first two years AIDS was almost wholly represented in non-figurative terms as a depersonalized medical conundrum as opposed to a health condition experienced by real people.[3]

Until 1984, people with AIDS could be legally discriminated against in the United States in terms of medical care, jobs and housing; understandably people diagnosed with AIDS were reluctant to put themselves at risk by making themselves publicly visible.[4] However, a small number did speak to the media, often in the hope of adding a human dimension to the emerging narrative. Kenny Ramsauer became one of the earliest 'faces of AIDS' after appearing on *ABC* network's May 1983 coverage of the unfolding epidemic. The show's researchers had contacted Gay Men's Health Crisis in New York and found several eloquent HIV-positive men. Deciding that these men looked insufficiently sick, the search continued until they found Ramsauer, whose previously handsome face was spectacularly disfigured by an AIDS-related skin condition. Following the broadcast, Ramsauer's image was disseminated internationally, with articles appearing in *Paris Match*, *Photo* (Paris) and the British *Sunday People*. The same photograph appeared in all three publications and pictured Ramsauer celebrating his twenty-eighth birthday from a wheelchair, accompanied by his male partner. In the spread of *Photo,* the distinction between 'healthy' and 'sick' is clearly delineated by the inclusion of two snapshots of Ramsauer taken a few years previously, one depicting a luxuriously moustached young man staring seductively into the camera and the other displaying his handsome physique in a pair of bathing shorts. The use of 'before' and 'after' images would subsequently become a standard feature of AIDS reportage, while the extreme virility conveyed by Ramsauer's earlier images also implied a covert moral judgement: AIDS as the outcome of sexual excess. Contextualized by the caption 'Taken four days before his death',[5] the triptych of images confirmed the network researchers' initial preconceptions of AIDS as a radically debilitating death sentence.

The media coverage of Ramsauer, and later, of other people with AIDS, served to strengthen the imaginary boundary between the ill or at-risk and what the media disingenuously referred to as the 'general population'. Writing in the late 1980s, Sander Gilman argued that images of AIDS should be understood as part of an ongoing psycho-social attempt to control disease by situating it within a rigid cultural framework.[6] For Gilman, the Western conception of disease is shaped by the fear of one's own potential disintegration, projected out onto the world in order to domesticate it by othering it.[7] In his dramatic facial disfigurement, his disability (signalled by his wheelchair), even in his sexual orientation (implied by the presence of his partner), Ramsauer represented the ultimate 'other' onto which an international media could displace a vast range of cultural anxieties about AIDS.

Visual conventions used to protect the privacy of people with AIDS in the media often had the effect of reinforcing their perceived otherness. It was common practice to obscure the subject's identity through the use of backlighting and silhouette; since the same convention was often used to protect the identities of convicted criminals, it had the unfortunate consequence of reinforcing the latent notion that being an HIV carrier was a form of criminality. This effect was often achieved by photographing the subject in a darkened room in front of a brightly lit window, further implying the complete exclusion of the person with AIDS from everyday life. Grover suggests that in such encounters, contrary to the media's stated intention to 'humanize' AIDS, the person with AIDS 'did not become *more like "us"*: his status as pariah was, if anything, reinforced'.[8]

The media's emphasis on gay men served to further stress the supposed binary distinction between those who were and were not at risk.[9] Simon Watney has suggested that the 'spectacle of AIDS' was almost exclusively played out upon the 'homosexual body' – not as an ontological reality but as a phantasm constructed through AIDS representations and commentary.[10] Writing in 1987, Watney described the dominant visual representation of AIDS as a diptych: on one side, the scientific image of the microscopic HIV retrovirus 'made to appear, by means of electron microscopy or reconstructive computer graphics, like a huge technicolor asteroid', and on the other, the over-determined figure of the 'AIDS victim', '"withered, wrinkled and loathsome of visage" – the authentic cadaver of Dorian Gray'.[11] As Watney noted, such images had an 'ideally interpellated spectator', who already 'knows' all he needs to know about AIDS. The purpose of such images was thus not to educate, nor to elicit sympathy, but to 'ensure that the subject of AIDS is "correctly" identified and that any possibility of positive sympathetic identification *with* actual people with AIDS is entirely expunged from the field of vision'.[12]

Stuart Marshall's 1984 video *Bright Eyes* (made for British television but widely exhibited in the United States) situates AIDS representations in relation to the historical usage of photography in the construction of the deviant gay man as an object of medical knowledge.[13] The video opens with a parodic sequence of a speeding ambulance and a masked orderly rushing a man on a trolley down a hospital corridor, pushing bystanders out of the way and shouting, 'Stand back! This man has AIDS and is highly infectious'. Red letters spell out 'MORAL PANIC PRODUCTIONS PRESENTS . . . BRIGHT EYES', before the camera cuts to a montage of newspaper clippings of AIDS coverage, including the *Sunday People's* article on Ramsauer, complete with before-and-after pictures and titled 'What the Gay Plague did to Handsome Kenny' (Figure 3). The scene then changes to feature a Victorian doctor, who proclaims that 'photography is the art of truth' and 'the camera presents things as they are', making it an ideal medium for the needs of medical science. Black-and-white photographs of pathologized 'types' are matched with a voice-over discussing the attempts of the nineteenth-century criminologist Cesare Lombroso to classify criminals by their physiognomy.[14] When the camera returns to the *Sunday People's* coverage of Ramsauer, the imagery is accompanied by an off-screen voice reading from Havelock Ellis' *The Criminal* (1890), a text which details the characteristics attributed to certain criminal types.[15] As this disembodied voice declares that

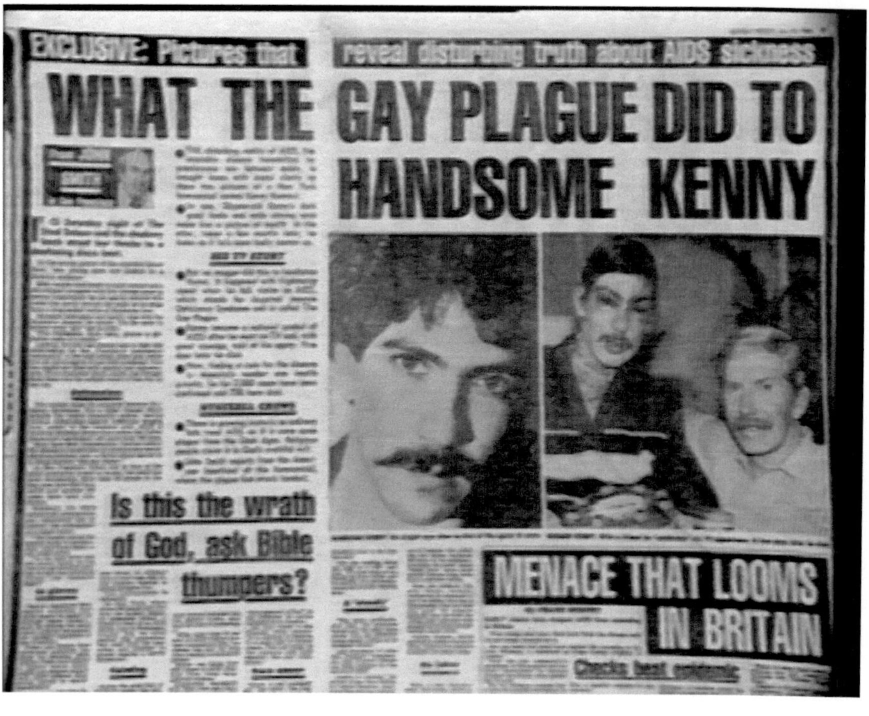
EXCLUSIVE: Pictures that reveal disturbing truth about AIDS sickness
WHAT THE GAY PLAGUE DID TO HANDSOME KENNY
Is this the wrath of God, ask Bible thumpers?
MENACE THAT LOOMS IN BRITAIN

Figure 3 Still from Stuart Marshall, *Bright Eyes*, 1984. Stuart Marshall c/o LUX.

'in those guilty of sexual offences Lombroso finds the eyes nearly always bright', the camera cuts to a close-up of Ramsauer's eyes in the 'before' photograph and then slowly pans down to the caption: 'Handsome Kenny: his bright eyes show no hint of the agony to come'. The voice-over continues to read from Ellis' text: 'the voice either rough or cracked; the face generally delicate, except in the development of the jaws, and the eyelids and lips swollen', as the camera moves back to the 'after' image of Ramsauer, his face puffy and engorged with illness.

When the media did depict heteronormative people with AIDS, their 'innocence' was conveyed via the inclusion of family members, pets and cuddly toys. Gay men were rarely depicted being cared for by friends and lovers but more frequently photographed in a suburban family environment: as Grover noted, 'it was only after being shorn of his sexuality and his identity as a gay man that he could be returned, neutered, to his mother and father, enfolded once again within the nuclear family, and die in peace'.[16] Grover's observation relates to the cultural difficulty of reconciling the sick body with the sensual one.[17] Douglas Crimp suggested that the reason so many people with AIDS, and especially gay men, were portrayed as desperately ill, was not that the images are intended to overcome a cultural fear of death and disease, nor merely to reinforce the status of people with AIDS as pariahs. Nor was it simply a straightforward question of homophobia, although that undeniably played a part. Rather, pictures such as that of Ramsauer constituted 'phobic images' that communicated a collective terror of imaging the person with AIDS as still sexual.[18] This phobia finds its ultimate expression in the figure of 'Patient Zero' in Randy Shilts' 1987 bestseller *And the Band Played On*: aware that he carries a highly contagious disease, the fictional Patient Zero continues to frequent the promiscuous milieu of the bathhouses, taking a pantomime villain's delight in bringing the visible signs of his illness to his victims' attention.[19]

The images discussed thus far presume a normatively heterosexual and healthy audience: as Grover put it: '*Whose* picture of health/sickness? and *for whom*? and in the service of *what*?'[20] Grover proposed that 'intra-community' images might offer a corrective to dominant media stereotypes. Jane Rosett's photographs typically represent people with AIDS in empowered and active roles, and were used to illustrate community literature such as the *PWA Coalition Newline* and *Surviving and Thriving with AIDS: Hints for the Newly Diagnosed*.[21] An image taken in 1987 depicts a tanned young man dressed in a white T-shirt and shades, his muscular arms holding aloft a sign which reads: 'Living with AIDS, 2 years, 3 months and counting! No thanks to you Mr Reagan'. The caption informs us that this is an ACT UP demonstration, held outside one of New York's officially designated AIDS Treatment Evaluation Units. Another image takes the form of a portrait, depicting (the caption informs us) 'Joseph Foulon, board member of the PWA Coalition and National Association of People with AIDS, with his lover Mark Senak, 1986. Foulon died in June 1987'. Taken in profile, the image reveals a smiling man in apparently good health, with tanned skin and a lustrous head of hair. His partner is crouched to his far side, his head inclined against Foulon's body, making Foulon appear strong and protective. The image is in stark contrast to earlier images of AIDS: not only is it of two men in a demonstrably caring relationship but Foulon is depicted as active and healthy and described in terms of his political work rather than simply labelled as a passive sufferer. Gregg Bordowitz and David Deitcher have described the distinction between media and activist imagery as part of a cultural transformation of the person with AIDS from passive victim to empowered street fighting guerrilla.[22] This rebranding was not without its difficulties in that it simply replaced negative images with positive ones, substituting 'the good PWA for the bad, the apparently healthy for the visibly ill, the active for the passive, the exceptional for the ordinary'.[23] As Crimp's remark shows, by the late 1980s more nuanced representations were desperately needed. Yet, as the case studies of Nixon's and Solomon's work demonstrate, documentary art photography would ultimately be deemed unable to rise to that challenge.

Nicholas Nixon's *Tom Moran* series and Rosalind Solomon's *Portraits in the Time of AIDS*

Nicholas Nixon was an established mid-career photographer by the time his first portraits of people with AIDS portraits were shown in *Pictures of People* at the Museum of Modern Art in late 1988. Prior to conceiving the idea for *People with AIDS*, Nixon had no previous association with anyone HIV positive. In the foreword to their book he and his wife admit that 'when we began the project, we did not know much about illness' and reveal their difficulty in acquiring potential subjects: 'we didn't know how to find those people even to begin with. They were hidden, undercover, private'.[24] Eventually the Nixons contacted the AIDS Action Committee in Boston; it was agreed that they could print an appeal in the committee's newsletter if they undertook a week-long training course. Over fifty people replied to the call, although many of these respondents dropped out when they learnt more about what the project entailed. The remaining fifteen that agreed to be photographed cited a range of motivations. Some wanted to show that it was possible to live well with AIDS, others wanted to gain control over a disease that had rendered them otherwise powerless; one simply stated that he wanted to be famous.

For *Pictures of People* Nixon had chosen to display what he described as 'the richest of the sequences' from this project, which was then still a work in progress.[25] These twelve pictures trace the decline and death of Tom Moran, a 37-year-old single white man from the Boston suburbs. Taken at approximately monthly intervals between July 1987 and February 1988, the images communicate a narrative of deterioration, with Moran becoming visibly weaker as the sequence progresses. The series starts with a closely cropped double portrait of Moran and his mother, who appears to be physically supporting him. The older woman's face dominates two-thirds of the composition, and her hand cups her son's chin to allow his gaze to meet that of the camera; in doing so, she obscures part of his face. Subsequent images show Moran alone and usually seated, either encased in bulky layers that make him appear tiny and childlike or partially dressed so as to reveal his wasted frame. Nixon is clearly keen to accentuate the extreme frailty of his subject's body; in the five shots that are taken unclothed, light and shadows are used to highlight a painfully protruding spine or emphasize a sunken ribcage and hollow chest. By the final three frames Moran is horizontal and corpse-like, barely able to turn his head towards the lens. The concluding shot, a finely focussed close-up of Moran's face, fetishes grim details such as the flaking skin around his eyebrows and the black lesion above his fungus-coated lips.

ACT UP responded to Nixon's *Tom Moran* series with a demonstration held inside the galleries at MOMA. The protesters claimed that Nixon's pictures sensationalized AIDS by portraying the condition as an automatic death sentence. By the late 1980s, this was no longer necessarily the case: in 1983, the life expectancy of a person with AIDS had only been eight months, while by 1989 it was over twenty.[26] A leaflet distributed by the protesters acknowledged this improved prognosis, attributing it to 'experimental drug treatments, better information about nutrition and health care and the efforts of PWAs engaged in a continuing battle to define and save their lives'.[27] To emphasize this in visual terms, many of the demonstrators carried snapshots of friends or relatives living with AIDS, effectively establishing an alternative gallery of personal AIDS portraits. A typical example was a photograph of a smiling, ostensibly healthy man, contextualized with the caption: 'this is a picture taken of my father when he'd been living with AIDS for three years'.[28] Their leaflet made the point even more unambiguously: 'We demand the visibility of PWAs who are vibrant, angry, loving, sexy, beautiful, acting up and fighting back.'[29]

A second facet of the protesters' critique of Nixon's photographs relates to the contextual framing of people with AIDS as visual objects, and even more problematically, as *art* objects. The curators at MOMA had chosen to let Nixon's AIDS images 'speak for themselves', displaying them untitled and without any contextualizing information. Rejecting a singularly visual representation of people with AIDS, the protesters demanded, 'NO MORE PICTURES WITHOUT CONTEXT', and 'STOP LOOKING AT US; START LISTENING TO US.'[30] The institutional setting of a major art museum further exacerbated the situation, effectively transforming people with AIDS into a spectacle for a museum audience with little first-hand knowledge of the concrete realities of the condition. The geographical location of MOMA in wealthy 'uptown' Manhattan provided an additional spatial metaphor separating Nixon's intended audience from those communities most afflicted by an epidemic frequently associated with the environs of 'downtown'.

A few months previously, Rosalind Solomon's small solo exhibition *Portraits in the Time of AIDS* was displayed at New York University's Grey Art Gallery. Like Nixon, Solomon had no previous connections with the AIDS community and had recruited her subjects through a church group.[31] *Portraits in the Time of AIDS* comprised seventy-five photographs, produced as large-scale gelatin silver prints pinned to the gallery wall, unframed and untitled. The pictures range from single figures to group portraits, and from close-up face shots to almost abstracted images of body parts. Not all of her subjects are visibly ill; some are pictured with their lovers (one pair is kissing passionately), and many meet the eye of the camera with expressions of wry humour rather than the melancholic countenance that is a hallmark of Nixon's *Tom Moran* series. In contrast to Nixon's formalist emphasis on the contours of the wasted body, the individuality of Solomon's subjects is frequently signalled by the inclusion of personal effects such as family snapshots, artworks and interior décor. (Indeed, Solomon had taken the deliberate decision not to photograph her subjects in hospital for fear of repressing their personalities.) In one such image, a young man (with no visible signs of illness) sits contemplatively beneath his own portrait. His apartment is hung with further paintings; taken together with his tan loafers and expensive watch, the image seems to suggest the epitome of yuppie good taste. If Nixon's *Tom Moran* pictures are over-earnest in their desire to communicate the dismal solemnity of dying from AIDS, several of Solomon's photographs are astute in the parallels they draw between the fragile human bodies that comprise the content of her images and the artworks that these bodies might become. In one such image, a bearded man is stripped to the waist, both arms raised above his head so as to draw attention to the cancerous black abrasions that mark his chest. Displayed next to him is a photograph of two young men (the viewer is led to assume that this is the sitter and his partner), two small busts resembling the men in the photograph, and two tiny sculpted torsos whose pose echoes that of the subject of the image. Solomon's picture draws parallels between contemporary representations of people with AIDS and established artistic motifs that denote physical suffering and social stigmatization: with his trunk twisted and his lesions on display, the bearded man recalls a Saint Sebastian, or a Christ revealing his wounds.

Solomon's exhibition produced a less pronounced reaction than Nixon's; no protest was held, although this may relate to the higher public profile of MOMA in comparison to the Grey Art Gallery, rather than specifically to the pictorial content of Solomon's images. However, in Crimp and Grover's influential essays, the same broad criticisms are addressed to both Nixon and Solomon's work. Grover dismisses Nixon and Solomon's work as 'inadequate' and 'irrelevant', claiming 'their crude emphasis on physically debilitated or disfigured PWAs most closely resembles the choice made by popular media three and four years ago emphasizing their difference from the rest of us'.[32] Similarly, Crimp writes: 'what we see first and foremost [in these] photographs is their reiteration of what we have already been told or shown about people with AIDS: that they are generally alone, desperate, but resigned to their "individual" deaths'.[33] Crucially, however, the iconographic content of these photographs is not the sole focus of Crimp and Grover's criticism: instead, the real target is a modernist conception of art that privileges the emotional experience of the artist over that of the depicted subject. The source of Crimp and Grover's anxiety at such outdated modernist practices, I shall argue, can be located in two ideas dominant at the time of their writing: first, a scepticism of the liberal discourse that equates visual representation with political power, and second, a critical framing of photography as an ethically suspect medium.

'Putting a face to AIDS'

The curatorial discourse that supported Nixon and Solomon's projects repeatedly anticipated, and then diffused, the charge of exploitation. In his catalogue essay for *Pictures of People*, Peter Galassi argued that Nixon's work avoids any implication that 'the photographer is superior to the subject [. . .] His pictures persuade us that we see individuals, not symptoms of a problem or, worse, heroes of the solution.'[34] Similarly, Thomas Sokolowski emphasized that Solomon's images should be understood as a 'collaborative endeavor, between sitter and artist'; comparing Solomon's prints to those of August Sander and Diane Arbus, he declares, 'the rather unique situation of Rosalind Solomon's portraits, done in the time of AIDS, is that the subjects *have been asked*.'[35]

The ethical case for the necessity of Nixon and Solomon's portraits, made by curators, art journalists and the photographers themselves, relied on the assumption that the visual depiction of a community might automatically lead to greater empathy and political change. Peter Galassi stated the case for photography's capacity to make an international health crisis comprehensible at a human level. Quoting from a recent interview with the artist Gary Indiana, Galassi wrote, 'One terrible thing about this epidemic is that it has taken away the concept of having one's own death, and made thousands of deaths into this kind of generic tragedy, which is not even perceived as a tragedy by the culture at large, which is pretty horrifying.'[36] If as Galassi suggests, 'the vastness of the epidemic tends to overwhelm even the most genuine concern', photography is able to return this universal experience of tragedy to that of the individual.[37] Galassi's text exemplified what Douglas Crimp labelled as 'the typical liberal position', that is, the dominant belief, 'from very early in the epidemic, that one of the central problems of AIDS, one of the things we needed to combat, was bureaucratic abstraction. What was needed was to "give AIDS a face", to "bring AIDS home"'.[38]

In Thomas Sokolowski's introduction to Solomon's exhibition, the face offers a mechanism by which AIDS can be known and thus conquered:

> Since it had no name by which it could be called, nor no known face by which it could be recognized, it was allowed to grow in strength almost simultaneously as our public awareness of it grew. And even after it was finally named AIDS, some dare not speak it, even though it was only a syndrome and not a real disease; not a disease like those which ravaged mankind throughout history. Yet, as our awareness of it grew through the accumulation of vast amounts of numerically derived evidence, we still had not seen its face. We could count it, but not describe it. Our picture of AIDS was a totally conceptual one [. . .][39]

This rhetoric of 'putting a face to AIDS' resonates with the theoretical model offered by Emmanuel Levinas, who posits the face as 'the most basic mode of responsibility' and as a foundation for the possibility of a truly inter-subjective relation.[40] Read through Levinas, Nixon and Solomon's images might be assumed to accomplish the laudable task of eliciting the compassion and action of the viewer. However, this constitutes an overly simplistic reading of Levinas' theory. To date, the ethical potential of the 'face to face' relation has been mentioned in the context of AIDS and representation primarily in relation to textual rather than visual materials.[41] There is good reason for this: Levinas rejects vision as a way of describing the authentic relation with the other:

> I wonder if one can speak of a look turned towards the face, for the look is knowledge, perception. . . . You turn yourself towards the Other as towards an object when you see a nose, eyes, a forehead, a chin, and you can describe them. The best way of encountering the Other is not even to notice the color of his eyes! When one observes the color of the eyes one is not in a social relation with the Other. The relation with the face can surely be dominated by perception, but what is specifically the face cannot be reduced to that.[42]

There is thus a difficulty in applying Levinas' ideas to the visual image. The Levinasian face is not necessarily physiognomic, and in fact the visual medium increases the likelihood of objectification: 'when you see a nose, eyes, a forehead, a chin, and you can describe them', 'you turn yourself towards the other as towards an object'.[43] For Levinas, the face is not strictly a visual object but a *relation*: rather than being 'seen', the Levinasian face 'speaks' so that 'face and discourse are tied';[44] vision is hence deemed insufficiently reciprocal to adequately mediate a truly reciprocal relationship with the other. The strictly visual nature of Nixon and Solomon's pictures, exhibited without captions or other written context, could only reinforce their sitters' status as 'other', objectified and made alien by the very medium that claimed to represent the 'truth' of their condition.

Anti-photography criticism

In her 2004 essay 'Precarious Life', Judith Butler suggested that the photographed face appears to 'conceal or displace the face in the Levinasian sense'.[45] Butler was writing in the context of visual representations of the United States' post 9-11 war on terror and was concerned with modes of address that appeared to produce a moral obligation on the part of the viewer. Butler argued that rather than having a humanizing effect, certain photographic representations of the face can actually perform a dehumanizing action. Citing numerous media images, including those of Osama Bin Laden, Yasser Arafat and Saddam Hussein, Butler claimed that in such instances 'the paradigmatically human is understood to reside outside the frame; this is the human face in its deformity and extremity, not the one with which you are asked to identify'.[46] This media evacuation of the human through the image must, Butler argued, be understood as establishing 'what will and will not be human, what will be a liveable life, what will be a grievable death'.[47]

Butler's text alludes to (although does not explicitly cite) a rich literature of 'anti-photography' photography criticism published in the late 1970s and early 1980s. This literature begins with Susan Sontag's essays gathered in *On Photography* (1979), which branded the medium as 'treacherous', 'voyeuristic', 'predatory' and 'reductive'.[48] Famously, Sontag proposed that 'to photograph is to appropriate the thing photographed. It means putting oneself in a certain relation to the world that feels like knowledge – and therefore, like power.'[49] While painted, drawn or written representations of people can be easily understood as subjective interpretations, photographs give the impression of being direct transcriptions of the external world, 'miniatures of reality that anyone can make or acquire'.[50] For Sontag, photography is especially ethically complicated when it is used to capture suffering, as 'to take a picture is to have an interest in things remaining as they are, in the status quo remaining unchanged [. . .] to be in complicity with whatever makes a subject interesting, worth photographing, including, when that is the interest, another person's pain or misfortune'.[51]

Sontag's sceptical attitude towards the photograph is developed by a subsequent generation of anti-photography writers, including Allan Sekula, who excoriated the medium as 'primitive, infantile, aggressive' in *Photography against the Grain* (1984).[52] In his important essay 'The Body and the Archive' (1986), Sekula described the dual genealogy of documentary portrait photography, which draws, on the one hand, from the honorific tradition of portrait painting and, on the other hand, from a set of repressive practices designed to identify and regulate criminal, deviant or non-normative bodies.[53] Looking through photography's archive that contains 'both the traces of the visible bodies of heroes, leaders, moral exemplars, celebrities and those of the poor, the diseased, the insane, the criminal, the non-white, the female and all other embodiments of the unworthy', Sekula suggested that *every* photographic portrait necessarily takes place within a social and moral hierarchy.[54] This 'shadow archive' of aberrant bodies is backed up by the paradigm offered by the nineteenth-century 'sciences' of phrenology and physiognomy, which were informed by the belief that the body's exterior (especially the face and head) could signify aspects of inner character. Photography proved an ideal medium for the documentation of the appearance of particular 'types'; Sekula's best-known example is the late nineteenth-century eugenicist Francis Galton, whose composite photographs aimed to scientifically establish the physiognomy of criminals and other deviants.[55] Turning his attention to the contemporary arts scene, Sekula noted a preponderance of 'neophysiognomic concerns' and observed that this linage is most apparent in the medium of photography.[56] For those that shared Sekula's critical position, by the late 1980s the medium of portrait photography had come to delimit the terrain of the 'other'; this theoretical framework inevitable shaped the way in which photographic depictions of people with AIDS would be received within a theoretical and intellectual context.

Working within the same theoretical terrain as Sekula, Martha Rosler's text and photo-based artwork, *The Bowery in two inadequate descriptive systems* (1974-5) delivered both a rejection and a critique of the tradition of 'victim photography'. As Craig Owens has noted, Rosler refuses to represent those 'twice victimized: first by society, and then by the photographer who presumes the right to speak on their behalf'.[57] For Sekula (who was a close friend and colleague of Rosler's), the work has 'an unrelenting *metacritical* relation to the documentary genre [. . .] The title not only raises the question of representation, but suggests its fundamentally flawed, distorted character.'[58] Sekula reads Rosler's refusal to depict the inhabitants of the Bowery not only as a direct criticism of the 'expressionist liberalism of the find-a-bum school of concerned photography' but also as an 'anti-humanist' strategy that is supported by the text's own failure, despite its signifying richness, to adequately explain the material reality to which it refers.[59]

The Bowery is reproduced in Rosler's book *3 Works*, where it is accompanied by an essay that traces the history of documentary photography from the work of social reformers like Jacob Riis and Margaret Sanger, to the 'new documentarians' Gary Winogrand, Diane Arbus and Lee Friedlander.[60] Rosler attributes the term 'new documentarians' to John Szarkowski, the influential Director of Photography at MOMA between 1962 and 1991, and suggests that documentary photography has taken a particular line under his guidance, exemplified by the work of Winogrand, 'who aggressively rejects any responsibility for his images and denies any relation between them and shared or public human meaning'.[61] Rosler reads liberal documentary as an essentially conservative medium that is more moralistic than progressive: it reassures its viewers about their relative wealth and position, 'putting a face on fear and transforming threat into fantasy, into imagery'.[62]

Crimp would have been familiar with Rosler's work and with the 'anti-photography' arguments of Sontag and Sekula, and their influence can be readily detected in his writings on AIDS images. Crimp asserts that his initial reaction to Nixon and Solomon's exhibitions was 'incredulity. [. . .] I had naively assumed that the critique of this sort of photography, articulated over and over again during the past decade, might have had some effect'.[63] To make his point, Crimp cites from Sekula's 1978 essay 'Dismantling Modernism':

> At the heart of [the] fetishistic cultivation and promotion of the artist's humanity is a certain disdain for the 'ordinary' humanity of those who have been photographed. They become the 'other', exotic creatures, objects of contemplation . . . The most intimate, human-scale relationship to suffer mystification in all this is the specific social engagement that results in the image; the negotiation between photographer and subject in the making of a portrait, the seduction, coercion, collaboration, or rip-off.[64]

Crimp and Grover's critiques of Nixon and Solomon's images focus on the balance of power that structures this negotiation. Noting that all positive art-world responses to the *Tom Moran* series presupposed the relationship between photographer and subject to be one of equals, Crimp deconstructed this assumption to expose the disturbing sub-text to Nixon's practice.

In the catalogue for *Pictures of People*, Peter Galassi framed Nixon's project explicitly as documentary, contrasting this to a more expressive 'artistic' approach and describing the project as one 'whose significance outweighed Nixon's private artistic mission. With this came the hope that if the pictures were good they might matter, not in the sense that all good art matters, but in a specific sense having to do with AIDS'.[65] The claim to a lack of 'artfulness' is supported by Nixon's choice of equipment: an old-fashioned, eight-by-ten-inch view- camera mounted on a tripod. As Galassi explains:

> At the back of the camera is a ground glass on which the photographer selects and focuses the inverted image, its dimness made bright by the shade of a dark cloth draped over the photographer's head. The photographer then inserts into the camera, just in front of the ground glass, a flat case holding a sheet of film; henceforth he cannot see the image. He removes the plastic slide covering the film and releases the cocked shutter in the lens to make the exposure. Even in skilful hands the equipment is cumbersome. It resists rapid revision and punishes sloppiness. Consequently view-camera work conventionally is confined to immobile subjects, which allow the photographer time to study, consider, adjust: to perfect.[66]

The view-camera produces an unusually large negative from which contact prints may be taken directly rather than enlarged, resulting in a precisely detailed image that offers 'an uncanny, sometimes hallucinatory presence.'[67] Other art-world professionals were similarly keen to emphasise the images' lack of artfulness.

For Andy Grundberg, photography critic of *The New York Times*, Nixon 'relies on the photographic images' ability to convince us that what we are seeing is the truth.' Grundberg suggested that Nixon's 'translucent' images eschew any stylistic reflections that would divert the viewer's attention from the subject to the photograph itself.[68] This ostensible lack of 'artfulness' is important: as Susan Sontag has observed, 'people want the weight of witnessing without the taint of artistry.'[69]

Nixon's choice of camera was also seen as significant in supposedly guaranteeing the collaborative nature of the photographic encounter; its sheer size and obtrusive appearance ensure that Nixon's subjects cannot be anything other than fully aware that they are being photographed. Galassi writes:

> Nixon has said that most of the people with AIDS that he has photographed are, perhaps because stripped of so many of their hopes, less masked than others, more open to collaboration.[70]

Galassi's evaluation is premised on an understanding of successful portraiture as a genre that penetrates the surface appearance of the sitter to reveal the inner truth of the essential self. Problematically, however, the precondition for this is the diminished health of Nixon's subjects. Grundberg's review in *The New York Times* was even more direct in its equation of the sitters' wasted bodies with a lack of self-possession:

> The result is overwhelming, since one sees not only the wasting away of the flesh (in photographs, emaciation has become emblematic of AIDS) but also the gradual dimming of the subjects' ability to compose themselves for the camera. What each series begins as a conventional effort to pose for a picture ends in a kind of abandon; as the subjects' self-consciousness disappears, the camera seems to become invisible, and consequently *there is almost no boundary between the image and ourselves.*[71]

In Grundberg's evaluation any potential distance between the subject and the viewer is apparently negated by Nixon's skill and determination in capturing the 'truth' of AIDS. Galassi's text made clear the absolute assimilation of Moran's experience with Nixon's, concluding 'the life and death of Tom Moran were his own.'[72] As Grover remarks, Nixon (and Solomon) 'use these images to foreground *their own experience* in photographing PWAs: they make it sound as if they were stalking rare animals at great emotional cost to themselves. The photographs then become the evidence of their bravery.'[73] This promotion of artist over subject matter is inherent in the genre: Nixon and Solomon both speak 'the central discourse of modernist art photography – that the subject of art is the artist's feelings.'[74]

In 1974, Sekula suggested that contemporary art was in a state of 'crisis', relating this specifically to the problem of modernist closure, which 'is larger than any one intellectual discipline and yet infects them all'.[75] In order to find its way out of this predicament, it was deemed necessary for art to overcome both 'a naïve faith in both the privileged subjectivity of the artist, at one extreme, and the fundamental "objectivity" of photographic realism, at the other'.[76] Thus Crimp and Grover's difficulty with Nixon and Solomon's work must be understood not simply in relation to the pictures' iconographic content (although both acknowledge that this is problematic) but also in the context of a specific intellectual heritage that addresses the exhaustion of the modernist art practice of liberal documentary photography.

Intimate images? Nan Goldin's portraits of AIDS deaths

In 2008, Chris Townsend lauded Goldin's images of the late 1980s and early 1990s as 'a passionate, political and ethical response to the AIDS crisis',[77] reading the work in terms of a universal experience of bereavement 'regardless of the cause of death'.[78] Townsend argued that Goldin's AIDS images illustrate 'the response to the death of the individual by the collective',[79] quoting Levinas: 'What we call, by a somewhat corrupted term, love, is par excellence the fact that the death of the other affects me more than my own'.[80] In a passage that could equally be applied to Nixon's *Tom Moran* series Townsend writes, 'Perhaps because the face of the slowly dying man is a face we would rather not see, but a face that, precisely because it makes us uncomfortable, because it tells us where responsibility lies, that we must see.'[81] Townsend's reading recalls the utopianism underpinning Nixon and Solomon's AIDS portraits, denying the political specificity of an AIDS death by instead insisting that the images are about a universal 'human experience'.

Goldin works in the tradition of intimate social documentary, and the perceived value of her images is often predicated on their ability to bear witness to the experiences of a specific community in a particular time and place. Goldin's camera is frequently described as a mirror to the soul (the mirror is a recurring motif in her oeuvre), and her pictures are invested with the power to portray not just physical but also spiritual or essential likeness.[82] While Goldin's work differs from Nixon's and Solomon's in terms of process, content and reception, it nonetheless rests on the same 'rhetorical commitment to photographic truth'[83] as underpins Nixon and Solomon's practices, with most commentators choosing to read her anthology of images as a direct transcription of lived experience.[84]

Goldin's early work comprises an intimate extended portrait of what she refers to as her own 'family', a group of friends that lived, worked and played together in Boston and New York in the late 1970s and early 1980s. Originally intended to help recover hazy memories of riotous all-night parties, Goldin's photographs soon became known for their vivid chronicling of an era-defining subculture. Her prints were not initially intended for the art market or for museum audiences but were circulated among the community of friends that they depicted.[85] In the late 1970s, this informal distribution of prints developed into slide shows, first at the Boston Museum School and then later in the downtown clubs of New York, where the audiences were again largely comprised Goldin's immediate circle. This format gave the work a narrative or cinematic quality that would continue to define Goldin's preferred approach to portraiture as an accretion of images over an extended time period: 'I don't believe in the single portrait. I believe only in the accumulation of portraits as a representation of a person. Because I think people are really complex.'[86] During the early 1980s the slideshow began a process of solidification, acquiring the title *The Ballad of Sexual Dependency* in 1981 and a permanent format as a book in 1986.

In the introduction to the print version of *The Ballad,* Goldin describes the camera as an extension of her own body, using terms that recall Galassi and Grundberg's positive framing of Nixon's work:

> People in the pictures say my camera is as much a part of being with me as any other aspect of knowing me. It's as if my hand were a camera. If it were possible, I'd want no mechanism between me and the moment of photographing. The camera is as much a part of my everyday life as talking or eating or sex. The instant of photographing, instead of creating distance, is a moment of emotional clarity for me. There is a popular notion that the photographer is by nature a voyeur, the last one invited to the party. But I'm not crashing: this is my party. This is my family, my history.[87]

As with Nixon and Solomon, responses to Goldin's work can be divided along two lines: admirers praise the brutal honesty, emotional directness and formal beauty of her images, while critics proffer the charges of voyeurism, exploitation or plain bad taste.[88] Also in common with Nixon and Solomon, the curatorial discourse framing Goldin's work frequently anticipates and diffuses these accusations. Writing in the catalogue for Goldin's 2002 retrospective at London's Whitechapel Gallery, Catherine Lampert takes great pains to distinguish Goldin's practice from the imbalances of traditional portraiture:

> Two assumptions underpin her attitude to portraiture, distinguishing it morally and visually from the tradition of the genre. First, that portraiture requires complicity with the subject, and secondly, that it is about the exchange of gifts – the moment, the consent, the print, and even the future path of the art object.[89]

In fact, as Goldin's work has become increasingly desirable to museum curators and private investors, it is its impressive trajectory precisely *as art object* that has fuelled criticism. Writing in 1996 for *Frieze* magazine, David Deitcher suggested that Goldin had exploited her subjects, not in the initial act of taking the pictures but in her subsequent re-appropriation of the images for a commercial audience: 'Now that so many of the individuals Goldin pictured have passed away, it is upsetting to see their images recycled as large-scale cibachromes or, even worse, clustered together as composites within a single frame where they coalesce into sexy, brutal and/or tragic narratives for a market that is now so hot for her work.'[90]

Many of the images included in *The Ballad* can with hindsight be categorized as pictures of people with AIDS, and indeed, in an afterword included in the book's 2012 reprint, Goldin offers an extensive list of those lost to the epidemic. Goldin has stated unequivocally, 'AIDS changed everything in my life. There's life before AIDS, and life after it. [. . .] In a large part, my work is about AIDS.'[91] In real terms, however, AIDS is not directly acknowledged by Goldin's work until 1990, when she exhibited her first explicitly AIDS-related piece, *The Cookie Portfolio*, based on pictures taken of her close friend Cookie Mueller between 1976 and 1989, and grouped together after Mueller's death to form a retrospective memorial. Subsequent works that address AIDS directly include a grid of images devoted to the Berlin-based curator Alf Bold (1991–3 and 1995) and a sequence dedicated to Goldin's Parisian dealer Gilles Dusein (1991–3). The images of Mueller, I shall argue, present quite a different set of issues to those of Bold and Dusein; if the former largely resist the visual stereotypes of AIDS, then the latter awkwardly embrace them.

The Cookie Portfolio comprises portraits of the actress and writer Cookie Mueller, 'queen of the whole downtown scene'.[92] The pictures were taken between 1976, when the two women first became close, and Mueller's death in 1989 at the age of forty. The portfolio was first exhibited at the Photographic Resource Center in Boston in 1990, where the images were installed as a grid (thus resisting a linear narrative of decline and death); a few months later they were shown at Pace/MacGill in New York, this time displayed in a chronologically ordered row. Pace/MacGill also produced a limited edition book, matching the images with a handwritten text by Goldin and a 'last letter' by Mueller.[93] Since then, the

Portfolio has only been displayed in its entirety a handful of times, including Goldin's retrospectives at the Whitney in 1996 and London's Whitechapel Gallery in 2002.[94] Approximately half of the images present Mueller in youthful good health, laughing and dancing, in the company of friends, lovers or her young son. Several are extremely intimate: in one Mueller is seated in a nightclub toilet stall chatting with another woman, legs apart and underwear around her ankles. These early images are all dated prior to 1986; between 1987 and 1988, Goldin was treated for drug addiction in a rehabilitation clinic and had little contact with the outside world. When Goldin left the treatment centre and returned to New York, Mueller was desperately unwell. These later pictures show Mueller faded and gaunt, her infirmity signalled by the walking stick at her side; weeping at the funeral of her husband, Vittorio Scarpati; bed-bound and cared for by her ex-lover Sharon; framed by the eerie light of an X-ray machine (Figure 4); and finally, at rest in her own coffin. The concluding image in the collection shows Mueller's empty living room, glamorous portraits of the actress poignantly displayed behind the vacant sofa.

Goldin's later images of Mueller use few of the prevailing visual clichés of AIDS: while Mueller looks aged and exhausted in prints such as *Cookie with Her Cane* or *Cookie at Vittorio's Casket* (both 1989), there is no recourse to the standard motifs of dramatic wasting or lesions. (In contrast to Nixon's pictures of Tom Moran, Mueller, appropriately for a woman who defined herself through her

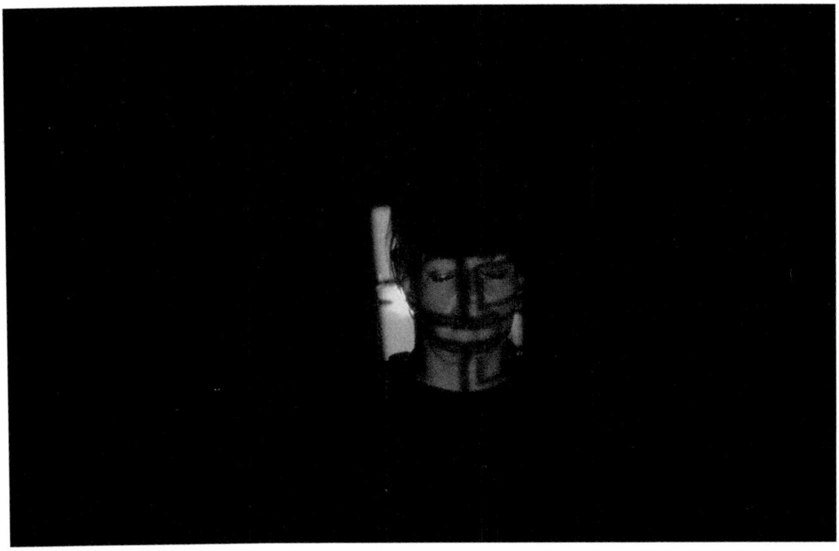

Figure 4 Nan Goldin, *Cookie being X-rayed, NYC, October*, 1989. Courtesy the artist and Marian Goodman Gallery. Copyright: Nan Goldin.

'look', is fully clothed in all of Goldin's images.) To some extent, the early pictures make Mueller's decline all the more shocking, but perhaps more importantly, they also celebrate Mueller as a unique individual rather than simply as an invalid and victim. If the intended subject of Nixon's *Tom Moran* series is 'AIDS: The Disease', the subject of *The Cookie Portfolio* is unmistakably Mueller herself. In the words of Elizabeth Sussman, curator of Goldin's solo exhibition at the Whitney in 1996: 'The Cookie Project is not about AIDS, about reifying the disease into a subject, but, like all Goldin's work, about restoring the narrative of a life for history.'[95]

In a handwritten text exhibited alongside the pictures in the *Portfolio*, Goldin describes photography as a means of both deferring and exposing the pain of bereavement:

> I used to think that I couldn't lose anyone if I photographed them enough. I put together this series of Cookie from the 13 years I knew her in order to keep her with me. In fact they show me how much I've lost.[96]

Goldin's observations on the bittersweet associations of photography with love, loss and memory resonate with Roland Barthes' celebrated text on the same subject, *Camera Lucida*, published in French in 1980 and translated into English in 1981 (thus making it more or less contemporary with Goldin's own practice). For both Barthes and Goldin, the ability of photography to preserve memory is closely connected to what Barthes refers to as its *noeme*: 'That-has-been'.[97] A painting can counterfeit reality: when confronted with a photograph, however, the viewer cannot deny that 'the thing has been there'.[98] Focussing on his own phenomenological experience of photography, Barthes' influential text provides an appealing and authoritative counter-discourse to the deconstructive approach of Sekula and Rosler outlined earlier in this chapter.

Goldin frames her later images of Gilles Dusein in similar terms: 'I photographed him and I was witness to his death. Gilles had shown *The Cookie Portfolio*. He and his lover, Gotscho, understood that it was important that I make the same kind of record of Gilles's life so that he wouldn't be lost. It was about trying to hold onto people, making sure they didn't disappear without a trace.'[99] However, Goldin's pictures of Gilles and Gotscho, as well as those of Alf Bold, are arguably more problematic than those assembled in *The Cookie Portfolio*. Goldin's images of Bold (1991–3/1995) employ the same visual motifs as Nixon and Solomon's prints: Bold is pictured in a dressing gown looking out of a window, lying on a hospital bed and, finally, as a corpse draped in a white sheet and with a single rose laid upon his chest; the sequence is intercut with images of tombstones and a solitary mourner. Similarly, in the sequence devoted to Gilles

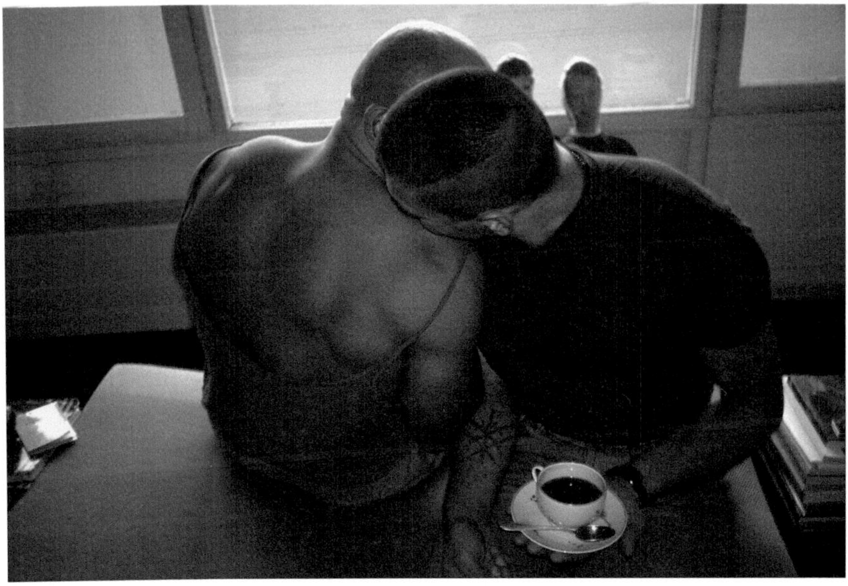

Figure 5 Nan Goldin, *Gilles and Gotscho embracing, Paris*, 1992. Courtesy the artist and Marian Goodman Gallery. Copyright: Nan Goldin.

Dusein (1991–3), Goldin juxtaposes the fragile frame of her subject against the bodybuilder physique of his partner Gotscho (Figure 5): consider, for example, the divergent size of the two men's necks in the image of Gotscho leaning over the bed to bestow a last kiss upon Gilles forehead, or the way in which Dusein's puny arm, isolated from the rest of his body, contrasts with Gotscho's pumped biceps.

If in *The Cookie Portfolio* AIDS enters the scene 'as a happenstance tragedy', in the words of Liz Kotz, then in the images of Dusein and Bold AIDS becomes both the subject and the narrative.[100] Kotz dismisses the sequence leading up to Dusein's death as 'pat and formulaic', presenting his death as 'heroic, exemplary, and fully spectacularized'.[101] In Kotz's critique, Goldin's work is contrasted against that of two of her contemporaries, Jack Pierson and Mark Morrisroe. Kotz's first example is Pierson's photo-book *Angel Youth* (1992), which is filled with sumptuous, pathos-steeped images of 'pretty boys, flowers [and] sun drenched meals with friends'. Kotz suggests that the death and disease that is made explicit by Goldin's work is completely invisible as a subject in Pierson's, yet is nonetheless strongly present as an emotional undertow. Her second example is a photograph taken by Morrisroe less than a year before his own death, which depicts an out-of-focus seagull hovering in a sickly yellow sky. For Kotz, this also 'speaks' of a life lived against the constant presence of AIDS, but it is far removed from the explicitness of Goldin's documentary images. Rather, Morrisroe's image insists on the importance of that which remains outside of representation; as such, it challenges the documentary tendency to provide *too much* visual information that typifies the work of Goldin, Nixon and Solomon. For Kotz, social documentary photography (as exemplified by Goldin's work) is too enmeshed in the awkward histories of social surveillance and coercion, too caught up in a tendency to exoticize, too *spectacularizing* to be an appropriate medium for conveying anyone's experience of AIDS. Hence Goldin, despite her familiarity with her subjects, is criticized by Kotz for the same problematic inclinations as Nixon and Solomon: for an uncomfortably clichéd iconography of AIDS (in the images of Dusein and Bold, if not of Mueller), and ultimately for a naïvely romantic attitude towards the photographic medium that is curiously out of step with the theoretical tendencies of her time.

* * *

The reception of these images testifies to the complexities of representing AIDS in photographic form. Writing in 2018, Lukas Engelmann notes that 'the history of AIDS photography resembles and reinstates the "epidemic of signification" as the medium could not resolve the ambiguities, uncertainties and unusualness of the emerging epidemic'.[102] Using Nixon's images of Tom Moran to contextualize a discussion of clinical AIDS photography, Engelmann draws attention to the different (and sometimes not-so-different) expectations placed on photographs in clinical versus fine art settings, observing that Nixon's images were 'broadly conceived to exhibit a clinical gaze'.[103]

Today, there is increasing recognition that Nixon and Solomon's images, while imperfect, are significant in being the earliest formal portraits in the art world to grapple with the complexities of representing people with AIDS. In 2013, the Bruce Silverstein gallery mounted a contemporary rehanging of Solomon's *Portraits in the Time of AIDS*. The press release noted the initial critical reception of the work, and argued for the historic significance of the original show in provoking debate about the polemical nature of representing people with AIDS as graphically ill at a time of widespread terror about the evolving epidemic.[104] The release further observed that twenty-five years later, expectations around photography as a medium have changed; now less immediately tethered to documentary, the camera is more readily understood as a technology that not only bears witness but also actively transforms. Reviewing for *The New York Times*, Holland Cotter also noted the negative press received by the initial show, situating that criticism in relation to the work of groups like ACT UP, who were at the time trying to alter the focus around the disease: that activism worked, but 'if you want to get a sense of what spurred that activism, and of the daily realities experienced by many people in homes and hospitals at that time, Ms Solomon's unflinching pictures are where to look'.[105]

In a 2016 interview with Linda Yablonsky, Solomon also recalled the reception of *Portraits in the Time of AIDS*, noting that 'the people who were still alive that I'd photographed came to the show and they loved the show, but the show was panned'.[106] Yablonsky concurs that, in her view, the pictures are 'not exploitative, by any stretch of the imagination', and the two reflect on the many reasons for the show's reception, including Solomon's outsider status in the AIDS community, her positioning as a woman in a male-dominated art world, the impact of long-standing taboos around photographing illness and death, and the fact that the pictures were produced so early in the epidemic (in an art-world sense) that nobody knew how to read them. Solomon and Yablonsky further observe that Nan Goldin's images were received very differently – promoted as a kind of diary, people came to them with a different set of expectations. Yet this notwithstanding, for some writers (such as Liz Kotz), Goldin's photography, like Nixon and Solomon's work, cannot shake its associations with social documentary, a genre enmeshed in histories of repression and surveillance.

A critical history of portrait photography as repressive, exploitative and othering informed contemporaneous readings of Nixon's and Solomon's work. Despite this troubled or troubling critical framework, artists seeking to convey their own subjective experiences of AIDS through self-portraiture did not eschew the medium entirely. Indeed, some of the most memorable and moving examples of AIDS self-portraiture are photographs: Robert Mapplethorpe's celebrated 'death's head' image (1988); David Wojnarowicz' burial 'rehearsal', which depicts his body submerged in the earth, his body barely visible (1990); or later, the autobiographical photographic practices of Albert J. Winn or the British artist Richard Sawdon Smith. The following chapter explores the photographic self-representation of the AIDS-afflicted body in the work of the artist and photographer Mark Morrisroe: as I shall presently argue, Morrisroe's late self-portraits are deeply complex works which fuse the apparently opposed discourses of documentary 'truth' with creative self-fashioning, critical illness with tangible sensuality and visual objectification with a sense of subjective empowerment.

3

Mark Morrisroe

A grandiose aesthetic encounter

Eroticism is assenting to life even in death.[1]

During the last year of his life, Mark Morrisroe (1959–89) produced a series of compelling black-and-white Polaroid self-portraits. Clad in a hospital-issue dressing gown and tie-waist pyjama pants and standing next to an unmade bed, the artist grips an intravenous pole; lines of plastic tubing tumble from bags of unidentified fluids, snaking across the infusion pump, which occupies the centre of the frame. In another Polaroid, Morrisroe – dressed in the same gown – clasps a shutter release cable, producing an unexpected but persuasive analogy between his medical care and the act of care taken in composing his images. In other pictures he is unclothed: curled elegantly upon a faded floral bed sheet as slices of light fall across his naked body, his head resting lightly on one arm in a mime of sleep, he performs both vulnerability and aesthetic appeal, bringing to mind one of Lord Leighton's slumbering pre-Raphaelite heroines.

The most widely reproduced of these late Polaroid self-portraits is a seemingly dispassionate depiction of Morrisroe naked on that same bed, taken just days before he passed away (Figure 6). The camera has been positioned somewhere towards the ceiling of the room: observing Morrisroe's fragile frame from this elevated viewpoint, we see thin legs folded artfully to one side, wasted buttocks, concave stomach and skeletal ribs. The atrophying of his body is echoed in the mess that gathers on the surfaces next to the bed – crumbled clothing, empty drinks bottles and a half-consumed cup of coffee. The most compelling detail of the image is the directness of Morrisroe's gaze, which seems to penetrate the camera lens and emerge from the photographic frame to challenge the viewer. His look is enigmatic and unsettling, its inscrutability hinting at the indeterminate status of the image itself.

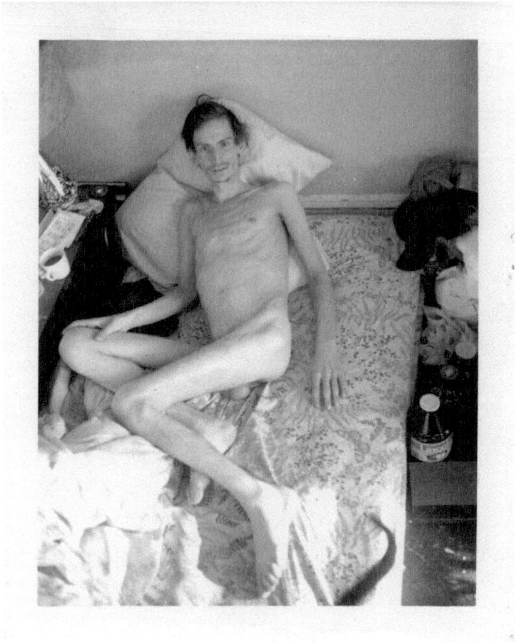

Figure 6 Mark Morrisroe, Untitled [Self-Portrait], 1989. T-665 Polaroid, 10.7 × 8.5 cm. © The Estate of Mark Morrisroe (Ringier Collection) at Fotomuseum Winterthur.

Morrisroe was one of the first artists to offer a personal account of the 'AIDS experience'.[2] Artists' images documenting the deaths of friends and lovers emerge as a sub-genre of AIDS portraiture from 1989 onwards: well-known early examples include David Wojnarowicz's photographs of Peter Hujar (d.1987) and Nan Goldin's photographs of Cookie Muller (d.1989), addressed in the previous chapter. However, Wojnarowicz and Goldin's images are necessarily structured by a different subject-viewer dynamic to that of Morrisroe's self-portrait. Robert Mapplethorpe's haunting photograph of himself clad in black and clutching a skull-topped walking cane is one of the few self-authored images to appear before 1989; Mapplethorpe aside, it is clear that Morrisroe's arresting first-person representations of AIDS are remarkable in both their timing and their candour.

At the time of his diagnosis in 1986, visual representations of people with AIDS varied according to intended audience. 'Positive' images, such as the photographs taken by Jane Rosett for use in the *PWA Coalition News-line* (the June 1987 copy 'Surviving and Thriving with AIDS' was found among Morrisroe's possessions after his death), were on the whole concerned with imparting an optimistic message about living with AIDS and had little to offer in terms of conveying the phenomenology of enduring a seriously debilitating and life-threatening condition. At the other end of the spectrum the sensationalist images disseminated by the popular media depicted people with AIDS as monstrously disfigured sub-humans awaiting their deaths; activists such as Douglas Crimp and Jan Zita Grover criticized the way in which this iconography was appropriated for a fine-art audience by Nicholas Nixon's (and to a lesser extent, Rosalind Solomon's) problematic AIDS portraits, examined in detail in the previous chapter.

On first acquaintance Morrisroe's self-portrait suggests a similar iconographic approach to Nixon's: the artist appears to be dying alone, his body wasted by disease, the rubbish that surrounds him mirroring the moral and physical decrepitude of his own person. Yet the self-authored status of Morrisroe's image complicates the binary logic that underpins critical accounts such as Crimp's and Grover's, which typically imply that the objectification of the person with AIDS arises as a direct result of the photographer's or intended viewer's personal situation as an outsider to the AIDS community.[3] A similar logic informs praise of Rosett's 'intra-community portraits', which are construed as representations of active and empowered individuals in control of their own subjecthood.[4] Morrisroe's self-portrait suggests a simultaneous adoption of both positions, passively inactive as the focus of the camera's gaze, and vibrant sovereign subject as the image's author.

In addition to the Polaroid self-portraits, between 1987 and 1988 Morrisroe also produced a series of strikingly beautiful, brightly coloured prints based on photograms of his X-rays, hand-tinting each image as if to map the effects of AIDS on his internal organs. If the Polaroid pictures imply a re-appropriation of the popular iconography of the AIDS victim, then the X-ray prints, produced in a temporary darkroom rigged up in Morrisroe's hospital bathroom, suggest a similar arrogation of medical spaces and technologies. Making visible the body's tangible surfaces and uncanny interiors, these two groups of work draw attention to a self that is both creative subject and abject other, played out across the fragile boundaries of Morrisroe's critically ill body.

Truth-telling and myth-making

References to Morrisroe's compelling personality and propensity for self-mythologizing frame almost all existing readings of his work. Indeed, for Morrisroe art and life were inextricably entangled. His primary subject matter was a life shared with his friends and collaborators in the punk and art worlds of 1980s Boston and New York. A significant proportion of his works are self-portraits that depict the artist in a variety of semi-autobiographical guises; the estate also includes numerous prints and Polaroids of friends and lovers, often unclothed and posed in dingy domestic spaces made strange and beautiful through his skilled re-workings of the original images. His physical manipulations of the negative, coupled with his habit of incessant lying and constant self-reinvention, invite questions about the photographic medium's complex relationship with truth-telling (on one hand), and myth-making (on the other).

Morrisroe was born in Boston in 1959, where he was raised by a single mother who struggled with alcohol addiction; Morrisroe was prone to embellishing the details of his unstable childhood, frequently exaggerating his mother's addiction issues and claiming that he had been fathered by the infamous Boston Strangler.[5] He left home at sixteen and supported himself with sex work; at eighteen a gunshot wound to the spine from a client left him hospitalized for several months, with doctors unsure if he would ever walk again. A note penned by clinical staff during this period gives a vivid sense of Morrisroe's compelling yet difficult personality:

> He speaks in an affected manner and theatrical gestures, which are effective in drawing people towards him. However, his obnoxious, acting-out behavior also alienates the staff at times and has made management [a] problem.[6]

With characteristic obstinacy, Morrisroe did walk again, although he was left with a pronounced limp that restricted his mobility and caused him chronic pain. It also enhanced his distinctive charismatic appeal. His gallerist, Pat Hearn, once described how Morrisroe would 'wobble, with much presence, into every social gathering [. . .] When he was not looking, he was being looked at. His clumsy gestures and whining voice commanded the attention of those around him'.[7] According to many accounts, Morrisroe desired nothing more ardently than to be looked at; his entire adult life was dedicated to producing a spectacle of which he was the star. His drive to be seen persisted even as he was dying: as his former tutor at the Boston Museum School recalls, 'Mark was a drama queen, so that was his final gesture: being a drama queen. To make art of his death . . .'.[8] Through his practice he embellished and reconstructed the life that underpinned it: initially known as a documentarian, he is now predominantly understood as master of postmodern self-fashioning.

The initial categorization of Morrisroe as a documentarian of 1980s' Boston subculture arose partly out of Morrisroe's association with Nan Goldin, who like Morrisroe had also studied at the Boston Museum School before moving to New York's East Village in the 1980s. In the introduction to the catalogue for the 1995 exhibition *Boston School*, Lia Gangitano refers to the young artists' sense of alienation from the documentary tradition that was prevalent at the Museum School in the late 1970s. The photographer Shellburne Thurber recalls taking pictures that her teachers might have 'made on the side' rather than for the purposes of art: her tutors' professional work depicted situations and people outside of their own lived experience, often in geographical or economic locations far removed from their everyday lives.[9] Yet at the same time, the School was well known for its permissive attitude and tolerance of unconventionality. Jane Hudson, who in the late 1970s taught the video and film class attended by Morrisroe, recalls that 'there was a great effort made to refrain from judgement, to be flexible in the face of radical departure from tradition'; tutors 'gave technical instructions, but [. . .] were pretty open to whatever anybody wanted to do [. . .] that was part of the Museum School's ethic: not to be directive, but almost like a mind reader, to figure out what it was that made someone tick and then support that, help them develop that'.[10] Such an environment made it possible for Morrisroe and his contemporaries to develop highly personal, often autobiographical artistic practices that suggested a break with the disinterested documentary tradition favoured by their tutors.

Goldin and Morrisroe occasionally appear in each other's work: one of Morrisroe's early prints, *Untitled (Nan)* (1980), shows the young Goldin in a black bra, pearls and dark eye make-up, leaning back on her hands and gazing sleepily downwards at the camera. Goldin's image (*Mark Morrisroe*) (1982) similarly captures Morrisroe shirtless and in repose, slumped against a wall with his eyes closed, his wiry and tattooed arm cradling a bottle of spirits. Yet the physicality of Morrisroe's work is a crucial point of difference with Goldin's; Goldin claimed to be uninterested in the darkroom, and early versions of *The Ballard of Sexual Dependency* were characterized by the physical immateriality of her images, which were displayed by being projected onto the walls of clubs. In contrast to Goldin's pictures, Morrisroe's prints are often highly tangible as objects: his signature techniques involved manual inference in both negatives and prints, and his works often bear the traces of these manipulations in the form of fingermarks, flecks of dust and stray hairs.

The messy physicality of these prints echoes the alluring chaos of a life once concisely characterized as 'romantic squalor, unbearable suffering and above all, incessant lying'.[11] Morrisroe was well known for creating outrageous stories that fused fact and fiction into one unstable yet utterly compelling narrative.

This strategy for self-(re)invention has been interpreted as overtly performative: Linda Yablonsky describes Morrisroe as an artist who 'seems never to have started the day without a role to play',[12] Fionn Meade notes 'an obvious and overt theatricality to Morrisroe's portrayal of himself and his friends',[13] and José Esteban Muñoz labels the work a 'melodrama'.[14] David Joselit's essay 'Mark Morrisroe's Photographic Masquerade' has been particularly important for a re-evaluation of Morrisroe's work in these terms.[15] By emphasizing how Morrisroe's physical interventions in the medium challenge notions about the 'truth-telling' capacity of the photographic image, Joselit's reading addresses the blurred lines between the apparently opposed categorizations of Morrisroe as either compulsive liar or chronicler of facts. Surprisingly, Joselit's text barely touches on Morrisroe's representations of his illness: this chapter will ultimately argue that the tension between 'fact' and 'fiction', authenticity and performance, self-objectification and creative self-(re)presentation can provide a powerful framework for considering Morrisroe's final self-portraits.

Seeing spectres

The previous chapter addressed the difficulties of documentary photography in adequately representing the experiences of people with AIDS. As read through critical accounts such as Douglas Crimp's and Jan Zita Grover's, the documentary genre was considered unable to shed its objectifying tendencies, and artists working in this mode were seen as overly prone to reproducing the clichéd iconography of the AIDS victim. These criticisms of fine-art documentary AIDS photography were traced to an 'anti-photography' discourse exemplified by texts by Allan Sekula and Martha Rosler. The present chapter draws on an approach to photography that is contemporaneous with Sekula and Rosler's critical methodologies, but markedly different: a phenomenology of photography with its roots in continental theory.

Roland Barthes' highly influential text *Camera Lucida* (1980; trans. 1981) initially appears to support an understanding of the photograph as necessarily objectifying: the instant at which the camera shutter falls into place denotes an act of violence; the photograph 'parcels out the body', making its referent into a 'passive victim'.[16] However, closer attention to Barthes' text reveals a greater subtly to his position. For Barthes, the experience of having one's picture taken induces the sensation of being neither subject nor object, but momentarily poised between both; through this indeterminate state of 'becoming an object' the photograph heralds 'the advent of myself as other'.[17] It is this moment of becoming object/other that Morrisroe's images evoke so successfully. Hanging in the instant when the photographer-referent is neither subject nor object, Morrisroe's images (and perhaps all photographic self-portraits) glimpse a liminal position where self and 'other' can meld and merge without compromising the subject's fundamental agency.

With its emphasis on death and desire (it is often understood as a lamentation for the author's dead mother), *Camera Lucida* is a compelling text to consider in relation to Morrisroe's work. Barthes' evocative characterization of the photograph as 'the return of the dead'[18] is related to its apparently indexical nature: the essence of the photograph is to show *what-has-been*; it is a 'certificate of presence' that guarantees the existence of an object or person. Yet the moment at which the referent is captured is always already in the past, and it is not the thing itself that is recorded but its *eidolon*, suggesting an image-double, phantom, apparition or ghost.

Although *Camera Lucida* is an obvious point of reference for theorizing Morrisroe's late work, this chapter attempts to diffuse its almost talismanic influence by supplementing it with a second body of writing. Hervé Guibert's collection of reflections on photography, *L'Image Fantôme* (1981; trans. 1996) was published in French within a year of *Camera Lucida*, although a number of articles included in the book had already appeared in print elsewhere.[19] Its relative lack of impact on Anglophone photography theory may be accounted for by the fact that the English translation *Ghost Image* did not appear until 1996, fifteen years after *Camera Lucida*. If *Camera Lucida* looks mainly to the past (Barthes' most significant case study, the 'Winter Garden' photograph, is a picture of his mother as a young girl), then *Ghost Image* is situated firmly in its own moment. A filmmaker, actor, photographer and journalist, Guibert was diagnosed HIV positive in 1988, documenting his experience of AIDS in the auto-fictions *To the Friend Who Did Not Save My Life* (1990), *The Compassionate Protocol* (1991) and *Cytomegalovirus: Journal of a Hospitalization* (1992) and in the documentary *La Pudeur ou l'Impudeur* (made between 1990 and 1991 and aired posthumously on French television in 1992).[20] Like *Camera Lucida,* Guibert's *Ghost Image* considers photography in the context of familial relations, death and pleasure ('How can you speak of photography without speaking of desire?', Guibert asks rhetorically).[21] If Barthes describes looking at an image in passive terms as *being* touched, Guibert imagines photography as an active mechanism for making physical contact with otherwise forbidden bodies: asked by a friend 'why do you photograph me so much?' Guibert replies, 'it's easier to ask to take your picture than ask to caress you.'[22] Guibert writes about not only taking pictures but holding them, kissing them, taking them into his bed and, in an extreme case, wearing a photograph taped against his skin until the image becomes transferred to his flesh; Guibert's phenomenological understanding of photographs as erotic objects proves particularly useful in relation to Morrisroe's work.

The title of this chapter, 'Becoming a Specter', alludes to the condition of spectrality that is explicit in the title of *Ghost Image* and implicit in both *Camera Lucida* and Morrisroe's photographic practice. This 'spectrality' is not intended to suggest the social, political or cultural invisibility of the person with AIDS: unlike Robert Blanchon or Felix Gonzalez-Torres, both of whom served as members of ACT UP and made politically motivated work (albeit in a subtle and often indirect manner), Morrisroe does not appear to have been politicized by AIDS. Instead of critiquing cultural and political reactions to AIDS or exploring the emotional dimensions of illness, Morrisroe's work belies an enthralled fascination with his changing body. Morrisroe's 'spectrality' thus suggests the transitory moment between subjecthood and objecthood, a moment of becoming rather than being, a pivotal instant where existential boundaries are briefly dissolved.[23]

Photographs and flesh

Morrisroe frequently photographed himself nude, often in sexually suggestive poses. *Sweet Sixteen: Little Me as a Child Prostitute* (*c.* 1984) (Figure 7) is a tongue-in-cheek reference to his history of sex work. Based on a Polaroid print initially used as a calling card, the image depicts the naked young artist sprawled provocatively across a bed. His legs are spread apart, and his semi-erect genitalia is at the centre of the image: one hand supports his head in a classic Odalisque pose and the other lingers teasingly on his inner thigh. Similarly, in *Self-Portrait (To Brent)* (*c.* 1982) (Figure 8), Morrisroe, fresh from the shower, his skin still gleaming with moisture, meets the camera in a full-frontal stance: one arm is raised with his hand out of frame, presumably so as to activate the shutter. In image after image, Morrisroe poses – often naked, occasionally outfitted (a black bustier and stockings make a regular appearance) and almost always gazing directly into the lens of the camera: a man who knows the value of his erotic and photographic appeal.

Morrisroe also photographed his friends, a group of camera-friendly young artists and performers including Steve Tashjian (aka Tabboo!), the Starn

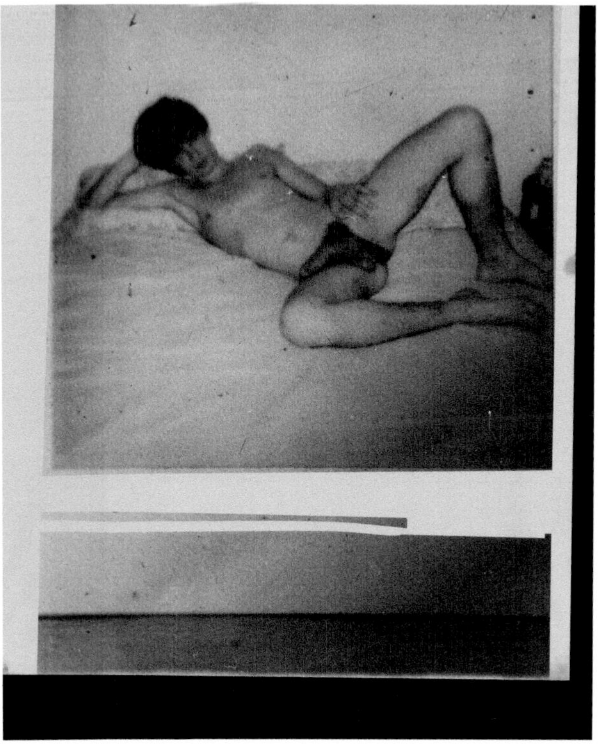

Figure 7 Mark Morrisroe, *Sweet 16, Little Me as a Child Prostitute*, 1984. C-print, negative sandwich, 50.5 × 40.4 cm. © The Estate of Mark Morrisroe (Ringier Collection) at Fotomuseum Winterthur.

Twins and his then-boyfriend Jonathan (Jack) Pierson: he was well known for persuading people to undress, and many of his subjects are fully nude.[24] The sensual appeal of these images, however, derives not necessarily from the subject matter but from the material physicality of the prints. Many of Morrisroe's works were designed to be handled: pictures like *Sweet Sixteen* were used to drum up work, while others were gifted to friends or lovers. In the margins of the print *Self-Portrait (To Brent)*, Morrisroe has scribbled a dedication: 'To Brent, a little something for all those words of wisdom that you've been offering me all these years, Mark xx.' Usually matted out in early exhibitions of the work, these inscriptions and other marks are now understood as part of Morrisroe's unique response to his medium.

Morrisroe's tactile approach to photography is also evident in his innovative treatment of the negative. He would produce two for each image, one in black and white and the other in colour, which he would then 'sandwich' together and re-photograph. At least 350 known works were produced using the sandwich

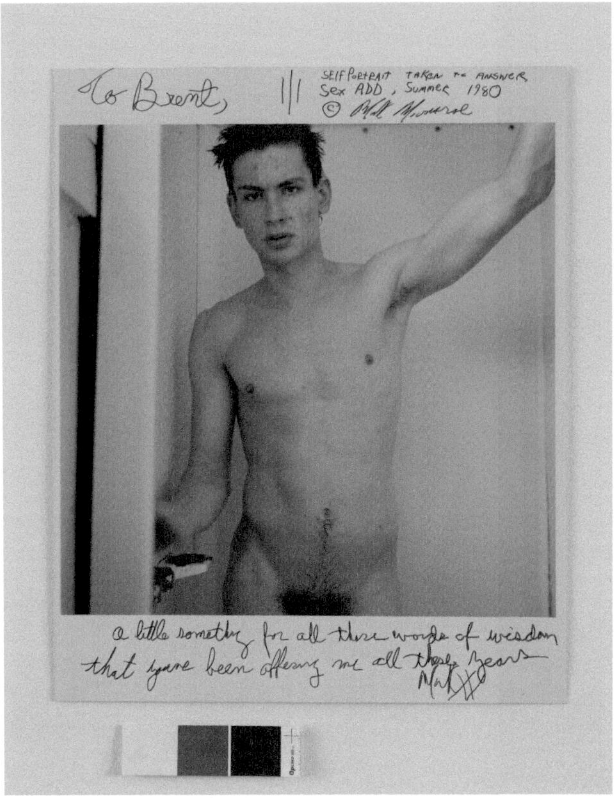

Figure 8 Mark Morrisroe, *Self-Portrait (to Brent),* 1982. C-print, inscribed with marker, 50.7 × 40.5 cm. Collection Brent Sikkema, Whitney Museum of American Art © The Estate of Mark Morrisroe.

technique, including *Sweet Sixteen* and *To Brent*, as well as a significant number of nude figure studies. These prints are lushly textured with a steamy, vaporous quality; skin is rendered dewy, tactile and inviting. The technique involved a significant degree of handling, meaning that prints are often marked with dust, hair and, occasionally, the artist's own fingerprints. *Rose's Back* (1983) (Figure 9) is a smoky-hued study of a woman's spine; a fingerprint on the negative has embossed her skin with swoops and whorls of ink, retouched by Morrisroe as if to emphasize the deliberate nature of this personal mark, which integrates his own body into the corpus of the photograph.

Elisabeth Lebovici uses the term 'erotogenicity' to describe Morrisroe's sandwich prints, referring to the 'insidious sexual pulse throbbing through each and every one'.[25] She borrows the term from Freud,[26] who uses it to denote the way in which erotic potential is distributed through the whole body, with

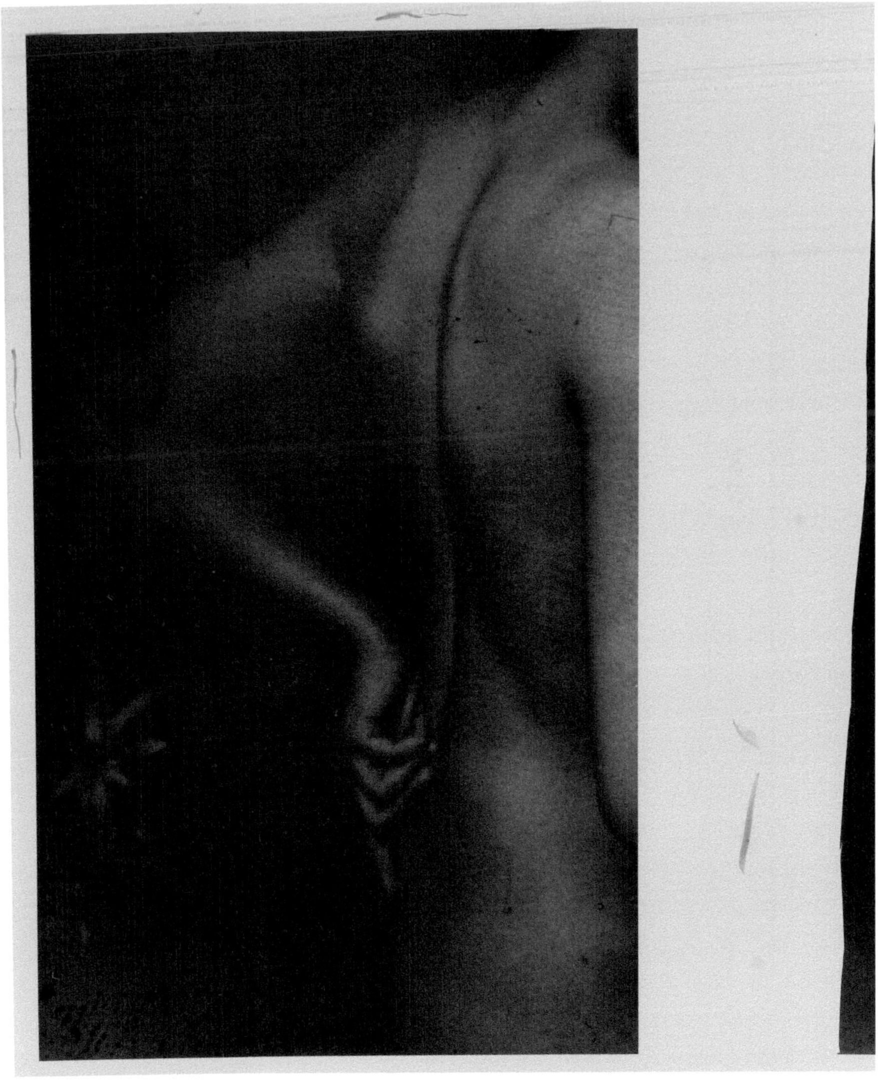

Figure 9 Mark Morrisroe, *Rose's Back*, 1983. C-print, negative sandwich, retouched with ink, 50.6 × 40.5 cm. © The Estate of Mark Morrisroe (Ringier Collection) at Fotomuseum Winterthur.

pleasure experienced not only by external sensory receptors such as the skin and mucous membranes but also by the internal organs.[27] Elizabeth Grosz has similarly drawn on Freud to emphasize the distinction between the sexual drive, which is directed towards an object, and erotogenic desire, which is not object-directed but instead exists as a series of layered intensities.[28] This is evident in Morrisroe's nudes, which are not so much objects of desire as spaces where photographed flesh coalesces with the traces of the artist's own tactile engagement. (Morrisroe's nudes do not suggest a specifically homoerotic gaze, with female bodies rendered with as much erotogenic appeal as male ones.)[29]

Grosz (drawing on Alphonso Lingis' reading of Lyotard, Deleuze and Guattari)[30] suggests that the object-directed sexual drive and more diffuse phenomenon of erotic desire each correspond to two different frameworks for conceptualizing carnality. The first approach, broadly psychoanalytic, imagines the erotic subject in terms of psychic interiority, emphasizing reasons, motives, causes, intentions and fantasies. The second approach is phenomenological, accentuating the externality of desire and in Grosz's words, privileging 'the erotogenic surface, the body's "outside", its locus as a site for both the perception of the erotic [. . .] but also for the inscription and intensification of the sensitivity of bodily regions'.[31] Yet the 'outside' of the body – put in scare quotes by Grosz – is not only external but also regional, confusing the usual topological organization of the body into surface and depth. Here, as in Morrisroe's sandwich print nudes, the erotogenic surface is not merely superficial; both the skin and the photograph itself are the meeting place where interior and exterior caress and (con)fuse.

Hervé Guibert's short story 'The Cancerous Image' describes a ghostly converging of photograph and flesh that is particularly evocative in relation to Morrisroe's work.[32] Written a decade before Guibert died from an AIDS-related illness, it prophetically weaves together death and desire, merging real and representational bodies, flesh with photograph. Guibert treasures a photograph of a young man. Over seven years, the picture assumes an almost unnatural supremacy: 'it chased away all others that wanted to take up residence in the bedroom, it was always the only possible photograph'.[33] One day Guibert notices that the image has begun to decay: the glue that fixes it to its cardboard mount is eating the photograph from behind. The boy's face is 'attacked with sores and pustules'; he looks 'syphilitic'.[34] No longer able to look at him, Guibert instead keeps the image in his bed: 'beneath the sheets that welcomed my body [. . .] I crushed him and heard him whimper'.[35] After a while Guibert decides to wear the decaying figure 'directly against my skin, directly against my torso, attaching him with bandages and tape'.[36] When finally Guibert decides to remove him, he sees that the limp cardboard is empty. The image, however, has not disappeared: 'in a mirror, I verified that it had stuck to my skin, like a tattoo or a decal. Each of the paper's chemical pigments had found its place in the pores of my skin. And the same image formed itself identically in reverse. The transfer had saved him from his illness'.[37] Guibert's text suggests a crisis of the representational image: disease threatens the photograph's materiality as object, but it is saved by becoming 'real' through prolonged contact with living flesh.

The symbolic associations between human skin and the photographic surface have been noted by scholars working in a number of different disciplines. The film theorist Laura U. Marks uses skin as a metaphor to emphasize the way film signifies through its materiality, via contact made between perceiver and represented object.[38] In a series of similes that could equally be applied to photography, Marks describes film and video as 'impressionable and conductive, like skin', and cinema as 'tactile and contagious'.[39] Marks' theory of haptic visuality suggests that if optical perception privileges the image's representational power, then haptic perception privileges its material presence. For Marks optic visuality invokes perspective and pictorial depth; haptic implies surface. 'Haptic' well describes Morrisroe's sandwich prints: despite their mode of production suggesting multiple layers and three-dimensionality, their luscious surfaces are never more than skin deep. Similarly, the psychoanalyst Didier Anzieu has drawn attention to the linguistic affinity between skin and photograph in French, where *pellicule* refers both to the membrane that covers the human body and to the photograph's base layer upon which is laid the chemical coating that receives the impression of the image.[40] Skin and photograph are both conceptualized as sensitive surfaces, capable of receiving traces and inscriptions. Yet, as Morrisroe's practice makes clear, the photograph is not simply a surface but far more complex: 'both permeable and impermeable, superficial and profound, truthful and misleading'.[41]

The photographic masquerade

The propensity of the photographic medium to be both 'truthful and misleading' is at the heart of David Joselit's 1995 analysis of what he identifies as Morrisroe's 'photographic masquerade'. The locus of this masquerade is the negative, conceptualized by Joselit as a borderland where an object can cross over to become an image, a marginalized zone that accommodates the subject's own splitting. Focussing on Morrisroe's sandwich prints, Joselit points out how the doubling, cutting and layering of the negative invests the depicted figures with a strange duality (perhaps even a spectrality): 'certain people in these photographs . . . seem to escape the ordinary comfortable fleshliness of human existence, being compounded instead out of something like the ethereal translucence of angels and the all-too-solid stone of statuary.'[42]

Joselit's argument about the 'performative' nature of Morrisroe's practice draws on three canonical texts: Joan Riviere's 'Womanliness as a Masquerade', Mary Anne Doane's 'Film and the Masquerade – Theorising the Female Spectator' and Judith Butler's *Gender Trouble*.[43] Riviere's text was ground-breaking not only in its proposal that femininity might be worn as a mask but also in the suggestion that no distinction could be drawn between genuine womanliness and its masquerade, the two being in effect the same thing. Joselit draws attention to the implicitly art-historical metaphor of figure and ground used by both Doane and Butler. If Doane imagines the female body as the ground upon which the figure of 'womanliness' can be displayed, Butler suggests that gendered identity is produced through a shifting interplay of figure and ground that destabilizes both terms. This subtle distinction illuminates the difference between performance and performativity: if 'performance' suggests a surface act that masks the real beneath, then 'performativity' suggests that reality is not distinct from performance but is generated through a shifting set of figurations.

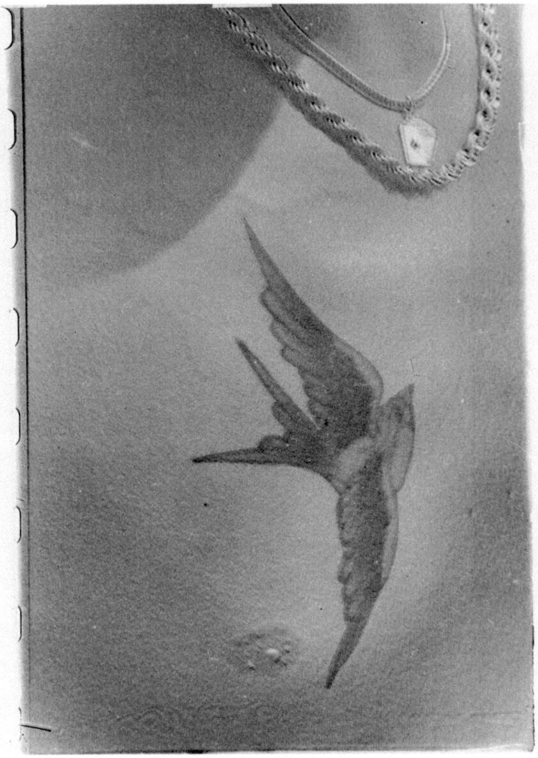

Figure 10 Mark Morrisroe, Untitled, *c.* 1988. C-print, negative sandwich, 50.5 × 40.5 cm. © The Estate of Mark Morrisroe (Ringier Collection) at Fotomuseum Winterthur.

Reading one of Morrisroe's furrowed, shadowy sandwich print nudes (Figure 10), Joselit points out how figure and ground lose their distinctness, each spilling over onto a single destabilized surface. Tellingly, Joselit imagines this through a metaphor of photograph as skin: 'If we imagine this surface *as a kind of skin*, then it is possible to understand the body, in a vivid metaphor for masquerade, *as a photograph*.'[44] By way of example, Joselit takes an untitled image, which depicts a man's chest from his neckline to just below his right nipple. His body fills the frame, rendering the figure almost indistinguishable from the frame. Details such as a tattoo of a bird, two gold chains and soft shadows playing over his skin prevent the flesh from becoming unambiguously a 'ground', confusing the relationship between figure and ground. Following Butler's argument, Joselit suggests that Morrisroe's sandwich prints reveal all identity to be a masquerade, a complex interplay of masks. Joselit shows how Morrisroe's photography undoes the assumed binary opposition between documentary realism and performance, fact and fiction: 'If, as Jack Pierson reported, Morrisroe was a chronic liar, the significance of this fact is rooted in his capacity *as an artist* to demonstrate that in truth, we are composed of lies.'[45]

The spectral uncanny: X-rays and photograms

Morrisroe tested positive for HIV in 1986, and his health began to deteriorate from this point onwards. He started to work with photograms: needing neither a camera nor a model, the medium was well suited to the temporary darkrooms that Morrisroe rigged up during periods of hospitalization. Many of his photograms de-familiarize the human form: found images (often figures sourced from pornographic magazines) are laid on photographic paper and exposed to light, then sliced, segmented and rotated, perhaps mimicking the violence being done to his own body. A second compelling source material for the photograms is Morrisroe's collection of X-ray images. Among the most captivating of the X-ray-based photograms are a trio of lungs tinted in pinks, yellows and inky blue, the dyes seeping from the chest cavity into the darkness of the body like a slowly spreading tumour (*Untitled (Triptych), c.* 1987) (Figure 11), and a frontal exposure of the thorax with the pulmonary organs marked in blocks of cyan and magenta and the body haloed with an unearthly yellow radiation (*Untitled, c.* 1987) (Figure 12). Vivid and gorgeous, these pieces seem strangely out of place in a corpus of work that emerges from an encounter with terminal illness. Perhaps more easily assimilated within this narrative are the large black-and-white prints

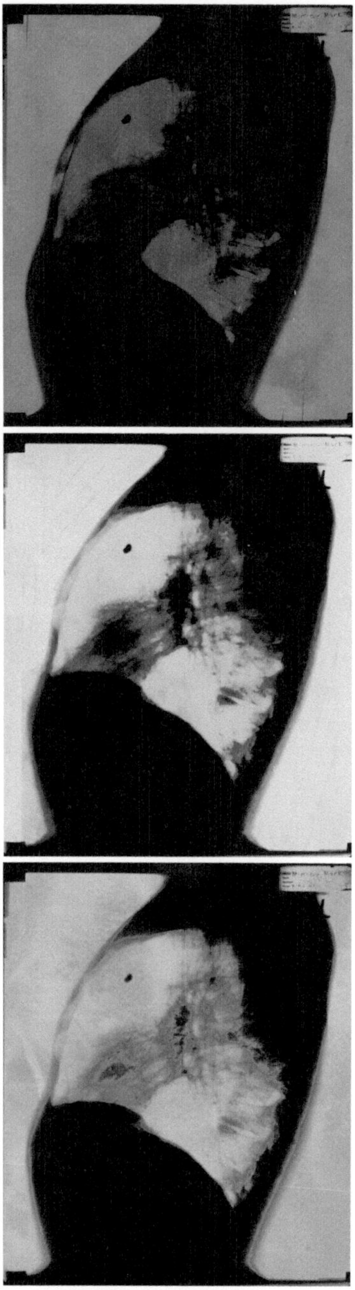

Figure 11 Mark Morrisroe, Untitled, 1988. Triptych, colourized gelatin silver prints, photogram of X-ray, each image 43.3 × 35.5 cm. © The Estate of Mark Morrisroe (Ringier Collection) at Fotomuseum Winterthur.

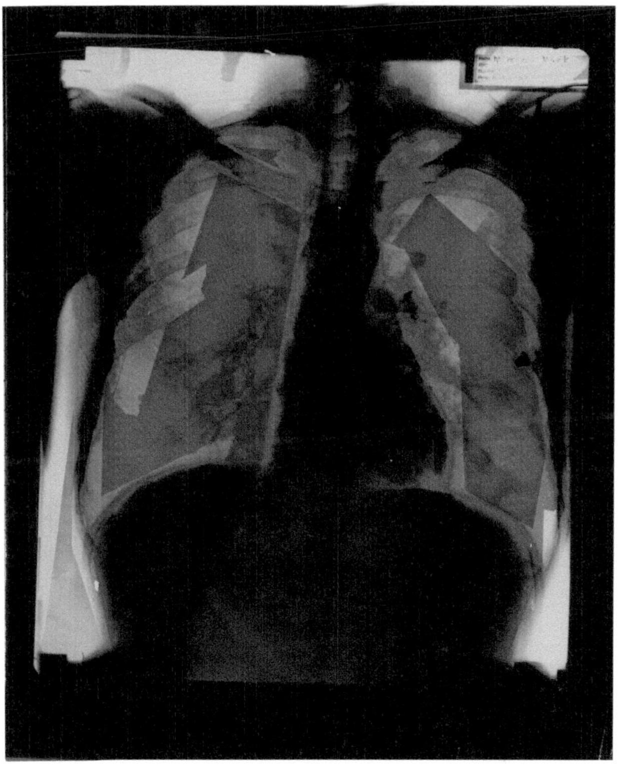

Figure 12 Mark Morrisroe, Untitled, *c.* 1988. Colourized gelatin silver print, photogram of X-ray, 50.5 × 40.3 cm. © The Estate of Mark Morrisroe (Ringier Collection) at Fotomuseum Winterthur.

made from dental X-rays, each threatening engulfment and annihilation, or the spectral images of ribs and skulls evoking the iconic personification of Death.

Morrisroe's partner, Ramsey McPhillips, has described the artist's enthusiastic response to the X-ray as source material:

> Once the doctor showed Mark his X rays revealing that he had pneumonia. Mark's response was 'THAT'S A MASTERPIECE!' He took it, added some of his concocted color photo chemicals, and made the X-rays into beautiful images.[46]

Morrisroe acquired an assortment of X-ray images of various body parts, from skeletal hands and feet, to femora, vertebrae and crania. The sheer volume of his collection is further evidence of Morrisroe's fascination with the medical medium, and to his eagerness to work with it, despite his failing health. Only a minority of these are unquestionable representations of Morrisroe's own body; those X-ray images that are indubitably his include the tinted triptych of lungs and frontal print of his chest described in the previous paragraph, all of which bear the institutional inscription of his personal details (name, date of birth and hospital number) in the top-right corner of the image. Many of the other X-rays in Morrisroe's archive have had this identifying information removed from the top-right corner; it is unknown by whom this excision was carried out. This means that only a minority of Morrisroe's X-ray photograms can be truly considered self-portraits; it is these that will be addressed in this section.

Artists have long been fascinated by the visual possibilities suggested by the X-ray, which turns the body inside out and allows for the portrayal of previously invisible corporeal spaces. X-rays spurred an interest in painted explorations of the body's interior, as in Frida Kahlo's *The Broken Column* (1944), where the artist depicts her spine as a fractured pillar inside her flayed torso, or Picasso's *Girl before a Mirror* (1932), which presents the model with her womb and ovaries exposed to view. The influence of the X-ray on Cubist vision has been noted by Stephen Kern, who hypothesizes that the 'X-ray must have had something to do with the Cubist rendering of the interior of solid objects'.[47] The Futurists showed a similar fascination with the changing relationship between inside and outside space: as their spokesman, Umberto Boccioni, asked: 'Who can still believe in the opacity of bodies . . . when our sharpened and multiplied sensibility allows us to perceive the obscure disclosure of mediumistic phenomena? What should we continue to create without taking into account our perceptive powers which can give us results analogous to the X-rays?'[48]

Other artists were similarly intrigued by the possibilities for self-portraiture offered by the X-ray print. In 1967, Robert Rauschenberg assembled the life-sized print *Booster* from a composite of five X-ray prints of his body, creating an image that is both specific to the individual (offering a privileged glimpse inside his own body) and at the same time depersonalized (the basic structure of the skeleton being similar for everyone).[49] Working in the same period as Rauschenberg, the surrealist artist Meret Oppenheim's self-portrait *X-Ray of My Skull* (1964; produced as a limited edition print in 1981) depicts the artist's head, shoulders and hand, the soft shadows of flesh and bone marked with the dense black forms of her jewellery. Often understood as a response to Man Ray's erotically charged solarized portraits (*c.* 1933) of the young Oppenheim nude in front of the printer's wheel, this image alludes to the sense of intimacy and sexual charge associated with the X-ray as an expressive medium; I shall return to this point shortly.[50]

As well as suggesting new pictorial possibilities for the representation of bodies and spaces, the X-ray also offered a means of re-conceptualizing the relationship between psychic interiority and the subject's tangible, visible exterior. Akira Mizuta Lippit has drawn attention to the historical convergence of psychoanalysis and X-ray technology, pointing out that the Roentgen rays were named in the same year as Freud and Breuer published *Studies on Hysteria* (1896); the convergence of the two, he suggests, inaugurates 'an epistemology of the inside'.[51] Lippit describes X-rays as 'radical photography' or 'photographs in reverse'; as with Morrisroe's sandwich prints, the X-ray collapses the 'essential divide between surface and depths [. . .] rendering the body a deep surface'.[52]

As Rosalind Krauss observes in 'Notes On the Index', the photogram is a subspecies of photography that forces the issue of the medium's existence as index.[53] Doing away with the need for a photographic negative, the photogram is produced by placing objects on top of light-sensitive paper, exposing the ensemble to light and then developing the result. Krauss describes the resultant images as resembling 'the ghostly traces of departed objects; they look like footprints in sand, or marks that have been left in dust'.[54] Writing in relation to Man Ray's photograms (or rayographs, to use his preferred term), Jane Livingston concurs:

> Operating both as an analogue to the cast shadow [. . .] and simply as the unmodeled residue of the thing's outer form registered through a simple photochemical action, the rayograph surpassed the camera-produced photograph in its univalent transformation of the real object into a sign or trace.[55]

The effect of the photogram, Livingston concludes, is to present the real object in such a way 'as to establish its self-evident corporeality and yet also to push it into the realm of the meta-real'.[56] This is exactly what Morrisroe's X-ray-based photograms achieve; the body is somehow real and yet not-real, based on a medical trace transformed into an uncanny, hallucinogenic form; rather than simply constituting the 'evidence' of Morrisroe's illness, these remade images express a breathtakingly imaginative and idiosyncratic response to it.

Morrisroe's X-ray-based photograms might be understood in terms of a resistance to the objectifying gaze that Michel Foucault has identified as part of the modern medical system. Foucault describes the pre-modern clinical encounter as a dialogic exchange between the patient and an accessible, community-based repository of medical knowledge: 'At the dawn of man', Foucault writes, 'medicine in its entirety consisted of an immediate relationship between sickness and that which alleviated it'.[57] This relationship was instinctual: the patient drew on a personal and local knowledge of what might improve his condition and acted accordingly. This kind of medicine was universally practised, with communities sharing knowledge without possession of it; Foucault describes this as 'a general form of consciousness of which each individual is both subject and object'.[58] The move to specular modern medicine comprises a shift from speaking to seeing, repressing the subjectivity of the patient in favour of the expertise of the clinician and constructing the patient's body purely as the object of the physician's gaze. Foucault suggests that this objectification is disturbingly violent and yet essential to the practice of modern medicine:

> to look in order to know [. . .] is not this a tacit form of violence upon a sick body that demands to be comforted, not displayed? Can pain be a spectacle? Not only can it be, but it must be.[59]

With their forceful and compelling colours, Morrisroe's photograms are powerfully suggestive of modern medicine's necessary display of pain as spectacle. They also strongly suggest the reduction of the individual patient to a series of diseased body parts. As the medical historian Bettyann Kevles points out, the clinical image operates according to a system of stand-in: the physician is accustomed to reading the partial image as a stand-in for the real body, and certain marks on the images as a stand-in for the disease itself.[60] Thus, the partial body is treated as a synecdoche of the total, unified body, and the visual fragment as a signifier for the patient as a whole.

Morrisroe's re-appropriation of his medical images, however, challenges the dominance of the medical gaze and re-presents his body as an expression of his own experience. Morrisroe's images are powerfully suggestive of a pre-modern medical understanding of the body, the unruly colours spreading across the surface of the prints recalling the four humours of blood, colourless phlegm, choler (red or yellow bile) and black bile. Humoral theory was the dominant paradigm of the inner body from the classical period until the start of a slow disintegration from the seventeenth century onwards.[61] The humoral body was understood as open, porous and in constant flux; external conditions such as the weather could affect the humoral balance within the body, and the humours themselves were fungible, shifting freely from one state to another. The language of the humours thus constructs a body that, even when in good health, is tumultuous and dramatic, possessing a 'strange alterity', with the internal organs frequently ascribed an agency at odds with the will of the subject.

Far from expressing his experience in necessarily negative terms, Morrisroe's photograms communicate the artist's awe and wonderment at the changes being wrought upon his body. In this they share something in common with earlier anatomical images, which from the Renaissance to the nineteenth century did not simply have a diagnostic or didactic function but were also aesthetic and theological statements about the nature of humans as God-created beings, designed to 'inspire awe in the public as much as they were used to educate'.[62] Morrisroe's images suggest a similar sense of near-religious veneration: installed in the white space of the Pat Hearn Gallery for Morrisroe's last solo exhibition during his lifetime, the coloured prints resembled nothing so much as the stained-glass windows of a place of worship, prompting one reviewer to describe the show as 'a clinical shrine'.[63]

Kevles has noted the long-standing historical associations of X-rays with sexuality and eroticism.[64] The first X-rays opened up the (usually female) body to new possibilities of voyeurism; early discourse is characterized by concern about the social propriety of the X-ray, expressing the fear that its penetrative power might render the female form improperly exposed. Clothing manufacturers capitalized on these fears by offering lead underwear to protect ladies from prying eyes, while cartoonists made sardonic proposals for other precautionary fashions.[65]

The erotic potential of the X-ray is curiously linked to its symbolic association with death. Lippit suggests that the very term 'X-ray' (especially its prefix) invokes 'a cultural semiology that includes pornography (adolescent notions of X-ray vision and "x" and "triple-x" rated movies), medicine, algebra, and erasure'.[66] Lisa Cartwright describes the X-ray as 'a highly charged site for the manifestation of anxieties about sexual difference, mutilation and death'.[67] This peculiar synthesis of the morbid and the erotic occurs in the reception of the first X-ray image to be circulated in the scientific and popular press, a photograph of the hand of Roentgen's wife. To Mrs Roentgen, as to many others later, this experience gave a premonition of death: when her husband showed her the picture, she could hardly believe that this bony hand was her own and shuddered at the thought that she was seeing her skeleton.[68] X-rays of female hands soon became a popular craze: in turn-of-the-century New York X-rays of female hands were exchanged as tokens of affection. It was fashionable for women to have X-rays taken of their hands covered in jewellery; married women gave X-rays of their hands with wedding ring affixed, to their relatives. In the early days of the X-ray, the female X-ray hand thus became 'a fetish object par excellence'.[69]

Thomas Mann's novel *The Magic Mountain* (1924), set in a tuberculosis sanatorium in Switzerland, has much to say about the deathly and erotic potential of X-rays, as well as the capacity of the X-ray to act as a 'portrait'. The inhabitants of the sanatorium each carry a miniature pulmonary X-ray in their wallets like an 'identity card';[70] the novel's protagonist Hans Castorp treasures such an image given to him by the woman with whom he is in love: 'Clavdia's X-ray portrait, showing not her face, but the delicate bony structure of the upper half of her body, and the organs of the thoracic cavity, surrounded by the pale, ghostlike envelope of flesh.'[71] When Castorp is first permitted to look at his own hand through the X-ray machine he sees 'into his own grave': 'the process of decay was forestalled by the powers of the light-ray, the flesh in which he walked disintegrated, annihilated, dissolved in vacant mist [. . .] for the first time in his life he understood that he would die.'[72] The sanatorium's director refers to the X-ray in directly erotic terms, showing his young patient a radiogram of a woman's arm and indelicately informing him, 'That's what they put around you when they make love, you know.'[73] His instructions to Castorp explicitly render the experience of submitting to an X-ray in terms of a sexual encounter: '"Put your arms about it," he said. "Embrace the board – pretend it's something else, if you like. Press your breast against it, as though it filled you with rapture."'[74]

The eroticization of pulmonary X-rays continues into the mid-twentieth century in the form of public health films designed to promote knowledge about tuberculosis.[75] *Mass Radiography*, a 1944 British government–funded film designed to teach industrial workers about the benefits of radiography, follows the story of Mary, a young, attractive factory worker who has reservations about getting X-rayed. By the end of the film, Mary has come to accept the benefits of X-rays: she presents her lover with two framed portraits, a photograph of her face and an X-ray of her chest, both signed 'to Tom, with all my love, Mary'. The final voice-over reassures factory girls like Mary of the usefulness of X-rays for confirming their own worth as targets for male desire: 'For you, an X-ray means that someone can say not only "Sure she's pretty", but "sure she's healthy."' Aligned with the personal snapshot or pin-up, the X-ray is thus transformed from an icon of death into a symbol of sexual value and attractiveness.

From the late nineteenth to the mid-twentieth century, X-rays were thus the locus of an erotic discourse of sexual availability and bodily commodification; in the late twentieth century, the X-ray remains similarly understood in terms of intimacy. There is a strong sense in which an X-ray is understood as a private image unsuitable for public display.[76] In a short story in *Ghost Image*, Hervé Guibert draws attention to the similarities between the X-ray and the nude:

> Several years ago in the flap of a portfolio, I came upon an X-ray of the left hand side of my torso. I stuck it onto the glass of the French window opposite my desk. The light passed through this blueish network of bony lines and blurry organs as through a piece of stained glass, but by placing this X-ray where anyone could

> see it (neighbors as well as visitors), I was displaying the most intimate image of myself – much more intimate than any nude, one that contained an enigma, and that a medical student could easily decipher. I no longer keep pictures of myself at home – it makes my skin crawl when I do – but there, with the pleasure of an exhibitionist, I display the image of a fundamental difference.[77]

Guibert might be describing Morrisroe's own pulmonary triptych, the body framed from the same angle and offering the same intricate network of delicate lines and shadows. Like the most erotic of nudes, Guibert's X-ray both conceals and reveals, offering a coded intimacy that is persistently displaced. The X-ray is for Guibert, as for Morrisroe, a source of sensuous exhibitionist gratification, of pleasure and wonder in one's own body, a mode of offering oneself up for public consumption while simultaneously holding something back.

The pin-up and the corpse: Late Polaroid self-portraits

If the photograph is 'an agent of death', this is doubly true for the Polaroid, which, as Guibert notes, has a throwaway quality. 'Backing away from time', the Polaroid also embodies a desire for immediacy: Guibert claims that the elderly photographer André Kertész (b. 1895) favours the Polaroid 'because he has arrived at an age when he can no longer wait for his film to be developed, out of fear that death might snatch the image away'.[78] A case might be made for the structural 'veracity' of Morrisroe's late Polaroid pictures, which clearly present a different proposition to the sandwich prints or X-ray photograms: these final images have not been manipulated at the level of the negative, written on, smudged with fingerprints, coloured with inks or otherwise worked over. At the level of iconography, they appear to reveal a man laid bare, no longer strong enough to compose himself for the camera.

In images such as the *Untitled (Self-Portrait)* of 1989 (Figure 6), Morrisroe's expiring form appears to be invested with an aura of incontrovertible facticity. Projecting a fantasy of total disclosure, the pictures are difficult to reconcile with a reading of Morrisroe as self-performer. Yet despite the images' intimations of an unmediated and authentic subject, there is something playful about Morrisroe's slight smirk, and a glint of mischievousness in his gaze that cannot fail to be noticed by anyone already familiar with his work. Given the historical associations of performance with disguise and dissimulation, this presentation of a simultaneously 'authentic' and 'constructed' self creates a fascinating tension, explored in a 2011 conversation between artists Sur Rodney Sur and Rafael Sanchez (who had helped care for Morrisroe in his final months). Sur reflects: 'The Polaroid of Mark, shot from above . . . my God, to bare yourself so. And all the while thinking of a good pose'.[79]

In his response, Sanchez recasts Sur's opposition of disclosure and 'pose' in terms of 'looking like death' and 'doing a pin-up shot':

> That picture . . . knowing that you look like death, and doing a pin up shot, like Marilyn for Playboy, is probably one of the most complicated gestures by any artist. He really faced it.[80]

This gesture is 'complicated' because, as Sander Gilman has argued, the sick body has historically been marked as ugly and undesirable: 'the healthy is the beautiful, is the erotic, is the good [. . .] that which is ill is therefore inherently anti-erotic'.[81] Morrisroe's late self-portraits wilfully challenge that formulation, investing the cadaverous AIDS 'victim' with the same erotic sensibility that permeates his earlier work.

What are the implications of the juxtaposition of 'baring oneself' and 'posing' implicit in Sur's remark? To bare oneself suggests both the presentation of one's naked body and the disclosure of one's innermost thoughts and emotions. Kenneth Clark's well-known art-historical distinction between nakedness and nudity argues that the former implies embarrassment and vulnerability, while the latter suggests a body that is 'balanced, prosperous and confident'.[82] The naked is actual, a sign of material reality; the nude is an idealization, 'the most complete example of the transformation of matter into form'.[83] Morrisroe's body, somehow both real and romanticized, clearly complicates this position. Other writers have sought to destabilize Clark's categories:[84] John Berger suggests that while the nude is subject to artistic conventions, to be naked 'is to be oneself'.[85] Yet arguably Morrisroe is most fully himself when he presents his body according to the pictorial principles of the art-historical nude. In his 1985 reading of Édouard Manet's *Olympia* (1865), T. J. Clark suggests that nakedness and nudity should be understood in terms of self-possession:

> By nakedness I mean those signs – that broken, interminable circuit – which say that we are nowhere but in a body, constructed by it, by the way it incorporates the signs of other people. (Nudity, on the other hand, is a set of signs for the belief that the body is ours, a great generality which we make our own, or leave in art in the abstract.)[86]

By simultaneously baring himself *and* posing, combining the conventional signifiers of nakedness *and* nudity, Morrisroe's body confuses all previous attempts to define the two categories. His body is both naked *and* nude: signalling AIDS 'victim', it assimilates 'the signs of other people'; by posing and levelling with the viewer's gaze, it communicates Morrisroe's steadfast assurance that the body, sick though it might be, is still his own.

Morrisroe achieves this equivocal position through the twin mechanisms of the look and the pose. The most striking detail of Morrisroe's 1989 self-portrait (some might call it a *punctum*, although this does not accurately communicate the universality of its power to 'wound') is Morrisroe's disconcerting gaze. A piece of text in the March 1987 *PWA Coalition Newline* provides a possible context for understanding this look:

> Some of us who've seen too many friends die [. . .] talk about 'the look' and 'the smell' which characterizes the terminal stages of AIDS. Although 'the look' varies from person to person, it's essentially the look of someone who has just seen clearly – perhaps for the first time – the image and immanence of his own death. The eyes are sunken with resignation and wasting, yet wide open with terror; vacant yet certain.[87]

Read in this way, the look is solipsistic, reflecting on the horror of death. Yet Morrisroe's look might also be interpreted as the return of the viewer's gaze: in art-historical writing, this is often assumed to signify the portrayed subject's resistance to the objectifying operations of visual representation. Perhaps the most celebrated text on this topic, Laura Mulvey's 'Visual Pleasure and Narrative Cinema', written in 1973 and published in 1975, has influentially addressed the power relations of spectatorship in terms of gender.[88] Its central thesis is that in mainstream cinema, woman is constituted as the object of the gaze, while man is constituted as a spectator. As Kenneth MacKinnon notes, Mulvey's argument does not seem to allow for the possibility of a male subject appearing in the position of erotic spectacle: 'According to the principles of the ruling ideology and the psychical structures that back it up, the male figure cannot bear the burden of sexual objectification. Man is reluctant to gaze at his exhibitionist like.'[89] Applying Mulvey's analysis to Morrisroe's self-portrait, we might conclude that the discomfort induced by the image is related at least in part to its erotic and indeed exhibitionist representation of the male body.

Perhaps an equally significant way of approaching Morrisroe's 'look', however, is through Foucault's concept of the medical gaze, outlined earlier in this chapter, which suggests that the visual objectification of the sick body is a necessary part of modern medicine's will to knowledge. Morrisroe's reciprocal gaze suggests his resistance to this objectification, and a refusal to be constituted in entirely passive terms as a terminally ill body poised on the ultimate object-like state of death. Morrisroe's strategy of reiterative posing can be understood as part of his efforts to retain control over his own representation. By the mid-1980s, the pose was increasingly understood as a strategy of 'mimetic rivalry', challenging the authority of official discourse by imitating and appropriating it.[90] The pose might also constitute a response to surveillance, transforming the objectifying experience of being observed into the personal pleasure of being watched.[91] A strategy of posing can thus challenge the passive position that is supposed to be assumed by the dying hospitalized subject.[92]

The rhetoric of the pose and the look is also discernible in Robert Mapplethorpe's famous 1988 *Self Portrait*, which conveys considerably more gravitas and statesman-like dignity than Morrisroe's raw and confrontational images.[93] Although dealing with similar subject matter, Morrisroe and Mapplethorpe were as different as two photographers can be. Their differences are elegantly summed up in a review article written by Vince Aletti for the *Village Voice*: 'Morrisroe revelled in the overheated and the handmade – in the serendipitous funk of crudely fixed Polaroids and photograms that looked like Man Ray on angel dust. Mapplethorpe strived for classic elegance, for balance, for sophistication, and a flawless finish.'[94] Yet the two men share an aesthetic that is most evident in a comparison of Morrisroe's late self-portraits with Mapplethorpe's early ones. As Aletti concedes, 'both photographers probed queer desire with an unflinching, consuming brilliance that's grounded in confrontational self-portraiture.'[95]

In Mapplethorpe's image, the artist faces the camera, his right-hand grasping a walking cane topped with a skull, the bony contours of which echo his own protruding cheekbones and wasted face. His trunk, clad in black, fades into the background, so that his head, hand and skull-topped stick appear peculiarly disembodied. The head is slightly out of focus as if to suggest that he is already fading away. Often reproduced by the popular press as 'evidence' of his illness, this image can be read as both a rehearsal of his own demise and a defiant attempt to stare death in the face: as with Morrisroe's self-portraits, Mapplethorpe's implied stance is halfway been passive acceptance and fiery insubordination.

Peggy Phelan reads Mapplethorpe's image in terms of a meeting and reflecting (or deflecting) of gazes: the eyeless skull meets the viewer's eyes, threatening to turn that gaze into a void.[96] In Phelan's reading, this meeting with alterity is not necessarily the result of an encounter with death but is implicit in all subjectivity: 'The image of the self, Mapplethorpe suggests, can only be glimpsed in its disappearance. To greet it, one risks blindness, vanishing.'[97]

Referring to Mapplethorpe's previous self-portraits where he poses in women's make-up (1980) or behind a machine gun (1983), Phelan suggests that these earlier works halt the slide of the self-image towards becoming an image of the other: 'The image ultimately captured by the camera is one which is performed in order to define the central absence of the image.'[98] In agreement with Phelan, Richard Meyer suggests that Mapplethorpe's portrait conveys the insufficiency of the visual field of photography to convey the experience of terminal illness: 'Robert Mapplethorpe confidently meets, even defies, the gaze of his own camera as though to signify the radical insufficiency of photography to narrate the experiences – and vulnerabilities – of the sentient body.'[99]

As Meyer notes, the photograph signifies anger as well as illness and asserts Mapplethorpe's authority over his own visual representation. Both Mapplethorpe and Morrisroe's images suggest the tension between authenticity and theatricality, the unmediated self and the pose. Richard Meyer notes the 'theatricality' of Mapplethorpe's portrait and suggests that it is this quality that allows him to avoid victim imagery.[100] Significantly, both Phelan and Mayer's accounts of Mapplethorpe's 1988 self-portrait make the connection between this image and his earlier body of S&M-related work. For Mayer, the S&M photographs explicitly refute the economy of victim photography and the tradition of documentary photography. Meyer argues that while Mapplethorpe's S&M images may at first seem to function within an economy of disengaged documentary, constructing the Other as a freak for visual consumption by an implicitly normative audience, their central point is that Mapplethorpe is a participant rather than just an observer. In the following section, I examine a further set of images by Morrisroe, suggesting parallels between these and the sadomasochistic images taken by Mapplethorpe.

A second group of images gives rise to further interpretative possibilities. The prints have been subjected to a deliberate process of destruction and decomposition, achieved by peeling apart the Polaroid print and negative while the film is still wet and sensitive, allowing patches of white light to leech over the film's surface and eat away at the image. All four images depict Morrisroe dressed in a hospital gown and positioned on a trolley-bed. Two are taken in quarter profile and are fairly unremarkable sick room images. The remaining two show Morrisroe from behind. In one (Figure 13), Morrisroe has almost disappeared under the sheets, glancing back over his shoulder with just a tiny amount of skin revealed by a gown casually falling from his shoulder. Given his previous predilection for nudity, this is striking, suggesting perhaps striptease, a spotlight angled at Morrisroe's head hinting at the staging.

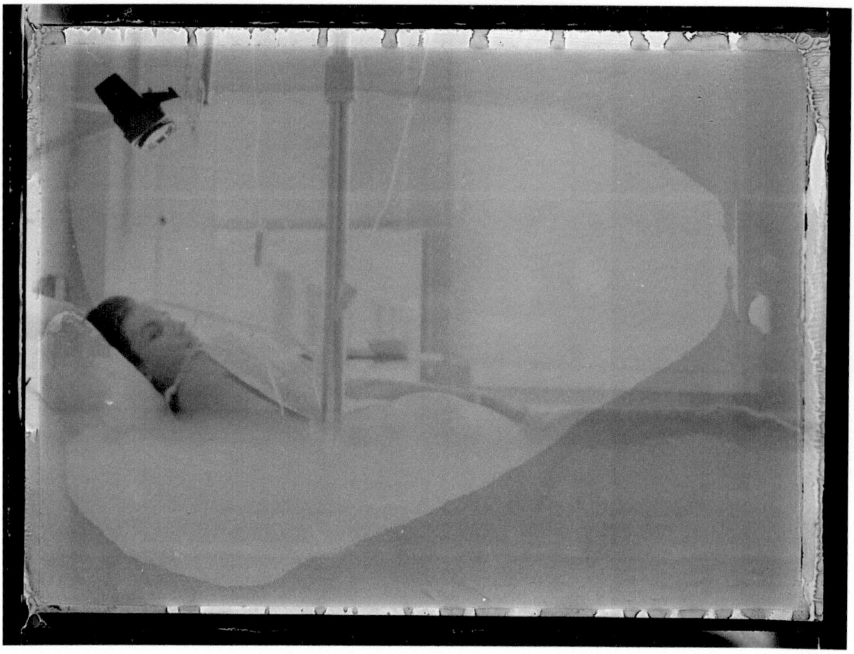

Figure 13 Mark Morrisroe, Untitled [Self-Portrait], undated. Instant-photographic negative, 10.5 × 8.3 cm. © The Estate of Mark Morrisroe (Ringier Collection) at Fotomuseum Winterthur.

The other image (Figure 14) also supports this interpretation of the hospital bed as a stage for Morrisroe's own strip show. Morrisroe is lying on his left-hand side, his torso twisted so that his lower half turns away from the camera, and his upper body rotates towards it, his right arm tethered to an IV line that hangs from a pole. His shoulders are covered, but his hospital garment (tied at the neck) falls away, revealing his buttocks, testicles and legs. Depictions from behind (e.g. in many images of Venus) are often shorthand for erotic vulnerability, but this image does not convey weakness so much as a sense of challenge or invitation.

The visual syntax of this composition not only uses the twisted form as shorthand for the body in pain but also employs an iconography of bondage that Morrisroe had explored in several earlier works. *After the Laone* (1983) shows Morrisroe's back and buttocks from behind, lain on his right-hand side, left arm draped back across his body towards the camera. *Untitled* (*c.* 1981) shows the head and shoulders of a person entirely encased in cellophane and packing tape, a black tube protruding from the mouth, presumably to enable breathing. Morrisroe's hospital bed images use the visual language of bondage to suggest a

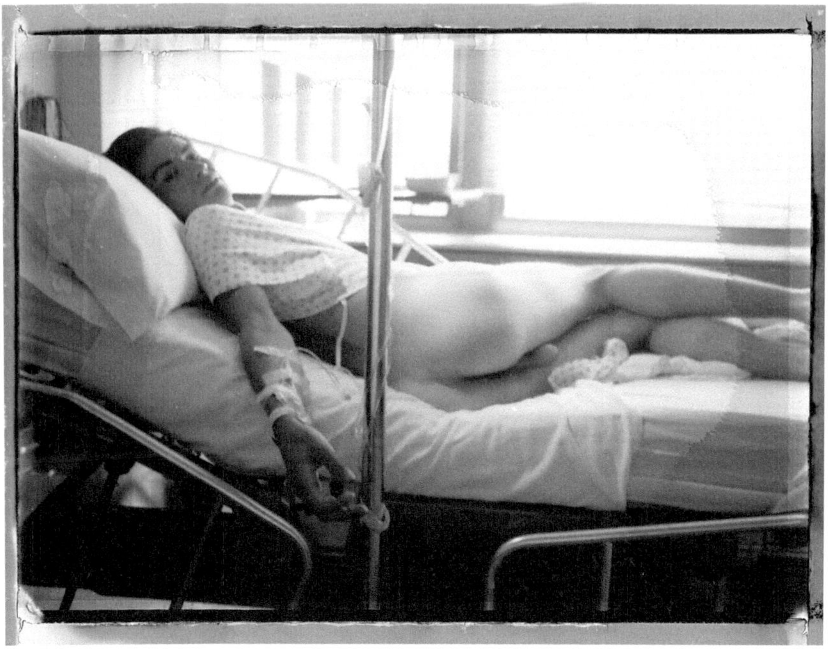

Figure 14 Mark Morrisroe, Untitled [Self-Portrait], undated. Instant-photographic negative, 10.5 × 8.3 cm. © The Estate of Mark Morrisroe (Ringier Collection) at Fotomuseum Winterthur.

position where one might successfully be both passive and active, in control and yet physically compromised.

There are some striking comparisons to be made between this set of images and a suite of Polaroid self-portraits taken by Robert Mapplethorpe between 1972 and 1973.[101] In several of these the artist's body is girdled with a slim black strap that cradles his buttocks, traverses his upper body and descends to cup his genitals, finally disappearing between his legs to return to its starting point. In one of these images, the entirety of Mapplethorpe's left flank is exposed to the camera, his elbow jutting out from the rest of his body as his shoulders pivoting to accommodate the hands tied behind his back. The pose echoes Morrisroe's: both men share the same somnolent, gentle gaze, a mixture of contempt and desire to be desired. Other images in Mapplethorpe's suite address the bondage theme more explicitly, with genitals twisted inside leather straps and metal rings. Some are more gently pornographic: like Morrisroe, the young Mapplethorpe poses on rumpled sheets, his body foreshortened, the images cropped or filmed from unusual angles.

The most immediately obvious point of comparison is Mapplethorpe's 1978 *Self Portrait*, which depicts the artist stripped from the waist and bent away from the camera with a bullwhip inserted in his anus. Richard Meyer has convincingly read the bullwhip as a visual metaphor for photography itself, representing the camera cord that needs to be pulled to capture an image. Extending this reading to Morrisroe's image, the IV line might stand in for the camera cord, becoming both a fetish object and a symbol of photography itself.

Meyer suggests that Mapplethorpe manipulates the 'intrinsic theatricality of s/m' to stage the artifice of photography.[102] In his reading of Mapplethorpe's S&M images, Richard Meyer points out that Mapplethorpe's own involvement with S&M is often cited as evidence of the authenticity of his images. Yet these very same images often emphasize their own theatricality. It also insists on Mapplethorpe's double position as both photographer and erotic participant. Meyer emphasizes the mobile subject position implicit in s/m: 'the masochism of the gay male body is [. . .] as much invitation as intimation, as much erotic object as dominating subject, as much psychic "bottom" as penetrating "top"'.[103]

Morrisroe's strategy of combining illness and sadomasochistic eroticism might be productively compared with the practice of the American performance artist Bob Flanagan (1952–96). Known as 'that performance artist guy who nailed his penis to a board', Flanagan was one of the longest-living survivors of cystic fibrosis, a debilitating congenital disease characterized by the overproduction of mucous in the lungs.[104] Flanagan led a sadomasochistic lifestyle and for over fourteen years was a slave to his mistress Sheree Rose; Flanagan and Rose documented their sexual experimentations in photography, video and writing, and collaborated on a number of art projects and performances. For *Visiting Hours*, a 1994 installation at the New Museum in New York, the exhibition space was arranged to resemble a hospital ward, the walls covered in small black-and-white close-up photographs taken by Rose, and depicting Flanagan in the throes of pleasure and pain. Flanagan is portrayed as an erotic object, the subject of Rose's visual pleasure; the relationship inverts the usual dichotomy of female-body/object, male-viewer/subject.

Most significantly for a consideration of Morrisroe's work, however, is the way in which Flanagan's practice transforms the physical pain of severe illness into positive masochistic pleasure. As Flanagan explains, 'I was forced to be in the medical world, so I turned that into something I could have control over instead of something that was controlling me.'[105] Flanagan frequently put medical equipment to sexual uses: in *Visiting Hours* he displayed a medical stool with a giant butt-plug nailed to the seat. In performance pieces he used needles and scalpels to sculpt his own genitals while laughing, joking and singing; Carrie Sandahl reads this as an open challenge to the symbolic castration conventionally assigned to the critically ill.[106] Over and again, Flanagan insists that he possesses sole jurisdiction over his own body: 'I am in control. I invented this.'[107]

The apparent paradox of a body that is simultaneously ill and eroticized is also presented by a number of AIDS autobiographies. In Hervé Guibert's *Compassionate Protocol*, one of the narrator's former lovers appears, wanting to see Guibert's ravaged body; after Guibert disrobes, he insists on making love to him. In his study of Guibert's video diary *La Pudeur, ou l'impudeur?*, which documents the final months of his life, Ross Chambers notes that Guibert's body, although gaunt, is still beautiful: it has no lesions, his facial bone structure is enhanced and illuminated by his thinness, and the elegant incline of his shoulder recalls the angularity of certain Picasso figures.[108] In her reading of Guibert's autobiographical AIDS memoirs, Emily Apter suggests that 'Guibert dares to explore the disturbing commonalities between *sida* treatment and rough gay sex – the rites of humiliation, the transgression of bodily limits, the submission to power, postures demanded and exchanged'.[109] In one scene, the forcing of a tube down Guibert's neck takes the form of an oral rape; in another, the tube thrust down the throat of his friend Muzil recalls the former pleasures of oral sex. Morrisroe's late images, like Guibert's text, suggest that disease and erotic experience might converge in surprising ways in and on the body of the critically ill subject.

In his essay on the power of the pose, Owens turns to a discussion of the sadomasochistic drive. The pose is neither entirely active nor entirely passive; Owens points out that it corresponds to what in grammar is identified as the middle voice or diathesis. If the active or passive voices indicate activity or passivity in relation to an external agent, the middle voice 'indicates the interiority of the subject to the action of which it is also the agent'.[110] Owens refers to the invocation of the 'middle voice' in Freud's discussion of the sadomasochistic drive:

> In addition to an active, externally directed stage, characterized by the desire to exercise violence or power over some other person as object [. . .] and a masochistic stage, in which the active aim is changed into the passive aim, and the subject searches for another person as object of the drive (but subject of the action), Freud posits a third, intermediary stage, a 'turning round of the drive upon the subject's self' (as in self-punishment, self-torture) *without the attitude of passivity towards an external object/subject* that characterizes masochism. [. . .] 'The active voice is changed,' Freud writes, 'not into the passive, but into the reflexive middle voice.'[111]

The reflexive middle voice well describes Morrisroe's images: his drive and indeed his gaze seem directed inwards, self-regarding but without the attitude of passivity towards the external viewer/camera. This mirrors the scopic structure of earlier works such as *Little Me as a Child Prostitute* or *Self-Portrait (To Brent)*, where Morrisroe is inviting but unavailable; the images suggest a plenitude brought about by himself as object and audience.

Bersani's essay 'Foucault, Freud, Fantasy and Power' concentrates on a desexualizing of eroticism, by which he means uncoupling it from an association with strictly genital pleasure. A key part of this investigation of the relation between pleasure and power is a reading of S&M bondage practices. Bersani reads Freud's use of 'erotogenicity' as connoting 'a degenitalizing of erotic intensities'.[112] Instead of being focussed on the genitals, erotic pleasure is suffused throughout the whole of the body. Bersani suggests that Freud appropriates the notion of sexuality to describe phenomena that until then were not thought of as sexual. Freud, Bersani writes, 'coerced the sexual into describing what I would call a certain rhythm of mastery and surrender in human consciousness'.[113] It is surely this 'rhythm of mastery and surrender' that describes the feeling conveyed by Morrisroe's *Untitled: (Self-Portrait)* (1989), with its equivocal position that simultaneously conveys passivity and active self-control.

* * *

The surrealist Georges Bataille – with whom Morrisroe would have had much in common – once declared that 'Eroticism is assenting to life even in death';[114] Morrisroe's late images give pictorial form to Bataille's claim and allow Morrisroe to find a visual language with which to express the experience of being delicately poised between life and death, photographing subject and photographed object.

In his study of AIDS memoirs, Ross Chambers quotes from Pascal de Duve's auto-fiction *Cargo Vie*:

> To look Death in the face, not only with open eyes but with eyes more open than ever, with a mixture of defiance and wonderment – perhaps there's a modest but genuine form of heroism in that, a pocket sized heroism that, in all humility I aspire to.[115]

Mark Morrisroe's photographic practice might be imagined as a visual equivalent to de Duve's writing: flamboyant and romantic, Morrisroe transforms his death into a grandiose aesthetic encounter. His final works are underpinned by an almost wilful sense of individualism and sense of self that contrasts markedly with the more widely discussed collaborative efforts of creative activist collectives such as Gran Fury, General Idea or Group Material, explored in Chapter 1 of this book. Similarly, Morrisroe's late self-portraits provide a fascinating counterpoint to the photographic depictions of people with AIDS produced by Nixon, Solomon and Goldin, examined in the previous chapter. Neither straightforward representations of victimhood nor activist-orientated pictures of an individual surviving and thriving with AIDS, Morrisroe's final self-images suggest something of the ambiguities and ambivalences that must characterize a first-person experience of an AIDS-related death.

4

Robert Blanchon

Abjection, 'absence' and autobiography

> *... the self-portrait's inaugural experience is one of emptiness, of absence unto himself.*[1]

Robert Blanchon's conceptual art practice offers a counterpoint to the powerful personal presence conveyed by Mark Morrisroe's prints and Polaroid pictures. Blanchon rarely depicts himself directly, instead signposting images, objects and installations as self-portraits, either through the choice of title; by the incorporation of 'personal' effects such as letters, clothes or bodily fragments; or, in text-based pieces, by the use of the first person. Even in his most intimate works, Blanchon's presence is rarely made explicit, and at times the artist seems maddeningly absent from his semi-avowed self-representations. On the infrequent occasion where he does appear to represent himself directly, either pictorially or in a first-person text, the subject put forward is enigmatic and unstable, at risk of slipping away before it can be grasped. The director of the Robert Blanchon Estate Project, Sasha Archibald, who collated and catalogued Blanchon's work between 2003 and 2006, describes the artist's personal voice as 'part of a complicated performance of improvised mythology'.[2] Blanchon's performative self-presentation rivals Morrisroe's, but whereas Morrisroe's practice suggests an exposed first-person subject that is immediately 'knowable', Blanchon's 'self-portraits' frustrate any attempt to get to grips with their supposed referent. Other archivists working on the Estate Project draw attention to the difficulties that Blanchon's characteristic evasiveness posed for their own research. Noting that 'his writings, personal documentation and artistic statements were incomplete, with many twisted signposts', they conclude: 'His conceptual practice and his lived experience thumbed its nose at truthfulness, preferring a blend of wit, parody, and imagination. In essence, he embodied the trickster.'[3] Frequently signposted as autobiographical, yet structured around a series of strangely elusive subject positions, Blanchon's work thus represents an intriguing paradox.

Blanchon (1965–99) discovered that he was HIV positive at almost the very beginning of his artistic career: he received his diagnosis in 1989 or 1990 while a graduate student at the School of the Art Institute of Chicago. While Morrisroe's work can be fairly neatly divided into 'before' and 'after' AIDS, Blanchon's long-term awareness of his seropositivity (as distinct from symptomatic AIDS) provides the biographical context for virtually the entirety of his practice. Furthermore, in contrast to Morrisroe's dramatic decline over approximately three years, the relatively prolonged ten-year period between Blanchon's diagnosis and eventual death afforded him time to consider the consequences of his passing and the nature of the artistic legacy that he would leave behind. These differences in viral chronology are reflected in the tone of the two men's works: if Morrisroe's late self-portraits suggest urgency and immediacy, Blanchon's practice is characterized by a meditative, melancholic quality.

In the introduction to his 2002 collection of essays *Melancholia and Moralism*, Douglas Crimp uses 'melancholia' to theorize the changing attitudes of the gay community towards the epidemic in the first half of the 1990s. Drawing on Freud's understanding of melancholia as defined by 'self-reproaches and self-revilings',[4] Crimp proposes a relation between 'devastation and self-abasement, between melancholia and moralism, between the turn away from AIDS and the turn towards conservative gay politics'.[5] Crimp suggests that conservative gay responses to AIDS are typically framed by a narrative of moral redemption, citing as an example Andrew Sullivan's article 'When Plagues End', published in the *New York Times Magazine* in 1996.[6] Crimp interprets Sullivan's text as follows: before AIDS, gay men were childlike hedonists who eschewed the responsibilities of normal, 'healthy' adulthood such as monogamy and children. Gay men were only interested in the selfish and transitory pleasures offered by parties, sex and drugs. AIDS made gay men grow up, deal with real life and accept moral responsibility for their own behaviour.[7] Crimp diagnoses Sullivan's view as 'melancholic, and his moralism its clearest symptom';[8] extending this analysis to form a critique of a wider psycho-social response to the epidemic, Crimp suggests that 1990s AIDS melancholia consists of the gay community's internalization of this homophobic discourse of abject gay identity.[9]

In the second half of his paper, Crimp acknowledges an alternative way in which melancholia has come to define the gay community's response to AIDS in the last decade of the twentieth century. While his initial reading of 1990s AIDS melancholia focusses on the repudiation of the crisis as a form of moralistic denial, he also acknowledges that 'turning away' may also be the natural response of those who *have* confronted the epidemic, but who have become overwhelmed and exhausted. If the first scenario involves the phobic denial of loss ('this isn't happening'; 'this can't affect me'; 'I have nothing in common with those people'), the second involves *too much* loss ('I can no longer bear this').[10] This reaction, Crimp concedes, may also be classified as melancholia.

It is in this sense that, in an article written for *Frieze* in 1996, the art critic David Deitcher uses the term 'melancholic' to describe the increasing fatigue of artist-led activist groups in the face of the continuing crisis.[11] ACT UP were exhausted, and their graphics were most likely to be seen in historical exhibitions such as Exit Art's *Counterculture* or the Drawing Centre's *Cultural Economies* than pasted onto buses or public billboards. Gran Fury disbanded in 1996, citing the changing circumstances faced by all involved in the epidemic: 'Embattled, fragmented and burned out, gay activists have adapted to the apparent permanence of the AIDS crisis [. . .] the drama of AIDS has been replaced by its normalization.'[12] This melancholic mood is also reflected in Blanchon's personal remarks. In a statement dated January 1996, Blanchon alludes to his personal 'difficulty with living longer than planned', clearly connecting this to an awareness of increasing public fatigue with the epidemic. He describes Magic Johnson, the basketball player who famously identified as HIV positive in 1996, as 'just another face in an overcrowded group of plague people', concluding wearily, 'Whenever Magic dies it won't matter. We are past the point of awareness and change. This DNA replicating virus is less talked about than *Melrose Place* or that really annoying show *Friends*.'[13] AIDS melancholia of the 1990s and the related themes of loss and abjection underpin this chapter's reading of Blanchon's practice of self-portraiture.

Blanchon was politicized about AIDS in a way that Morrisroe was not. In 1989 and 1990, he produced several activist posters in Chicago, including one of Richard Daley, the former Chicago mayor, emblazoned with the caption 'I will not get AIDS. Actions speak louder than words'. Blanchon hung the design around the city, and the poster's appearance was widely commented in the Chicago press. He also designed a billboard poster for Art against AIDS ('AIDS Is a Virus, Sex Is Natural', 1990), which was installed at bus centres and train platforms across the city. In 1990, he moved to New York, where he rented a studio on Canal Street, worked in the education department of the New Museum (where the installation *Let the Record Show* had been displayed in 1987) and became involved in ACT UP. It was at this time that he struck up a friendship with Felix Gonzalez-Torres, who was also collaborating with ACT UP as part of the collective Group Material.

Ultimately, however, Blanchon's interests lay not so much in the production of agitprop as in his conceptual investigations of the radical sexual politics of the pre-AIDS gay community. Archibald describes Blanchon's approach as 'a quasi-documentary style for a body of work that exposes the discreet history of gay sex culture',[14] relating this to Douglas Crimp's writing on the political dimensions of mourning and melancholia. Work made by Blanchon in this spirit include documentation of the different-coloured bandanas worn by men to indicate their sexual preferences, a tour of cruising places in New York and a series of photographs of public monuments, focussing only on the statues' buttocks and groins. Such projects had a deep political significance for Blanchon, who, as Archibald acknowledges, 'thought it imperative to defend and preserve this radicality, despite efforts at the time to mollify public discrimination by "normalizing" the face of AIDS'.[15] This is perhaps the final difference between Morrisroe's and Blanchon's work: while Morrisroe's work is erotic (or perhaps more accurately, erotogenic, as I have argued in the previous chapter), it is not concerned with sexual activity as such and does not address the sexual politics of the epidemic. Blanchon's work is not strictly erotic; the human body is only rarely represented and only very occasionally in sexually explicit situations. Its references to sexual activity are allusive rather than direct, suggesting (as this chapter will argue) both the AIDS-related disappearance of what Crimp describes as 'a culture of sexual possibility: back rooms, tea rooms, bookstores, movie houses and baths; the trucks, the pier, the ramble, the dunes',[16] and the fundamentally un-representable nature of such pleasures and practices in an art world stifled by the Helms Amendment and other 'culture wars' legislation.

Like many involved in AIDS activism, Blanchon was conversant with a range of critical debates about art and the politics of representation, evidenced both in his art and in his teaching, which was an integral part of his practice. Between 1995 and 1997, Blanchon lectured at the University of California, Irvine, and the California Institute for the Arts: his course syllabi bear witness to his passionate engagement with a number of contemporary critical issues. In spring 1997, he taught bell hooks' text on the 1990 documentary *Paris Is Burning*, which follows a community of Black drag queens.[17] hooks criticized the (white, female) director Jenny Livingston for a lack of awareness of the way in which her own privileged subject position had shaped the film; Blanchon's own interest in hooks' text related to questions regarding the right to speak for someone else versus the right to be represented. He often set extracts from *Blasted Allegories*, a collection of artists' writings published by the New Museum in 1987. In the spring term of 1997, he scheduled a discussion of Sherrie Levine's text 'Five Comments', which adapts Barthes' essay on the death of the author to ask questions about authorship, originality and authenticity in contemporary art:

> We know that a picture is but a space in which a variety of images, none of them original, blend and clash. [. . .] Succeeding the painter, the plagiarist no longer bears within him passions, humors, feelings, impressions, but rather this immense encyclopedia from which he draws. The viewer is the tablet on which all the questions that make up a painting are inscribed without any of them being lost. A painting's meaning lies not in its origin, but in its destination. The birth of the reader must be at the cost of the painter.[18]

Levine's text provides a useful starting point from which to engage with Blanchon's practice of self-portraiture. This chapter will ultimately argue that the authorial absence that is a hallmark even of Blanchon's most autobiographical works can be read as part of a deliberate strategy to foreground the role of the viewer in meaning making.

After providing an initial overview of the significance of absence and self-representation in Blanchon's work, this chapter focusses on the 1996 exhibition *[gum, waste, indentations, stains + envelopes]*, which it reads as both an elusive self-portrait and a collective representation of 'abject' homosexuality in the age of AIDS. I do not intend to suggest that Blanchon himself is maintaining an abject subject position, nor is he (or I) suggesting that the position of gay men is inherently abject. I propose instead that Blanchon is interested in the fantasmatic production of identity and that his installation explores the idea of self-portraiture from the outside (as opposed to the more traditional notion of self-portraiture from within). Mirroring the structure of the melancholic repudiation of the AIDS crisis identified by Crimp, the installation functions according to the logic of a series of displacements, substitutions and associations. Freud's work underpins many of the texts that provide the theoretical groundwork for this chapter. For an understanding of Blanchon's work as 'confessional', I turn to Foucault's treatment of the confession in *The History of Sexuality Vol. 1;* Foucault critiques psychoanalysis while barely mentioning Freud.[19] I use Julia Kristeva's writing on abjection and melancholy to situate Blanchon's installation in the context of the contemporaneous popularity of abject art; Kristeva's work builds on Freudian and Lacanian theories of the subject.[20] To understand Blanchon's references to abject homosexuality, I turn to Simon Watney's text 'The Spectacle of AIDS', which invokes Freud but does not engage with any of Freud's texts per se.[21] Finally, for an understanding of the positive value of self-shattering, I turn to Leo Bersani's essay 'Is the Rectum a Grave?', which is based on a Freudian perspective.[22] It is worth noting that these two final texts were published together in the 1987 AIDS special issue of *October*, edited by Crimp; Blanchon was certainly acquainted with Bersani's text, and given his familiarity with both AIDS activism and critical theory, it is no leap of the imagination to suggest that Blanchon may have read this special issue, or at the very least be casually aware of the work of the authors published within it.

Absence, AIDS and mortality

Sasha Archibald suggestively describes Blanchon's practice as an 'archive of absence', relating this primarily to his illness:

> [Blanchon's] work is about the profound vulnerability of the human form and its ego, about the anonymity of death to a physical body and the irreplaceable particular of a human subject, about the stains and smells of illness and the mortality they portend.[23]

In Archibald's reading, Blanchon's evocations of non-presence find their ultimate expression in the artist's death: 'the foreboding and terrifying blank, the absence that imagines all the others'.[24] Suggestive though it may be, this reading is too neatly reductive, and Blanchon himself was wary of interpretations that diminished his practice to a personal narrative of declining health: 'I think there's many levels to my work. I don't sit around and think I don't feel well and the work comes out, that's not how I work at all.'[25] He warned that AIDS was only one of many possible readings,[26] withdrawing a piece from an exhibition of work by HIV-positive artists when he learnt that it was to be installed semi-permanently. Explaining his decision to the curator he wrote: 'It will continue to contextualize and impact all upcoming work presented under the auspices of the AIDS forum. I believe this to be a grave disadvantage for myself, and can only assume similar effects for participating artists as well.'[27] Blanchon was acutely conscious that AIDS would overshadow other possible interpretations of his work, which would inevitably be read as autobiographical; his evasive position with respect to personal content is to some extent a reaction to this. Yet, at the same time, he recognized the strategic importance of the personal voice for responding to an epidemic where the private was also innately public and political.

Blanchon's ambivalence about the relationship between his illness and his work is revealed in his reaction to an obituary written for Gonzalez-Torres, who died in 1996. The author, the critic Roberta Smith, implied that if Gonzalez-Torres had lived longer, he would have continued to produce exceptional art.[28] Blanchon disagreed, suggesting that, on the contrary, Gonzalez-Torres' awareness of his own mortality was in fact the motivation underpinning his best work. Blanchon felt so strongly about this that he scheduled a class on Gonzalez-Torres as part of the 'Issues in Contemporary Art' course that he taught in the spring of 1997: the obituary was required reading.[29] It has been noted that a sustained engagement with mortality is more characteristic of Blanchon's work than of his friend's:[30] Blanchon's projection of his own anxieties onto Gonzalez-Torres suggests a disavowal of the degree to which his practice was influenced by his diagnosis.

Blanchon was undeniably fascinated by the prospect of his own death. He rehearsed his future passing in works such as the photo-series *Untitled (Death Valley Walking)* (1996), where the artist turns his back on the camera and walks away into the sands of California's Mojave desert, or *Situations 1, 2, and 3* (*c.* 1995), a trio of videos in which Blanchon depicts himself as a ghost-like presence in the middle of three busy social settings. The notion of death as a form of disappearance is suggested by one of his ultimate works, a performance piece created for a show of ephemeral art designed to vanish over the course of the exhibition.[31] Titled *Smackwater* (1998), the work consisted of the lyrics to a Carole King song written out in a crystal meth substitute on a long roll of white paper. The piece was 'completed' by scrapping off the lyrics with a razor blade and then cutting out the section and removing it from the gallery. In a letter to the curators, Blanchon drew a literal parallel between himself and the erased text:

> I am definitely interested and will follow up soon with more details (seems like I am going to propose a literal incarnation of the title and suggest, in lieu of disappearing into death, I would like to fall asleep after not sleeping for a week or more of such deprivation and then have two friends who remain my 'health proxies' and 'caretakers' in NYC remove me and bring me home to rest.) Working title: *wake*.[32]

Other aspects of Blanchon's practice blend a personal investment in exploring death with a more abstract concern for the phenomena of emptiness, absence and ephemerality. The significance of the empty textual space is obsessively investigated: Blanchon repeatedly photographed un-inscribed items such as nameplates, table settings and mass-produced greeting cards. The most moving of these impersonal missives express the sentiment that the unnamed recipient should 'get well soon' or offer condolences on a bereavement; framed and displayed, one such card reads, 'The family of _____ acknowledges with grateful appreciation your kind expression of sympathy'. Anonymity is related to erotic activity in *Untitled/We've Met* (1992/1996), a mixed-media installation incorporating seventy-eight identical, unused contact cards taken from a Los Angeles bathhouse, each bearing the line 'Remember Me? We Met At _____', with blank spaces for the user's name and details. Like the cards of condolence, these documents also imply bereavement: as Douglas Crimp wrote in 1989, gay men must mourn the loss of a culture of sexual possibility that AIDS has

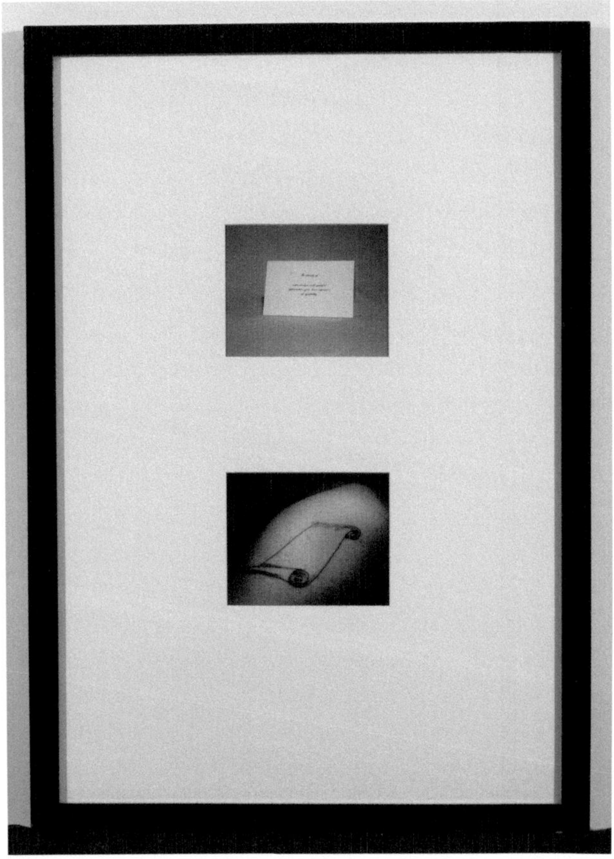

Figure 15 Robert Blanchon, *Untitled (sympathy)*, 1994. Two colour photographs in black lacquer frames, each 27.5 × 19 in. Courtesy of The Estate of Robert Blanchon/ Mary Ellen Carroll – MEC, studios © 1999 The Estate of Robert Blanchon/Mary Ellen Carroll – MEC, studios.

taken from them.[33] Absence takes on a political context in *Infected Wall* (1992), where a label on a blank wall explained that the work was supposed to have been completed by the Infected Faggots Collaborative, but that two members had died before it could be finished. The power of the empty space is reiterated by Blanchon's personal tattoos, which he photographed, framed and presented as art works. One image documents an ornate scroll at the nape of his neck, blank where a name would usually be added; another focusses on his bicep, decorated with an empty white ribbon twisted around two red hearts. In a diptych *Untitled (sympathy)* (1994), an image of a blank parchment inked onto Blanchon's upper right arm is paired with a photograph of a condolence card (Figure 15). This work's suggestive mix of the personal (Blanchon's own body as a medium) and the impersonal (a resistance to naming or perhaps to being labelled) provides a fitting metaphor for Blanchon's practice as a whole.

Blanchon's self-portraiture: An overview

It is clear that 'absence' does not only simply denote Blanchon's literal death but also describes an air of authorial opacity that permeates even the most self-referential works. To suggest that selected works by Blanchon might be read as self-portraiture is potentially problematic: while a portrait is traditionally considered to be the visual expression of a unique individual, the installations and conceptual works considered in this chapter frequently have little to say about either Blanchon's physiognomy or his essential self. Part of the aim of this chapter is therefore to argue for an expanded understanding of self-portraiture, released from historical association with the self-contained individual subject, and recast in terms of fragmentation, incoherence and contingency upon others (including the viewer).

Untitled (Self-Portrait) (1991) (Figure 16) is one of the earliest examples of Blanchon's unusual self-portrait practice. For this project, he commissioned a sketch of himself from fourteen different street artists. Drawn in pencil, pastel or crayon on paper sheets of differing quality and dimensions, the images are striking in the range of variations. The result is often interpreted as a reflection on typecasting; as one reviewer wrote: 'Blanchon blushes up as everything from smirky wiseguy to prissy prettyboy, to a very serious young man, to a sailor boy with clear Tom of Finland whispers, and finally to clear signs that the portraitist assumed Blanchon was gay . . . and painted him in the straight-world's worst way as gay, gay, gay.'[34] However, Blanchon was also interested in the idea that distortion

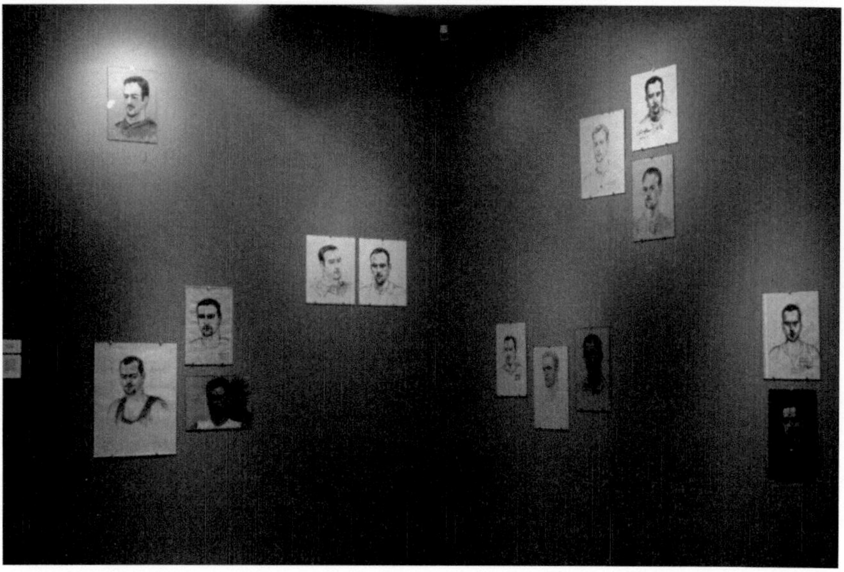

Figure 16 Robert Blanchon, *Untitled (Self-Portrait)*, 1991. Installation. Pencil, crayon on paper, dimensions variable. Courtesy of The Estate of Robert Blanchon/Mary Ellen Carroll – MEC, studios © 1999 The Estate of Robert Blanchon/Mary Ellen Carroll – MEC, studios.

is inherent in the very idea of portraiture, not only of reality by the artist but of the artwork by the viewer: the portraits were exhibited with a piece of text from Rudolf Arnheim's *Towards a Psychology of Art*, suggesting that variation is characteristic of how different people view the same work of art.[35] The artist's statement on the piece clarifies Blanchon's ideas about self-portraiture: 'Self-portraits, like autobiographies, are reflections of oneself through likeness via visual or literal composure. [. . .] Like photography, classified personals, letters of application and phone sex, these drawings anxiously anticipate the capture of individual character by using skills (talents) of interpretation and perception.'[36] While the project ostensibly relies on a traditional view of portraiture as likeness, the result is the revelation that likeness is an unstable concept open to the vagaries of individual perception. Importantly for a consideration of his later work, the project suggests that the self is a projection from the outside as much as from within; furthermore, when experienced through others this 'self' is characterized by a profound lack of unity. Blanchon's inventory of media that might 'capture' individual character is also revealing, apparently placing photography on a par with classified adverts and phone sex. His point is of course that all these media can only ever offer a partial view of their subject.

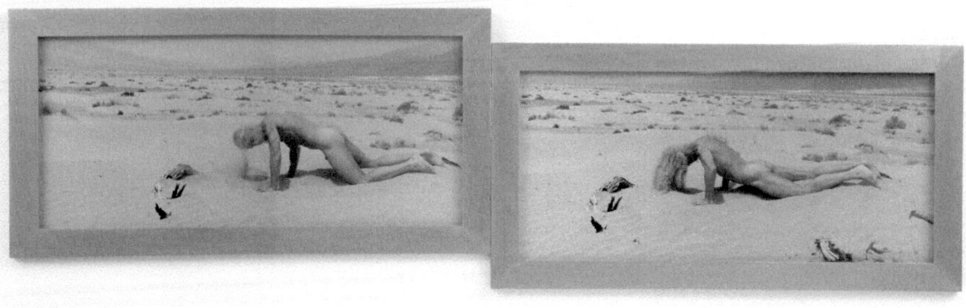

Figure 17 Robert Blanchon, *Untitled (Death Valley Horizon)*, 1997. Two cibachrome prints, wood frames, 35.5 × 45.4 in. each. Courtesy of The Estate of Robert Blanchon/ Mary Ellen Carroll - MEC, studios © 1999 The Estate of Robert Blanchon/Mary Ellen Carroll — MEC, studios.

In contrast to this project, several of Blanchon's later self-portraits are ostensibly extremely intimate. Among the most personal of his self-depictions are the photographs taken in the Death Valley desert between 1996 and 1997. The setting is, as Archibald notes, 'a classic one of masculine self-reliance, and even, in the allusion to Christ's fasting, messianic wisdom'.[37] In the diptych *Untitled [Death Valley Horizon]* (1997) (Figure 17), Blanchon aligns his naked body with the distant horizon, supporting himself on his hands and knees as he raises his head from the sand in a cascade of fine golden grains.[38] His body is held in tension, suggesting not the passivity traditionally associated with a horizontal position, but movement and energy. The diptych offers a contrast to (indeed, perhaps a response to) David Wojnarowicz's powerful self-portrait *Untitled (Face in Dirt)*, taken in Death Valley in 1990 shortly before his own death.[39] Where Wojnarowicz's image evokes burial, Blanchon's implies resistance, even resurrection. It also reverses the terms of Wojnarowicz's image: while Wojnarowicz's body is buried, his face remains (just) visible; in Blanchon's diptych, the body is placed on display, and the face obscured by a shower of sand. While adhering to many tenets of traditional portraiture such as visual likeness and intimacy, the lack of facial visibility marks this as different. In his book on portraiture, Richard Brilliant points out that we are so used to recognizing people by their faces that we feel disorientated when they are absent; the 'missing face' can function as a metaphor for the gap between a 'public' and a 'private' self or be used to express uncertainty about the relation of inner and outer identity.[40]

In the diptych *Untitled (Death Valley Self-Portrait)* (1995) (Figure 18), Blanchon faces the camera head on, nude, muscular (to extend an argument made in the preceding chapter, his is certainly not an 'ugly' body), eyes closed, feet planted firmly in the sand and hands resting behind his back. The effect is

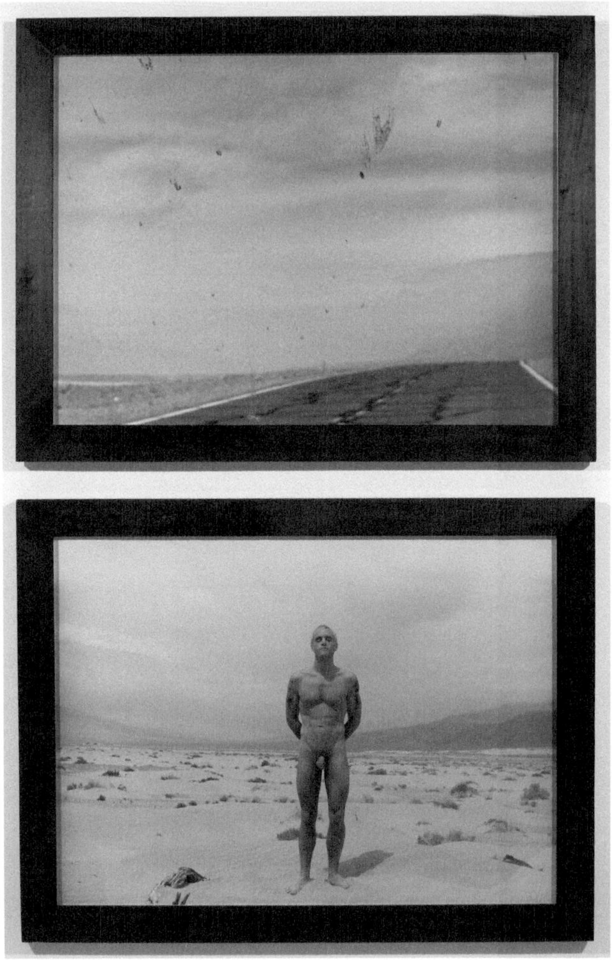

Figure 18 Robert Blanchon, *Untitled (Death Valley Self-Portrait)*, 1995. Two cibachrome prints, wood frames, 35.5 × 45.5 in. each. Courtesy of The Estate of Robert Blanchon/Mary Ellen Carroll – MEC, studios © 1999 The Estate of Robert Blanchon/ Mary Ellen Carroll – MEC, studios.

an aura of calm confidence and self-possession. In line with the monumentality of his pose, the cibachrome print is large, measuring thirty-five-and-a-half by forty-five inches. This image is paired with a second print of the same dimensions, taken from behind the blurred windscreen of Blanchon's car, also in the desert but mostly picturing the road ahead. It is, as Archibald notes, 'as if Blanchon introduces himself to us and then invites the viewer into his own skin.'[41] Representing Blanchon first from the outside and then from his own embodied viewpoint, the diptych recalls Stephen Spender's observations on autobiography: 'We are seen from the outside by our neighbors; but we remain always at the back of our eyes and our senses, situated in our bodies, like drivers in cars.'[42] Blanchon's double image follows Spender in acknowledging the singularity of embodied perception, the blurred graininess of the second print suggesting the impossibility of really seeing from inside someone else's skin. The diptych also realizes the inherent duality of the self-portrait: both an image of Blanchon as seen from the outside and his own view from inside his body. There is a possibility that the blurred screen might be an allusion to Blanchon's failing eyesight, also referred to by the work *Untitled (eye frame)* (1998) (Figure 19),

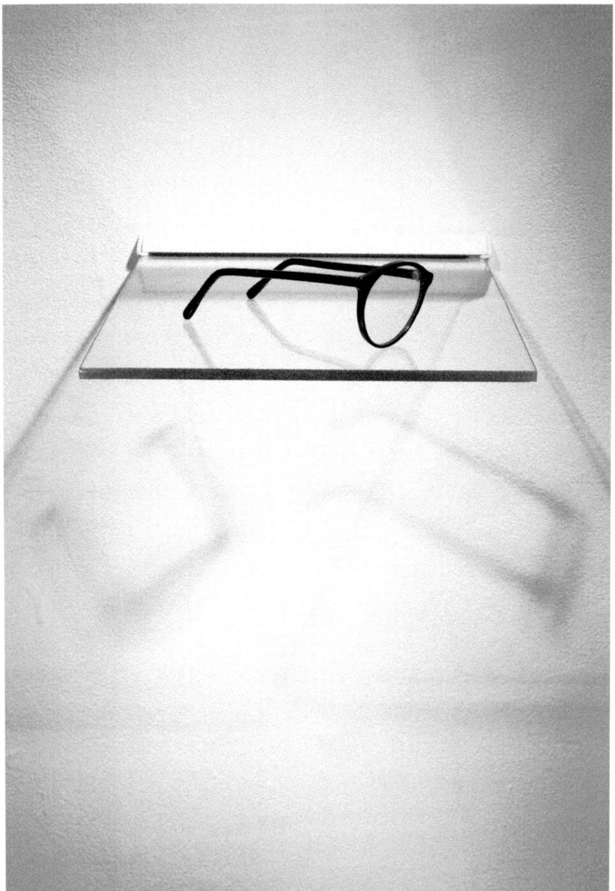

Figure 19 Robert Blanchon, *Untitled (eye frame)*, 1998. Prescription eyeglasses, custom frame, glass shelf, 2 × 9 × 10 in. Courtesy of The Estate of Robert Blanchon / Mary Ellen Carroll – MEC, studios © 1999 The Estate of Robert Blanchon/Mary Ellen Carroll – MEC, studios.

an eyeglass and frame made for a single eye, with the lens matching Blanchon's own prescription. Its unusual shape means that the eyeglass cannot be worn, suggesting an impossible invitation to the viewer to step into his body, but also, perhaps, the irreversibility of Blanchon's condition.

Blanchon's most intimate self-portrait is, however, not a photograph but a text-based work. The installation *Protection* or *Carcharodon Carcharias (Jaws)* (1992–5) was one of Blanchon's earliest works to explore his personal experience of AIDS. Its central component consists of a short letter written by Blanchon informing his parents of his HIV status and his religious mother's rambling sixteen-page reply. In its 1992 incarnation the letters' pages were framed and installed in a grid, accompanied by a twenty-dollar bill and clippings of religious text that his mother has enclosed with her missive.[43] Blanchon's own letter is weary and resigned: he says that he has long given up attempting to challenge his parents' attitude to his sexual orientation, but that it hurts him when they fail to acknowledge his partner as a significant other in his life. He finishes: 'But anyway, enough said. I'm too scared to call you. I still love you both.' The significance of personal history is brought to the fore in a 1995 reincarnation of the work, which displayed his mother's letter next to two further items.[44] The first was a painted mural of Blanchon, adapted from the front cover of Peter Benchley's novel *Jaws*, depicting the artist as a naked swimmer about to be ripped apart by the gleaming teeth of a Great White (Figure 20). The second item consisted of a silver-plated specimen of *carcharodon carcharias*, or fossilized shark dung, presented on a red velvet cushion. The image and object can be read as a double self-portrait: self as object of the shark's dinner, and the excreted result.

The installation was accompanied by a wall text, which clearly established the installation in the context of Blanchon's personal history:

> Set in fictional Amityville, *Jaws*, the original, was actually filmed in Martha's Vineyard where my mother grew up and I spent most summer vacations. At the age of ten, I was obsessed with the movie's production and would beg my parents or siblings to take me to the harbor or beach where filming took place. I wore my Jaws tank top everyday – dirty due to the fact that I never released it long enough to be laundered. A few years later, as part of family car trips across country, we were touring Universal studios past movie sets and devices in California. Still consumed with pride – I finally quit sucking my thumb while travelling through South Dakota – I paid little attention to the Studio until we came upon a small lake where my beloved Jaws lived. The tour trolley glided over the water on suspended tracks while the shark circled us. While preparing my Instamatic for

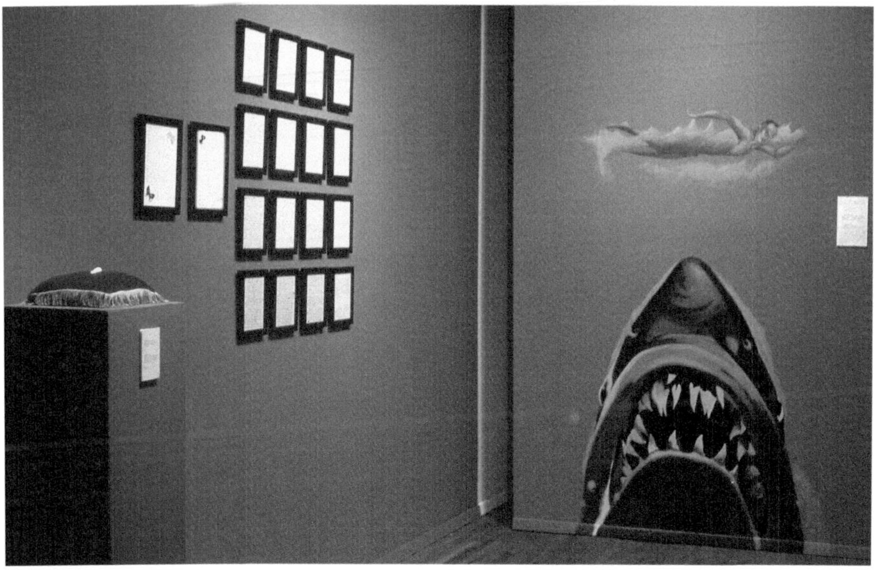

Figure 20 Robert Blanchon, *Protection* or *Carcharodon Carcharias (Jaws),* 1992–5. Fossilized shark dung, red velvet pillow, gold fringe and silver-plated dried faeces, dimensions variable. Courtesy of The Estate of Robert Blanchon / Mary Ellen Carroll – MEC, studios © 1999 The Estate of Robert Blanchon/Mary Ellen Carroll – MEC, studios.

> the photo opportunity of my little lifetime, the shark suddenly appeared aside my face. Shocked, I instinctively threw my camera in its artificial mouth.[45]

Blanchon fretted over the possibility that he was revealing too much of himself in this work; in a note to the curators, he wrote:

> Along with continuing in the vein of sharing too much personal information – a common thread in all my work these days, the inclusion of Jaws in the installation raises a variety of interesting, to me at least, issues regarding art about AIDS, art and photography, and the manner in which a person's life enters history, and how, practically and historically, this happens.

The installation suggests Blanchon's preoccupation with the problem of victimhood as related to AIDS; while he recognized that victim photography was problematic, he also wrote passionately about his right to call himself a victim. In this anecdote, photography is a mode of defence, but the tools of photography are destroyed or consumed in the process.

Blanchon addressed the problem of AIDS portraiture more directly in *[never realized]*, a small artist's publication, approximately five by five inches, and sixteen pages in length. In it, Blanchon distinguishes four major cultural representations of people with AIDS: the decaying, white homosexual male; the innocent victim; the celebrity; and (a category that Blanchon acknowledges overlaps with the others) the lunatic or deviant. He adopts the first person to decry the rejection of the 'victim' label:

> Victim, in our culture, became a swear word years ago. I find this alienating, since I am told not to use the word, yet I am planning on dying from a disease that I didn't invite into my body.[46]

Listing the reasons why he needs to call himself a victim, he accuses society of failing to care for the sick, drugs companies of holding back research, life insurance companies of encouraging him to cash in a policy that he doesn't hold and 'do-gooders, like Kathy Lee Gifford and her AIDS baby hospice scam on the Upper East Side' for failing to 'raise money for me or offer me a nice place to die'.[47] He suggests that he is a casualty of language and of labels and implies that the acronym AIDS might best be rejected altogether:

> I am a victim of you and you are a victim of me when we tossed away individual life choices to identify ourselves with words. In search of the unproven advantages of self-empowerment, we were People Living with AIDS, now we are People with AIDS, or just plain old PWAs.[48]

As a corrective to labels and images of people with HIV, Blanchon proposes a large-scale public art project that will make manifest the disease itself. Since AIDS is a disease comprising symptoms, the project, titled *4 opportunistic infections for public viewing and consumption*, will consist of sculptures of four body parts typically affected by AIDS-related conditions (Figure 21). Suggesting the inadequacy of verbal or pictorial attempts to represent the lived reality of AIDS, Blanchon claims that his project aims 'to elevate the physiological aspects of HIV to a level of reality that represents the pain, loss, and massive suffering caused by this plague'.[49] These inner body parts will be produced in plastic multiples: 10,000 brains, 10,000 spinal cords, 10,000 pairs of lungs and 10,000 tongues resting on jaw bones. In a scheme that is 'romantic at best, never realized at worst', the organs will be distributed among the sick of New York City, each accompanied by an invitation to throw the casting from a window at a set time. Upon the appointed hour, 'like rain, the falling body parts would shower the streets with the reality of this disease'.[50]

Who is the 'I' in Blanchon's text? The answer might seem simple: the artist himself, of course, speaking from a position as HIV positive, perhaps already

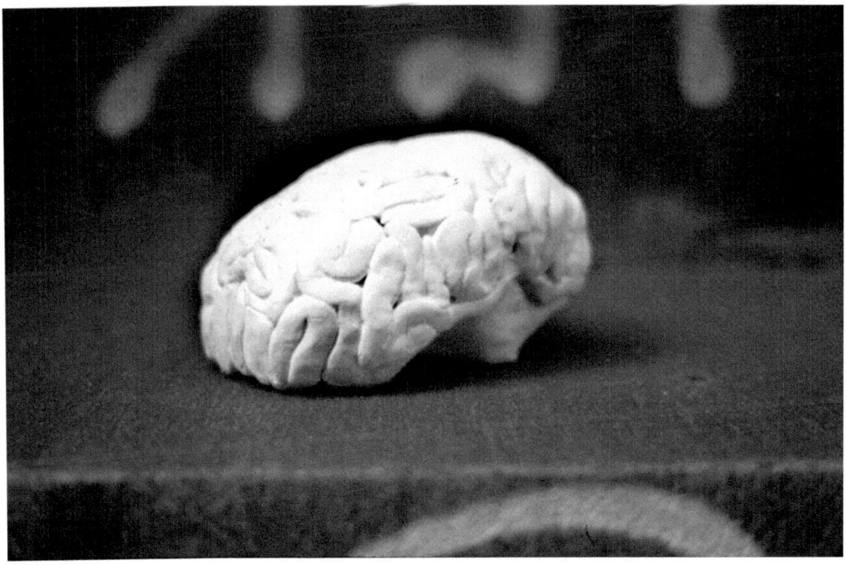

Figure 21 Robert Blanchon, *4 opportunistic infections for public viewing and consumption (Brain)*, *c*. 1992. Unrealized proposal, plaster prototypes, dimensions variable. Courtesy of The Estate of Robert Blanchon/Mary Ellen Carroll – MEC, studios © 1999 The Estate of Robert Blanchon/Mary Ellen Carroll – MEC, studios.

sick. However, the unrealized sculptural project that accompanies the text suggests a rejection of the political efficacy of individual identity. Blanchon implies that anatomy is universal, and the physiological portrait 'the only one that won't submit to discrimination'.[51] I suggest that a similar motivation is behind Blanchon's equivocal use of the 'I' in his work.

Given the text-based nature of much of Blanchon's work, I have found the distinction made by recent literary scholars between traditional autobiography and the broader term 'life writing' to be particularly useful. According to Sidonie Smith and Julia Watson, 'autobiography' denotes 'a particular practice of life writing that emerged in the Enlightenment and has become canonical in the West'.[52] Autobiography celebrates the autonomous individual and the universalizing life story; it is the 'master narrative of the "sovereign self"'.[53] If autobiography in this sense can be understood as offering a parallel to the traditional understanding of self-portraiture, then recent efforts to expand this literary category might be usefully applied to the visual field.

Roland Barthes argued that writing entails the loss of a singular voice, replaced by a special voice that consists of several indiscernible ones. The literary voice is a composite, 'that oblique into which every subject escapes, the trap where all identity is lost, beginning with the very identity of the body writing'.[54] This is extremely suggestive with regard to Blanchon's work: glossing Barthes, one might say that the very act of producing a self-referential artwork is the erasure of the self. The effect of this, Barthes suggests, is that meaning is generated not by a single God-like author figure but through the interplay between reader and text. I want to suggest that Blanchon's installation (and indeed, many aspects of his practice) deliberately interpolates the viewer as the source of the meaning of the work.

Recent scholarship has pointed out that 'autobiography' as traditionally understood excludes other forms of self-reflexive writing such as confessional texts, memoirs or diaries. In his study of AIDS memoirs, Ross Chambers proposes that AIDS diaries might resist the temporally backward direction that traditionally defines autobiography. AIDS diaries, Chambers suggests, are not orientated retrospectively (like classical autobiography or even narrative texts of witness); instead, they often look forward as enunciations 'to a future in which they will be read'.[55] This relation between writer and reader is implicitly ethical: 'The first effect of a textual authority derived from (the author's) death is thus to transmit a responsibility and, as it were, an obligation.'[56] This is the register in which I ultimately read Blanchon's work: as a practice that aims to elicit meaning from an interaction with the viewer. This process, I argue, necessitates the suppression of Blanchon's personal, 'authentic' voice; to misappropriate Roland Barthes' famous line, the 'death' of the artist, in Blanchon's case at least, is a precondition of the responsive viewer.

'An autobiographical show by an artist who has AIDS'

The remainder of this chapter focusses on the 1996 installation *gum, waste, indentations, stains, + envelopes* displayed at the Randolph Street Gallery, an experimental artist-run space in Chicago. At the time of the installation, Blanchon had been aware that he was HIV positive for at least six years; in a statement dated the same month as the show opened, Blanchon (in typically understated fashion) refers to himself 'not feeling so great'.[57] The show was widely interpreted as 'an autobiographical show by an artist who has AIDS'.[58] The more straightforwardly corporeal aspects of the installation support this interpretation: Blanchon's failing body is suggested by a (blood?) stained shirt, monogrammed with the artist's initials and arranged supine on the gallery floor, and by a plaster cast of the artist's decaying teeth (caused by 'crystal meth use and symptoms related to HIV', according to the exhibition literature).[59] Less easy to synthesize within this reading are two rather more enigmatic works. *Untitled [gum stains]* consists of four photographic prints of pavements stained with chewed gum, taken at popular cruising locations. *Untitled (self-portrait/waste)* comprises the fascia of a waste disposal unit inserted into the gallery wall at waist height and illuminated by a red light, suggesting a bodily orifice. The installation's final component, a towering pile of envelopes each containing an unaddressed, mass-produced 'with sympathy' card, recalls Blanchon's long-standing interest in anonymous communications and hints at the scale of the AIDS epidemic as a collective tragedy as well as a personal one.

If this installation is to be read as a self-portrait, the 'self' in question is a fragmented, unstable and contingent one. The subject of the work oscillates between the individual and the collective, between intimate bodily secretions and anonymous generality. Michel Beaujour suggests that, unlike a traditional autobiography, the literary self-portrait has no continuous narrative or any systematic history of the personality, instead subordinating linear narrative to a collection of thematic elements. According to Beaujour, the self-portraitist

> is forced into a detour that seemingly thwarts the intention of 'painting oneself', should we assume that the self-portrait is even bourn of such a naïve project: X by himself. That's improbable. The self-portrait is in the first place a found object to which the writer imparts the purpose of self-portrayal in the course of its elaboration. A kind of misprision or compromise, a shuttling back and forth between generality and particularity, the self-portraitist never has a clear notion of where he is going, of what he is doing.[60]

With its emphasis on haphazardness, fragmentation and authorial absence, Beaujour's text is wonderfully suggestive for a reading of Blanchon's work, and indeed a literary approach seems particularly apposite for Blanchon's practice. To some extent, this may be related to the text-based nature of some of Blanchon's works. In other terms, however, such comparisons implicitly raise questions about authorial identity similar to those posed by recent text-based approaches to self-representation.

Sidonie Smith and Julia Watson identify an ethnographic form of life writing that parallels self-study with the study of others, citing the example of the French Surrealist and ethnographer Michel Leiris' four-volume autobiography *The Rules of the Game* (of which only the first two volumes *Scratches* and *Scraps* have been published). They note: 'Confounding I and other, inside and out, language and ideas, Leiris makes the autobiographical a meeting point of exchange.'[61] Leiris' own text suggests the function of memory as an inter-subjective encounter:

> If I have a memory in my head, and it extends in all directions through emotional ramifications, it is not a foreign body to be extirpated. Even though it has come to me from outside [. . .] it is nonetheless an integral part of me; it has become my substance just like the food from outside me.[62]

Leiris' mapping of the body into inside and outside has strong resonances with Blanchon's installation, which, as I shall argue, functions according to a series of topological body metaphors. The entrances and exits of the body are suggested in various aspects: the mouth in the teeth, the chewed gum, and possibly in the allusions of the waste disposal fascia to a mouth or anus. The bodily traces explicit in the stained shirt and, less obviously, in the traces of saliva on teeth and gum, suggest the permeable boundaries between the outside of the body and its abject waste products, memorably and influentially outlined by Julia Kristeva in *Powers of Horror* (1981; trans. 1982).[63]

Just as Leiris uses a digestive metaphor to suggest the fluidity of inter-subjectivity, so *gum, waste, indentations, stains + envelopes* requires a revised understanding of a portrait as a fluid entity with a capacity to shift between the registers of personal and group experience. Writing in the catalogue for the contemporaneous exhibition *Face/Off: The Portrait in Recent Art*, Melissa Feldman proposes that the portrait might be divorced from its association with the individual subject to be re-imagined as 'an accumulation of its ethnocultural and socio-political circumstances'.[64] Her redefinition of the portrait provides a useful framework for understanding how Blanchon's installation interweaves personal and collective significance:

> Such works employ fictional or allegorical modes of representation that open themselves to multiple meanings and new art forms. In some cases the figure is replaced by object-based, sculptural or environmental assemblage. By posing as a symbol of a larger community, the portrait is forced out of its figural domain and into a body of evidence.[65]

Blanchon's resistance to an unambiguously autobiographical approach allows the work to bear witness to the collective experience of AIDS in the context of a homophobic society. His refusal to represent the body directly has a similar effect, liberating the work from the individualizing limitations of the purely self-referential and bestowing upon it social and political significance as an investigation into the social and psychical construction of the gay male subject at this critical historical moment.

Confessional fictions

The bloodied shirt *Stain #6* (1996) (Figure 22) is one of a series of soiled items of clothing either physically exhibited or photographically documented by Blanchon. *Stains #1 and #2* (1994) (Figure 23) comprise a photographic diptych that sets against a matt black background a white pair of men's briefs, the crotch and seat tainted with a pale, incriminating blemish of yellowish-brown. The two C-prints are handsomely framed in silver leaf, monumentalizing an

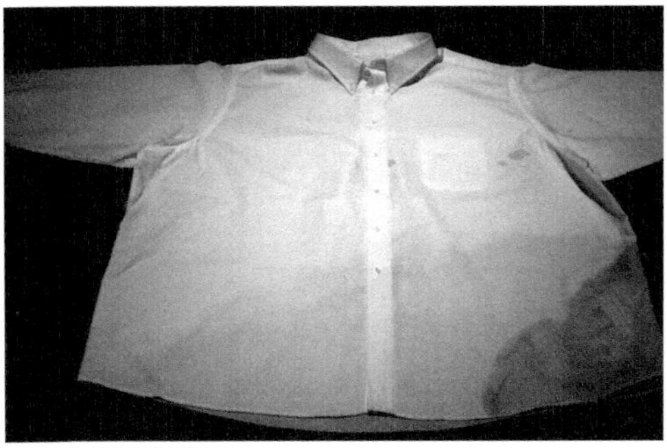

Figure 22 Robert Blanchon, *Stain #6,* 1996. Shirt, stain, monogram, men's size 22. Courtesy of The Estate of Robert Blanchon/Mary Ellen Carroll – MEC, studios © 1999 The Estate of Robert Blanchon/Mary Ellen Carroll – MEC, studios.

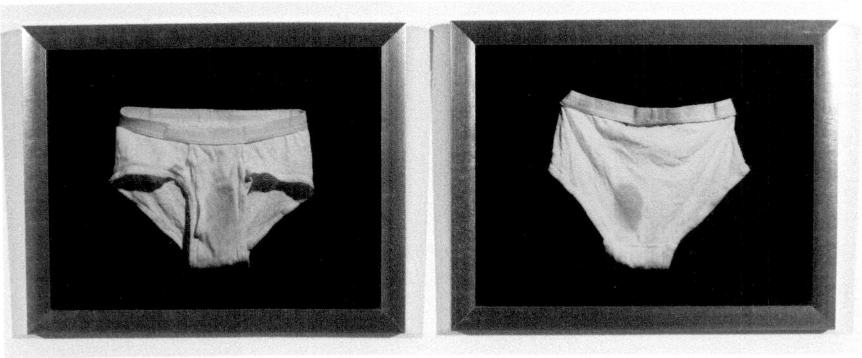

Figure 23 Robert Blanchon, *Stain #1 and Stain #2,* 1994. C-prints, 12.5 × 15.5 in. each. Courtesy of The Estate of Robert Blanchon/Mary Ellen Carroll — MEC, studios © 1999 The Estate of Robert Blanchon/Mary Ellen Carroll – MEC, studios.

embarrassing bodily moment that would more considerately be ignored. The mode of presentation further suggests an evidentiary role to be played by these dirty garments, witness perhaps to a body that will no longer stay within its proper boundaries, rendered incontinent and childlike by illness. *Stain #3*, also a framed C-print, is a closely focussed shot of the seam of another white garment. The fabric is softly creased and discoloured through multiple washes; the rust coloured blotch, suggestive of the slow seep of blood across cotton, is faded but stubborn. *Stain #4* (1995) depicts a dense black spot at the heart of a white T-shirt, its pale penumbra radiating softly outwards like a piece of tie-die. *Stain #5* (1995) reiterates the scatological theme of *Stains #1 and #2* on a crumpled pair of white boxer shorts.

Of all these items, only *Stain #6* is unequivocally identified with Blanchon, the association signalled by the artist's initials monogrammed into the cloth; read as a portrait it recalls Blanchon's fear of revealing too much of himself, particularly with respect to his illness. Literally and figuratively airing the artist's dirty linen in public, it evokes the two major influences of confessional and abject art. Writing with reference to what is perhaps the definitive work of confessional art, Tracey Emin's *My Bed* (1999), Christine Fanthome has noted that the confessional mode is capable of provoking questions about the relationship between the artist and observer that go beyond the artwork,[66] and Sidonie Smith and Julia Watson have similarly suggested that the work forces the spectator to 'enquire about an absent subjectivity whose traces surround us'.[67] Arguably, Blanchon's stains (and indeed the installation as a whole) operate in a similar manner, compelling the viewer to construct a narrative based on the absent figure whose presence and personal traces pervade the work.

In a discussion of autobiographical AIDS video works, Roger Hallas expresses concern that the confessional mode may be too overtly individualistic; its use risks reinforcing the notion that AIDS is a private, rather than historically and socially constructed experience.[68] Hallas identifies a heteroglossic quality in many examples of queer AIDS media, which mixes an autobiographical voice with other modes, including poetry, fantasy, testimony, political commentary and philosophical reflection. Blanchon's installation arguably does just this, questioning and subverting the ostensible truth produced by the confessional voice.

An understanding of the confessional as historically rooted in religious ritual raises certain powerful associations: *Stains #1 and #2* in particular are displayed like precious relics, their worn and dirty appearance clearly at odds with the status apparently accorded them. Stretching this analogy further, the artist (or the confessional persona of the artist) attains a saint-like quality (possibly even a martyrdom); this reading is reinforced by the supine position of the shirt in *Stain #6*, arranged on the floor with its arms outspread in a crucifix pose.

In the *History of Sexuality*, Foucault suggests that the modern-day practice of psychoanalysis is the secular heir to religious confessional practices. Confession has, since the Middle Ages, been one of the West's most important techniques for producing truth.[69] As Foucault points out, the 'truth' produced through the confessional is imbued with power relations. The spectator has an important function in confession: representing not only the interlocutor but also the authority who requires the confession, judges, punishes and forgives. If Blanchon's stains are read as confessional, this clearly raises questions about the role of the viewer; this is a point that I shall return to later in this chapter with regard to the minimalist vocabulary of other aspects of the installation.

Foucault's project is, in part, to find alternatives to the psychoanalytic subject. Blanchon's installation, with its emphasis on upper and lower body, mouths and anuses, seems to require a psychoanalytic reading. Yet it also resists, or perhaps gently mocks, this possibility. Blanchon's shirt raises the possibility of a confessional voice, but ultimately this position is a pose. The shirt is outsized, a US men's size 22 (roughly equivalent to a standardized XL). Despite the monogram, it is likely not Blanchon's own shirt, and there is no reason to believe that the fluid is either blood or indeed Blanchon's personal bodily excretion. The excessive dimensions of the shirt hint at the fictitious nature of the whole installation. If the viewer is the analyst and Blanchon the analysand, he refuses the production of truth through confession.

Abjection and melancholia

The *Stains* series and the more visceral aspects of *gum, waste,* etc. are strongly suggestive of Julia Kristeva's influential theory of abjection. Kristeva's text *Powers of Horror* (1980; trans. 1982) describes a subject engaged in a constant struggle to maintain the proper boundaries of his or her own physical and psychical self; the abject is the waste or excess that must be expelled by that subject in order that he or she might continue to exist. In a physical sense, this might include excretory products such as urine, tears or sweat; in a psychic register this not only is most often associated with the primal necessity of separation from the mother but also suggests an insurmountable fissure at the heart of all subjectivity.

Abjection is associated with the border between life and death, an interpretation that casts light on Blanchon's own interest in mortality. As Kristeva writes:

> This body fluids, this defilement, this shit are what life withstands, hardly and with difficulty, on the part of death. There, I am at the border of my condition as a living being. My body extricates itself, as being alive, from that border. Such wastes form so that I might live, until, from loss to loss, nothing remains in me and my entire body falls beyond the limit – *cadere*, cadaver.[70]

Falling, horizontality and gravitational pull – all feature strongly in Kristeva's account. It is noteworthy that unlike its predecessors, *Stain #6* is not a photograph, displayed in a frame and on a wall, but an object installed on the floor, low and corpse-like.

In the early 1990s, abjection (in the art world at least) had acquired a political dimension. As the introductory catalogue essay for the Whitney Museum's 1993 'Abject Art' show put it: 'the concept of abjection, encompassing investigations of discursive excess and degraded elements as they relate to the body and society, has emerged as a central theoretical impulse of 1990s art'.[71] Drawing on theories by Julia Kristeva and George Bataille, the catalogue introduction defined abjection as 'a blurring of boundaries between self and other'[72] (related to psychoanalytic ideas of the visceral unconscious and bodily ego), and the notion of base materialism. Abjection is assumed to be political: it incorporates elements 'deemed inappropriate by a conservative dominant culture', and is seen by the exhibition organizers as a reaction to the 'culture wars' attacks on artists such as David Wojnarowicz, Robert Mapplethorpe and Andres Serrano. While the majority of readings of abject art have focussed on the female body, the male body is also at stake. Simon Taylor's essay 'The Phobic Object' suggests ways in which works by Jackson Pollock, Andy Warhol, Mike Kelley and Robert Gober encourage a rethinking of the male form.[73] It is fair to suggest that ideas about abjection and its political dimensions were very much in the air at the time at which Blanchon was making his work.

The state of abjection also has inexorable links with melancholia, as Kristeva's subsequent book *Black Sun* makes clear. In a passage that echoes *Powers of Horror*, to suffer from melancholia is to be 'wounded, bleeding, cadaverized [. . .] on the frontiers of life and death'.[74] Drawing on the psychoanalytic theory of Freud, Abrahams and Klein, Kristeva identifies melancholia as an oral and anal phenomenon. The phenomenon of 'melancholy cannibalism' accounts for a passion for 'holding within the mouth' the lost, loved-hated other; vagina and anus can also lend themselves to this. This process is intended to keep a hold on the loved, lost object: 'better fragmented, torn, cut up, swallowed, digested . . . than lost'.[75] Applied to a melancholic person, Kristeva's logic is as follows: the melancholic loves the lost object but also hates it for having abandoned him/her; in order not to lose it, the melancholic incorporates it within him or herself. Since the object is hated, the melancholic experiences its incorporation as indicative of their own 'bad self'.

Similarly, abjection is also profoundly oral. One of Kristeva's earliest examples of abjection is food loathing, the way in which the skin on a glass of milk can cause retching, dizziness and nausea. A number of elements in Blanchon's installation suggest a similar fascination with orality. Most obviously, *My teeth as of November 23, 1995* (1996) (Figure 24), which consists of a silver-painted plaster cast of Blanchon's tooth decay. As with early items in the *Stains* series, the mode of presentation – the silver paint, the fringed velvet pillow – is at odds with the abject subject matter, suggesting a relic-like status, and as with the stained clothing, *My teeth* purports to offer a literal trace of the artist's body, this time not as mark but as the cast of a negative space. Other oral elements include the 'gum stain' photographs, which will be discussed in the following section, and the 'mouth' of the waste disposal unit, explored at the end of this chapter.

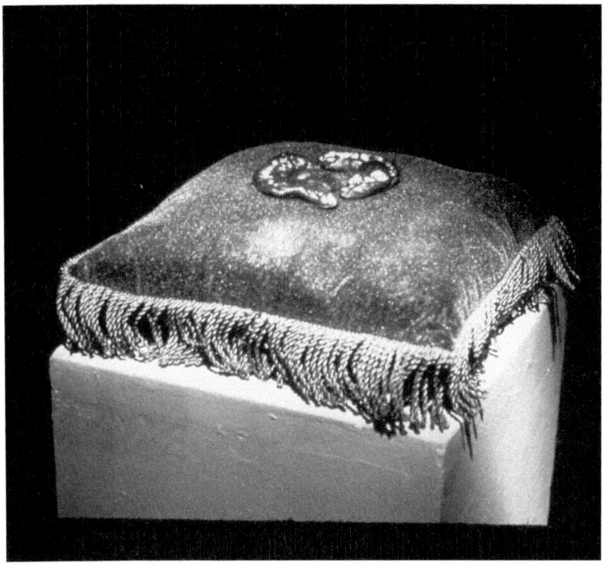

Figure 24 Robert Blanchon, *My teeth as of November 23, 1995*, 1996. Plaster cast, silver paint, velvet pillow, dimensions unknown. Courtesy of The Estate of Robert Blanchon/ Mary Ellen Carroll – MEC, studios © 1999 The Estate of Robert Blanchon/Mary Ellen Carroll – MEC, studios.

Blanchon was familiar with Freud, listing *Deviation in Relation to the Sexual Aim* as part of the core reading for the course he taught in the fall of 1996. He is likely to have been familiar with Freud's account of the functions of the mouth in 'Three Essays on Sexuality'. Freud was intrigued by the fact that, despite the kiss being held in high sexual esteem, the mouth is not part of the sexual apparatus but constitutes the entrance to the digestive tract. He concludes that certain regions of the body, such as the mouth and anus, are constantly appearing in sexual practices. It therefore seems logical to assume that they should be regarded and treated as genitals. Freud's treatment of the mouth is tied up with an investigation of perversions, defined as sexual activities which either extend beyond the regions of the body intended for sexual use or linger over the intermediate relations that should normally be quickly overcome in order to reach the final aim. In his writing *On Dreams*, Freud suggested that dreaming of teeth signified a displacement from the lower to the upper part of the body. Dreams with a dental stimulus were thus assumed to have a masturbatory meaning.[76] Finally, in his Dora case study, Freud suggests that that disgust caused by Herr K's kiss has caused the patient's symptoms to displace from the lower to upper part of her own body, resulting in a cough, hoarseness, loss of appetite and, most importantly, loss of voice.[77] The entrances and exits of the digestive tract – one might say, the inner topology of the body, are the latent organizing metaphor of Blanchon's installation.

Monuments to loss: The *[gum stain]* series

Abject bodily excreta also provide the subject matter for the four photographic prints *Untitled [gum stains 1, 2, 3 & 4]*, each of which depicts an irregular grey background mottled with dark spots and smears. These apparently non-referential images (Figure 25) borrow the visual vocabulary of abstract expressionism; two are punctuated with a tiny circular dollop of sky-blue, and one is bisected with a rough black horizontal line and streaked with red in its upper right-hand corner. Were it not for the parenthetic title, it would be difficult to determine exactly what – if anything – the images depict. The revealed subject matter – a sidewalk stained with chewed gum – suggests a connection between the grime of an urban pavement and bodily dirt implicit in the traces of saliva and molar imprints on the masticated, ejected material. This thematic of filth – or more specifically, a kind of tainted bodily residue – is echoed throughout the rest of the installation in the faintly repulsive silver cast of Blanchon's decaying

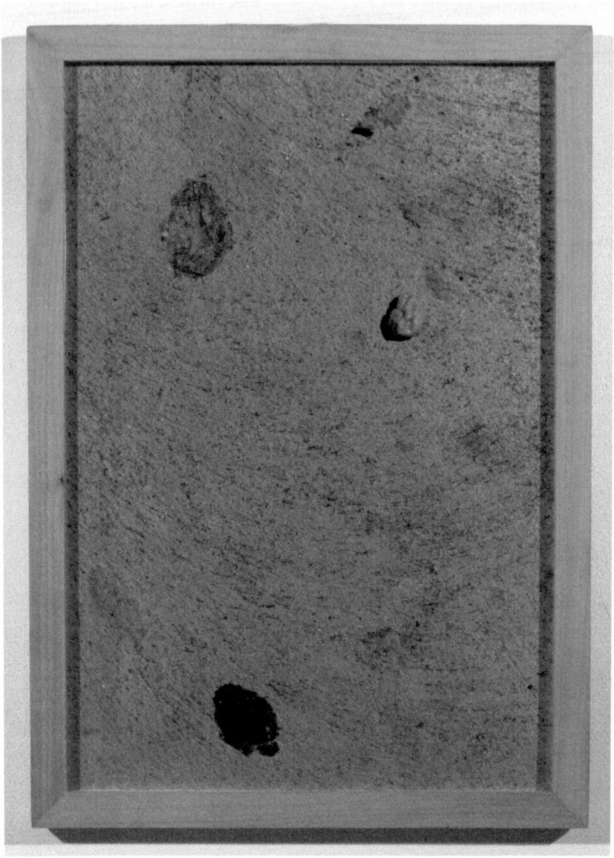

Figure 25 Robert Blanchon, *Untitled [gum stain 4], c.* 1995. C-print, wood frame, 32.25 × 22.5 in. Courtesy of The Estate of Robert Blanchon/Mary Ellen Carroll — MEC, studios © 1999 The Estate of Robert Blanchon/Mary Ellen Carroll — MEC, studios

teeth, the blemished shirt and in the waste disposal unit's suggestion of public toilets and private orifices.

An alternative set of titles for the gum stains evokes a further range of associations. *7985 Santa Monica Blvd, 7566 Melrose Avenue, 8722 Santa Monica Blvd,* and *9000 Sunset Blvd* are, according to the exhibition literature, all West Hollywood addresses of cruising places for gay men. Each mark acts as a 'trace' of an actual or potential sexual encounter, and indeed, the gum stains have been likened to wads of semen.[78] These bodily deposits are clearly intended to represent the unseen men who constitute the true subjects of this conceptual group portrait, an interpretation supported by the literature produced by the gallery to accompany the installation:

> Continuing a project begun on New York City subway platforms, documenting the chronological life-span of spat out gum, the color photographs in *[gum, waste, indentations, stains + envelopes]* represent isolated segments of West Hollywood sidewalks (a community known for its healthy and assimilated gay men). Depicted in various stages of decay these metaphorical images refer to the discarded, nameless victims of a number of social and medical ills.[79]

There is an unmistakeable pathos in these little marks: the lack of human presence raises the spectral possibility that each stain indexes an AIDS-related death. The images signal a double bereavement, not only memorializing the men themselves but also paying tribute to a post-Stonewall, pre-AIDS culture of sexual liberation. In 'Mourning and Melancholia', Freud suggests that the condition of mourning can occur not only in response to the death of a person but also to the loss of an abstraction or ideal.[80] This loss is memorialized by Blanchon's images, which communicate the multitude of bodies that once congregated on these patches of ground, while suggesting that such pleasures are a now a thing of the past. In *Black Sun*, Kristeva points out that Aristotle links melancholia to spermatic froth;[81] Blanchon's marks are emblematic of 1990s AIDS melancholia in their synthesis of abject bodily identification with nostalgic, silent mourning.

As monuments to loss, Blanchon's images are constructed on a diminutive scale that bears witness to the perceived expendability of the men whose traces they document. Simon Watney has observed how, in the context of the AIDS epidemic

> the 'homosexual body' continues to speak after death, not as a memento-mori, but as its exact reverse, for a life that must at all costs be seen to have been devoid of value, unregretted, unlamented, and – final indignity – effaced into a mere anonymous statistic. The 'homosexual body' is 'disposed of' like so much rubbish, like the trash that it was in life.[82]

Watney's polemic proposes that homosexual expendability is the necessary outcome of a political authority invested in the social institutions of marriage, reproduction and 'family values', institutions that can only be sustained by positioning homosexuality as the dangerous 'other' of normative heterosexuality. Watney describes the homosexual body as an 'impossible object'[83] – a popular discourse of 'family values' brands the homosexual as a threat, 'a monster that can only be engendered by a process of corruption through seduction', yet the heteronormative sexual economy that supports this discourse cannot account for the existence of any form of desire that does not conform to the needs of familial reproduction.[84] Within this heteronormative framework the homosexual is a logical impossibility whose real existence reveals the fragility of the dominant model of acceptable sexual desire.

The homosexual body can only enter public visibility on the condition that identification with it is rigorously refused. For Watney, the 'homosexual body' is not a tangible entity but a fantasmatic space where the consequences of resistance to heteronormative social practices are displayed and punished. The discursive construction of the homosexual body as a legitimate object of knowledge – for example, through nineteenth-century physiognomic photography – provides scientific 'evidence' of the homosexual's essential deviance. As Watney suggests, AIDS merely provides the most recent opportunity for the confirmation of what is 'already known' about the homosexual body: that its blemished outwards appearance mirrors its moral corruption:

> Reading AIDS as the outward and visible sign of an imagined depravity of will, AIDS commentary deftly returns us to a pre-modern vision of the body, according to which heresy and sin are held to be scored in the features of their voluntary subjects by punitive and admonitory manifestations of disease.[85]

Watney proposes that this fantastical body finds its ultimate expression in the over-determined image of the AIDS victim, a cadaverous bed-bound male whose physical condition announces his sexual guilt. The lack of direct bodily representation in *[gum stains]* suggests the anonymity and expendability of homosexual AIDS casualties; it also implies Blanchon's unwillingness to risk the inadvertent reproduction of the pictorial stereotype of the AIDS victim.

Rather than engage with hackneyed visual iconographies, Blanchon instead addresses the negative fantasmatic potential of the homosexual body. The stains reimagine the fantasmatic gay male body as a blemish on the city, untouchable, revolting and excluded from the proper social order. As Watney points out, within the realm of psychoanalysis the body is not a pre-given reality but a psychic projection that can be both internal and external. Like Blanchon's *[gum stains]*, the body itself is 'radically mute, yet rendered garrulous by projective, desiring fantasies all around it'.[86] By *not* representing the body, the gum stains open up a space that signifies far in excess of that generated by direct corporeal depiction.

Blanchon gum stains find an interesting parallel in the work of a well-known female artist: Cindy Sherman's 'disgust' photographs. Taken in the late 1980s, Sherman's images depict floors strewn with foodstuffs, vomit and other filthy substances. In common with Blanchon, Sherman's work entails a form of self-effacement: in those images where she is present, she is concealed behind masks, make-up and other props; in the 'disgust' photographs her likeness is barely visible, a tiny figure reflected on the mirror of a powder compact that lies buried in the waste. Using language that could equally describe Blanchon's installation, Laura Mulvey describes Sherman's work as a riddle or enigma.[87] Mulvey traces Sherman's work chronologically, from the soft-core pastiches of femininity in the 1980s *Untitled Film Stills*, through the harshly lit, theatrical parodies of the masquerade of womanhood in the *Untitled* series of 1983 and the 'monstrous' images of the mid-1990s, which often involve animal-like features, prosthetics and blurred gender identities, finally arriving at the 'disgust' photographs where nothing remains of the female body except detritus. In Mulvey's account this final transformation is announced by a shift in perspective to the downward camera angle: as this occurs, the body disappears or disintegrates. At the same time, Sherman's images become monstrously enlarged, each measuring in the region of seventy-two by forty-nine inches. At thirty-two by twenty-two inches, Blanchon's *[gum stains]* are not quite in this category, but the difference in size between representation and reality is enough to achieve an uncanny 'making strange' of the subject material. For Mulvey, Sherman's work is about the 'phantasmatic space' of the female body,[88] revealing the abyss that occurs when the female body is defetishized and deprived of its significance. If the female body has come to 'represent the shudder aroused by liquidity and decay',[89] then the gay male body is in Blanchon's work both feminized and constructed in similarly abject terms. Applying this reasoning to Blanchon's installation, we can say that the installation addresses the 'phantasmatic space' conjured by the gay male body. In the context of the gum stains, this body has become almost completely dematerialized, and as with Sherman's work, this is at least partly connected to the political difficulty in representing it.

According to Watney, the 'spectacle' of AIDS constructs the homosexual body through a 'studied emphasis on dirt, depravity [. . .] and above all, promiscuity'.[90] Promiscuity constitutes a central feature of AIDS discourse, both in the context of the popular conception of the homosexual as voraciously promiscuous and in the efforts of activists such as Douglas Crimp to de-problematize a proclivity for multiple partners and disassociate safe promiscuous practices from AIDS. Crimp argued that monogamy *in itself* was not a factor in preventing viral transmission: more significant was the use of appropriate protection and practising sexual activity in ways that did not involve the exchange of bodily fluids. Implying that homosexual activity was inherently more varied than heterosexual sex, Crimp claimed that gay men were in fact better placed to practice safe sexual activity than heterosexuals.[91]

The promiscuous homosexual body was popularly associated with a specifically urban environment littered with bars, clubs and cruising places. From the beginning of the epidemic, AIDS had strong metropolitan connotations. Jan Zita Grover claims that in 1986, the preponderance of reported cases in the United States were located in just five cities – New York, San Francisco, Los Angeles, Houston and Miami – and suggests how the popular imagination connected AIDS with a debauched urban lifestyle:

> For the majority of Americans living outside of those communities, AIDS appeared to be someone else's problem – something freakish and citified, related not only to an exotic homosexuality but to the corruptions of downtown city life.[92]

These last few words – the 'corruptions of downtown' – are a reminder of the way in which the city is mapped according to a bodily metaphor, with downtown having specific connotations of permissive sexuality; the association of promiscuity, contagion and the urban environment suggested by the *[gum stains]* gives weight to Grover's observation. It also echoes the language of nineteenth-century city reformers: Peter Stallybrass and Allon White have described the nineteenth-century city as something to be surveyed and mastered from a high window or other raised position.[93] The elevated viewpoint from which Blanchon captures the gum images, camera held high and pointed downwards parallel to the floor, recalls the charting of the city by such reformers. The city was thus 'mapped' in both moral and spatial terms according to the relations of high to low: this process drew a line between the surveyors themselves and the objects of their study, which were constructed according to metaphors of filth and sexuality, aligning moral depravity with disease, and disease with the dirt of the city slums. Recalling Freud's writings on the interchangability of the 'high' and 'low' parts of the body, Stallybrass and White suggest that the almost hysterical attention paid to the 'low' of the city is a transcoding of attention away from the repressed 'low' of the bourgeois body. In a similar move, Blanchon's *gum stains* map the socially low (promiscuous homosexual men) onto the low of the city (recall that the project was first started on the New York City underground), drawing a parallel between this and the low (sexual) part of the body. Mirroring this downwards trajectory, an oral deposit (gum) becomes misrecognized as a sexual one (ejaculate).

Earlier works by Blanchon suggest a more positive interpretation of the intersections of homosexuality and public space; for example, the performance piece *Cruising New York* (1993), an artist-led tour of popular meeting places for anonymous gay sex in the city. In another project, Blanchon drew attention to the homoerotic aspect of a series of public monuments, thus challenging any clear distinction between 'straight' and 'queer' space. *Untitled (Benjamin Franklin)* (1992–4) depicts the statue from a low vantage point, with the image closely cropped to fix the gaze on the patriarch's surprisingly well-proportioned genitals; in a similar vein are *Untitled (John Quincy Adams, Boston)* (1995) and *Untitled (Alexander Hamilton, Boston)* (1995). The low viewpoint afforded by the camera angle contrasts with the 'high up' of the authority figures depicted, offering a queer twentieth-century revision of Stallybrass and White's mapping of the city according to a vertical bodily metaphor.

George Bataille's notion of the *informe* is closely allied to the condition of spatial and metaphorical lowness: the *informe* is 'a term that serves to bring things down in the world'.[94] Certain qualities of the *informe* recall those of chewing gum: likened to spittle, the *informe* 'gets itself squashed everywhere'.[95] Since the early 1990s, Rosalind Krauss has used the *informe* as a theoretical alternative to abjection, developing her interpretation of the term in a series of papers on Jackson Pollock, to whose drips and splattered paintings (when viewed as photographic reproductions, if not in the flesh) Blanchon's *[gum stains]* bear a suggestive visual resemblance.[96] Krauss' account of Pollock's work focusses on the transition of the drip paintings from the horizontal to vertical plane and the implications of that axial movement for an embodied reading of the work.[97] Proceeding from Clement Greenberg's recollection of Pollock as 'a very respectable gentleman', Krauss proposes that Greenberg's comment should be understood as symptomatic of a wider process of 'sublimating' Pollock by denying the base bodily materialism of his practice. Contrasting early criticism of Pollock with the positive recognition that he enjoyed from 1950 onward, Krauss suggests that the rising status accorded to Pollock as painter is connected his canvases' journeys from floor to wall, low to high and disorder to order:

> *before*, it was on the floor: 'a child's contour map,' 'a flat, war-shattered city, possibly Hiroshima, as seen from a great height,' 'dribblings,' 'droolings,' 'a mass of tangled hair.' And *now*, it's on the wall. Where it takes on order, and the sophistication of tradition[98]

This raising of the work from floor to wall suggests to Krauss a disavowal of the work's abject bodily qualities. Krauss proposes a selection of works by Andy Warhol as a response to the essential horizontality of Pollock's drip paintings. In 1961 Warhol – a great admirer of Pollock – spread blank canvases on the pavement outside his house so that people would have to walk on them, leaving a network of tracks. In the same year, he executed what he referred to as 'piss paintings', specifying the materials as 'urine on canvas'. For Krauss the convergence of the footprints and the urine makes explicit Warhol's formal reading of the horizontality of Pollock's work: '[for Warhol] the pictures begged to be read as the residue of a liquid gesture performed by a man standing over a horizontal field'.[99] Krauss' reading of Pollock through Warhol suggests that the low and the horizontal are associated not simply with the body in general but more particularly with the genitalia. In a later paper, Krauss labels this horizontal impulse as *informe*: 'Pollock's importance was lodged in an axial rotation of painting out of the vertical domain of the visual field and onto the horizontal vector of what I begin to call . . . formlessness.'[100]

Like Pollock's drip paintings, Blanchon's gum stains suggest a trajectory from low and horizontal to high and vertical: in the journey from grubby pavement to gallery wall, the ground has been rotated into the vertical plane and elevated to eye level. Transposing Krauss' argument to Blanchon's prints, we might contend that this process sanitizes the abject subject matter by transforming it into an aesthetic object. The implications of this for the politics of sexual representation are clear: it is only through the sublimation of the gay male body that it can appear in representation at all, still less be raised to the category of fine art.

Interpolating the viewer: *Untitled (self-portrait/waste)*

Untitled (self-portrait/waste) (1995) (Figure 26) comprises a stainless-steel waste disposal ring four-and-a-half inches in diameter, lined with black rubber, inserted into the wall of the gallery and illuminated by a red light. The installation transforms the ring from a mundane object into a figurative metaphor for mouth and anus, with the red light evoking warm flesh as well as the more obvious suggestion of sex clubs, brothels and private cinemas. The work irresistibly invites a sexual interpretation: one reviewer emphasized its placement 'at crotch or anus height',[101] while for another it suggested the glory hole, 'icon of once-glorified anonymous bathroom sex'.[102] In its allusions to potential locations for the soliciting of gay sex, *Untitled (self-portrait/waste)* reprises Blanchon's interest in the often-invisible queer annexation of 'public' space for 'private' activity explored in the *[gum stain]* series and other works.

In a number of respects, this piece recalls the handmade sculptural forms based on domestic sinks, public urinals and drain grilles that were produced by

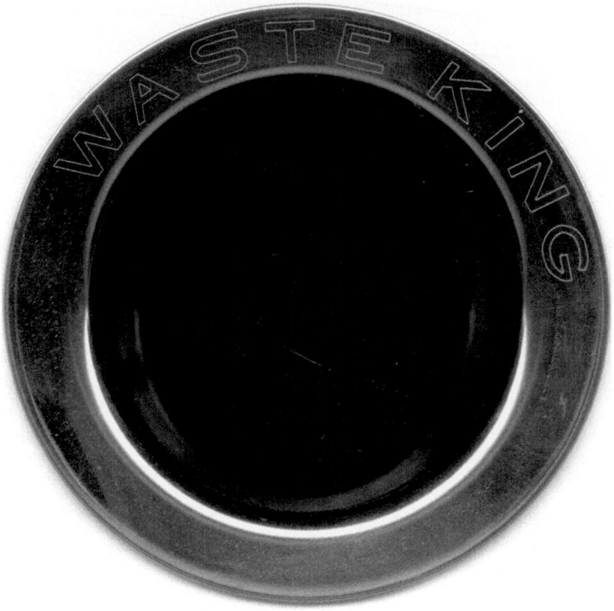

Figure 26 Robert Blanchon, *Untitled (self-portrait/waste)*, 1995. Metal, rubber, 4.5 in. diameter; 1.75 in. deep. Courtesy of The Estate of Robert Blanchon/Mary Ellen Carroll — MEC, studios © 1999 The Estate of Robert Blanchon/Mary Ellen Carroll – MEC, studios.

Robert Gober from 1983 onwards. Gober made over forty sinks between 1983 and 1992; fashioned from plaster over wire lathe and finished with white semi-gloss enamel paint, their lack of faucets or drainage holes emphasized their sculptural, non-functional quality. His urinals were produced between 1984 and 1988 using the same plaster and lathe technique. These were followed by a series of drain grilles, generally sculpted from metal; an edition of pewter sink drain holes, each four and a quarter inches in diameter, inserted at the height of the artist's breastbone into the wall of New York's Paula Cooper Gallery in 1989,[103] suggesting a clear visual similarity with Blanchon's *Untitled (self-portrait/waste)*.

Gober has described his drains as metaphors functioning in the same way as paintings, opening a window onto a dark and unknown world.[104] A drain (or a waste disposal unit) suggests multiple interpretations: a passage for waste liquid to pass through, away from our sight and our world, and a filter for rubbish; it can also be, as Gober suggests, the opening to an underworld, a boundary between the known and unknown, like the analogous bodily zones of the mouth and the genitals.[105] Helen Molesworth has noted how drains

> do not so much delineate the threshold between public and private as establish the very contiguous nature of public and private, the permeability between inside and outside [. . .], between oneself and others.[106]

In the light of Molesworth's observation, Blanchon's *Untitled (self-portrait/waste)* suggests two things. First, that the limits between public and private are not absolute; Blanchon was acutely aware that the AIDS epidemic had eroded the previously private nature of sexual preferences and activities. Second, it suggests the potentially limitless nature of the self and the way in which that self is inextricably bound up with others; Blanchon's expanded self-portraiture, with its consistent refusal to represent the artist as a unique or original individual, can best be understood in this sense, as a recognition of the significance of the part of his own identity that is collectively and externally constituted.

Interpretations of Gober's use of the sink, urinal and drain motif have tended to follow two main paths, both of which are relevant to a reading of Blanchon's work. The first approach is to view Gober's sculptures in their social context as responses to the AIDS epidemic; the second is to read them art-historically in relation to the influence of minimalist sculpture and the conceptual art of Duchamp. As Richard Flood has written,

> it is tempting to see the sinks, urinals, and drains cumulatively as surrogate portraits of gay men in the 1980s [. . .] When the sinks were begun in 1984, the gay community was already being sorely tested by the growing stigmatization of gay men as carriers of the AIDS virus, as pariahs being visited by a plague tailored to their heedless otherness.[107]

At this moment in time, Flood suggests, the slight archaic passive term 'gay' begins to give way to the more ambiguous term 'queer'. Flood reads Gober's sculptures as 'queer' in the most homespun sense of the word: designed to fail in their function, their very nature means that they simply cannot do what utility expects of them. Nonetheless, they remain complex, unique and beautiful in their otherness.[108]

In response to the tendency of reviewers to align the inoperative quality of his sculpture with the supposed 'non-functionality' of the gay male body, in 1992 Gober created a lavish installation at the DIA Arts Foundation in New York. A series of metal grilles were integrated into the floor, under which copious volumes of clean water flowed lavishly through open drainpipes. Referring to this installation in a later interview, Gober made explicit the role of his sculptures as self-portraiture:

> I think that making the sink functional wasn't only an internal imperative of expressing who I am, but maybe it was also a response to so much of the

> interpretation that had to do with the non-functioning sink and the epidemic and myself as a gay man. I think that I felt a need to turn that around and to not have a gay artist represented as a non-functioning utilitarian object, but one functioning beautifully, almost in excess.[109]

Blanchon's own sculpture might similarly be interpreted as a deliberate decision to represent himself 'in excess' with a sign that, despite his diagnosis, he is still functioning 'beautifully' as a gay man and sexual being. Blanchon's assumption of a position of sexual excess echoes an approach discernable in other of his works: for example, *Untitled (Robert)* (1993), which consists of eight photographs of himself accompanied by seven small blocks of text taken from the personal ads. One of these reads as follows:

> COCKSUCKING TOILET WHORE.
>
> I'm a cocksucking toilet whore. I'm the kind of guy you see in toilet stalls sucking one big dick after another. All races are welcome. Give me a location and I'll be there with my hot mouth.

This snippet of text clearly anticipates Blanchon's sculptural representation of himself as a 'hot mouth' in *Untitled (self-portrait/waste)*. In personal correspondence, Blanchon often described the work as the 'Waste King' piece, referring to the manufacturer's name printed on the metal rim; with its connotations of stately power, this alternative title suggests a positive, joyful embrace of sexual stereotypes.

The second dominant response to Gober's sculptures is to stress their art-historical lineage as reinterpretations of Marcel Duchamp's readymade urinal *Fountain* (1917), or as examples of a softer, more emotionally suffused response to the hard lines of minimalism. Gober himself was often resistant to the interpretation of his work in Duchampian terms,[110] and indeed the painstakingly hand-crafted nature of his sculptures would seem to resist its interpretation as a readymade. The comparison with minimalist sculpture is more compelling (and certainly more productive in relation to Blanchon's own work). Elisabeth Sussman describes Gober's sinks and urinals as

> sensuous, glowing and tactile, combining the tactility of painting and ceramics [. . .] they are completely unlike either the works to which they might be compared: the hard, industrially manufactured surfaces either of Duchamp's urinal or of the abstracted forms sent out for fabrication by, say, Donald Judd. Gober's sinks and urinals undoubtedly do somewhat reflect a Minimalist aesthetic, but, once again, closer in a way [. . .] to the body, to 'people engaged in various kinds of activities'.[111]

Many of Gober's pieces were untitled, but others were described by anthropomorphic adjectives such as *Sad*, *Silly*, *Scary* or *Mixed-Up*; according to Richard Flood, the sculptures' suggestive titles and uncanny presence invested the clean lines and thematic repetition of Minimalism with a 'haunting emotional resonance'.[112]

Minimalism has traditionally been understood in terms of the rejection of both thematic content and subjective presence. More recent re-readings of minimalism have drawn attention to the way in which subjective, embodied or emotional characteristics are repressed rather than eliminated.[113] Writing in 1996 (the same year as Blanchon's exhibition), Hal Foster notes, 'recently the status of minimalism has changed once more'.[114] Artists seeking alternatives to the practices of the 1970s and 1980s are offering alternative revisions of minimalism that 'refashion it in iconographic, expressive and/or spectacular themes';[115] it is in this sense that Blanchon's installation must be understood (as indeed must the work of Felix Gonzalez-Torres, which will be examined in this context in the following chapter). Foster argues that the minimalists' suppression of artistic expression and foregrounding of the spectator gives rise to the principles put forward by Roland Barthes in 1968 that the 'death of the author' is at the same time a birth of the viewer'.[116]

The way in which minimalist sculpture depends upon the viewer for the completion of the work is the central complaint of Michael Fried's influential essay 'Art and Objecthood' (1967). Fried refers to the 'anthropomorphic' quality of minimalist sculpture and suggests that the viewing subject experiences himself

> *as subject* to the impassive object on the wall or floor [. . .] being distanced by such objects is not, I suggest, entirely unlike being distanced, or crowded, by the silent presence of another *person*; the experience of coming upon literalist objects unexpectedly – for example in somewhat darkened rooms – can be strongly if momentarily disquieting in just this way.[117]

Arguably, Blanchon's *Untitled (self-portrait/waste)* can have just this effect on a viewer, appearing as both uncanny and threatening and demanding an almost physical response.

Following Freud's logic of displacement from the lower to upper part of the body (and of the idea that teeth falling out is a sign of castration), the sculpture can also be read as a castrating mouth with teeth.[118] When *Untitled (self-portrait/waste)* was displayed at the Los Angeles Center for Photographic Studies (LACPS) a few months later, a reviewer wrote that it takes 'the viewer's initially provoked desire and figuratively grinds it to shreds'.[119] Judith Butler has suggested that the fear of castration implies two possible figures of 'abject' homosexuality: the 'feminized fag and the phallicized dyke'.[120] If *Untitled (self-portrait/waste)* threatens to castrate, then it might threaten to turn the (heterosexual) viewer into what Butler labels the 'feminized fag'. Butler posits abjection as a strategy used by heterosexual culture in order to remove the threat that homosexuality poses to the heterosexual. The gay male therefore poses the threat of castration *through* its symbolic mark of absence or abjection. If 'the mark of castration, a mark which is, after all, a lack, . . . can precipitate a set of crises', then this unassuming little metal and rubber hole might be interpreted as capable of precipitating a crisis in the heterosexual psyche. Thus, its 'castrating' threat might be turned around, so that it does not represent a castration via the threat of AIDS but represents the psychic threat of castration that homosexuality constitutes.

In a letter to Marc Foxx (of the Marc Foxx Gallery),[121] Blanchon suggested that the 'Waste King wall piece' had been inspired by Leo Bersani's critical essay 'Is the Rectum a Grave?', published in the 1987 AIDS special issue of *October*.[122] Bersani's paper examines the popular fantasy of homosexuals as killers: in this context, *Untitled (self-portrait/waste)*, with its dangerous 'bite', might be read as a potentially lethal sexual encounter. Bersani describes AIDS as a public health crisis that has been reconfigured as a sexual threat, supporting Watney's view that AIDS involves a crisis of representation over the human body and its capacity for pleasure; like Watney, Bersani is concerned primarily with the 'fantasmatic potential' of the human body. The history of this potential has typically been told from a heterosexual male viewpoint, where powerlessness is understood as a radical disintegration of the self. He describes the gay sex act as having 'the terrifying appeal of a loss of the ego, of a self-debasement':

> The realities of syphilis in the nineteenth century and of AIDS today 'legitimate' a fantasy of female sexuality as intrinsically diseased; and promiscuity in this fantasy, far from merely increasing the risk of infection, is the *sign of infection*. Women and gay men spread their legs with an unquenchable appetite for destruction [. . .] the seductive and intolerable image of a grown man, legs high in the air, unable to resist the suicidal ecstasy of being a woman.[123]

Bersani re-thinks this self-debasement (which recalls the melancholic self-debasement with which this chapter opened) in positive terms. He is keen to promote the appeal or even the value of powerlessness, in what he describes as a 'radical disintegration and humiliation of the self'.[124] Bersani bases his argument in a reading of Freud's 'Three Essays on Sexuality', where Freud speculates that sexual pleasure is achieved when the subject is momentarily disturbed, somehow going beyond him or herself.

> From the Freudian perspective, we might say that Bataille reformulates this self-shattering into the sexual as a kind of nonanecdotal self-debasement as a masochism to which the melancholy of the post-Oedipal superego's moral masochism is wholly alien, and in which, so to speak, the self is exuberantly discarded.[125]

Bersani's words recall the sadomasochistic poses adopted by Mark Morrisroe in his final self-portraits, which convey an equivocal position of both passive surrender and controlled self-possession. In contrast to Morrisroe's images, however, Blanchon's *Untitled (self-portrait/waste)* seems to suggest a negation of the self rather than a productive reiteration of it.

Echoing Bersani, Lee Edelman has written about the value of recognizing 'queer negativity' as an ethically desirable force, on the grounds that it is capable of deconstructing the 'heteronormative' logic of political discourse. On both left and right, political rhetoric invokes the figure of the Child to suggest an ideological investment in the future ('We're fighting for the children. Whose side are you on?'); the effect of this, Edelman argues, is to effectively foreclose all other possible frameworks for imagining political space.[126] Queerness offers resistance to this dominant political mode of 'reproductive futurism', by figuring the social order 'outside and beyond its political symptoms'.[127] Often rejected by liberal politics due to its association with the 'abjection expressed in the stigma, sometimes fatal, that comes from reading [the figure of the queer] literally', queerness, Edelman argues, attains an ethical value precisely through its accession to that place of abjection, outside of reason, order or logic.[128] *Untitled (self-portrait/waste)* invokes this 'other' place, a negative space situated outside of the proper social order, and makes it visible via the framing device of the waste disposal fascia. The effect of embracing such queerness, Edelman claims, is to deliberately sever ourselves from any sure knowledge of who we are and 'afford an access to the *jouissance* that at once defines and negates us'.[129] Read through Edelman's text, *Untitled (self-portrait/waste)* can be understood as a meditation on the positive value of the symbolic embrace of emptiness or absence, suggesting a joyful liberation from a restrictive model of fixed and bounded selfhood.

* * *

Blanchon's work provides an important counterpoint to the activist graphics of the late 1980s, to the naïve photographic practices of Nicholas Nixon and Rosalind

Solomon and to the aggressively in-your-face Polaroid self-portraits of the dying Mark Morrisroe. Calling attention to the self-referential nature of selected works via naming or the inclusion of personal traces, while simultaneously rejecting the traditional function of self-portraiture as an expression of the artist's outward appearance or inner identity, Blanchon's practice constructs the artist's 'self' as an intriguing absence that might be interpreted in a number of ways. Blanchon himself indicated that this strategy of authorial or artistic absenteeism might be understood in a deeply personal register in relation to his own fears about mortality; his work has thus sometimes been read in a therapeutic context as a means of coming to terms with his illness and as a rehearsal for his prospective death. This chapter has argued that, compelling though this biographical reading may be, Blanchon's work (unlike Morrisroe's) is not primarily an individual narrative of sickness but instead blends suggestive personal allusions with attention to the social and cultural consequences of the AIDS epidemic, particularly in relation to the problematic (non-)representation of the gay male body.

In this respect, it brilliantly evokes the 'crisis of representation' described by Simon Watney: suggesting that the 'impossible object' of the gay male body cannot be represented through conventional pictorial means, Blanchon's work instead reveals the near-invisible 'presence' of this troublesome body in public spaces that include streets, squares, pavements and bathrooms. At the same time, Blanchon deconstructs the dominant view of this body as social detritus: by embracing the gay male body's connotations of filth or waste and identifying himself with an abject subject position, Blanchon is able to disrupt, problematize, and ultimately re-signify that position in more positive terms.[130]

Blanchon's tactic of inscribing himself into his work while ultimately denying the viewer any privileged access to that 'self' can be read both through the prism of literary theory as a 'death of the author' scenario that assigns the production of meaning to the reader and in art-historical terms as an appropriation of minimalist sculpture's foregrounding of the experience of the spectator over the subjectivity of the artist: Blanchon was certainly aware of both those genealogies. Ultimately, however, the origins of his self-effacing practice matter less than its effects. Refusing to play the role of either victim or survivor, Blanchon's expanded self-portraiture challenges the binary discourse of AIDS representation, exposing the porous boundaries between self and other, public and private and inside and out.

5

Felix Gonzalez-Torres

Falling out of time

> *Critical illness not only presents you with issues of finitude, but more importantly, it threatens the very foundation of time structuring by removing you from life's comforting rhythms. It becomes a struggle not to* fall out of time.[1]

In a 2007 interview Douglas Crimp stated, 'If there's an artist associated with AIDS who is now being chosen as the most representative and important artist of a period, it would be Felix Gonzalez-Torres.'[2] Five years previously Crimp had selected an image of one of Gonzalez-Torres' works to illustrate the front cover of his collection of writings on the AIDS crisis.[3] The work in question consists of two strings of white light bulbs suspended in parallel lines from a high ceiling in the corner of a neutral gallery space; approximately halfway down the two cables meet and become entwined, finally collapsing onto the floor in a knotted, tangled heap. Tellingly named "*Untitled*" *(Couple)* (1993), the work is sparse, elegant, latently erotic and – when read through the artist's biography – deeply moving. Gonzalez-Torres' partner Ross Laycock died from AIDS-related complications in 1991 and Gonzalez-Torres (1959–96) from similar causes five years later; a significant proportion of the artist's work invokes their relationship through an expanded portrait practice that uses quietly beautiful, pared-back sculptures and installations to suggest the physical bodies of the two men.

The relation between public and private in Gonzalez-Torres' is complex, but given that "*Untitled*" *(Couple)* symbolizes an essentially private act of remembrance, it is perhaps a surprising choice by a writer who had once criticized the art world's preference for 'personal, elegiac expressions' of grief over more didactic, militant works aimed at actively ending the crisis.[4] Crimp chose to explain his selection of cover image thus:

> I didn't want anything too specific, because my book covered a whole era of my writing about AIDS. I also did it, frankly, as a kind of gesture of reconciliation, I think, with regards to questions of the elegiac and so on, which I had sort of polemicized against in my early AIDS writing, and which I have come to value a lot more as time has gone on.[5]

Crimp's endorsement of Gonzalez-Torres' work in the mid-2000s acknowledges the appeal of a personal approach to representing the crisis, and signals a break with the overtly political aesthetic strategies that had characterized the relationship between AIDS and creative practice in the first decade of the epidemic. In a 1991 interview with the artist, Robert Nickas observed, 'a shift away from the "sloganeering" art that appropriated the media, towards a more personal voice'.[6] Gonzalez-Torres replies that while work by artists such as Jenny Holzer and Barbara Kruger had a very specific purpose in trying to transform the dominant order, that order has since changed, and thus requires new modes of contestation, which include a strategic use of the 'private' voice for addressing questions of sexuality and politics in the wake of AIDS.

In common with Blanchon, Gonzalez-Torres' use of the 'personal' or 'private' voice is not straightforward; like Blanchon's practice, Gonzalez-Torres' work consistently alludes to the existence of a concrete individual identity but simultaneously troubles that possibility. The work of both thus has an especially complex relationship to self-portraiture, hinting at authorial presence rather than portraying the subject directly. In one sense, Gonzalez-Torres' practice is even more self-effacing than Blanchon's; for example, he consistently refused to have his photograph taken by the press, insisting that it was the work that should be reproduced rather than his own image.[7] In another sense, however, the artist's biography is essential to the affective potential of the work and frequently informs critical readings of it. Gonzalez-Torres was well aware of the power of biography, preserving all his personal correspondence with Laycock and donating it to an archive upon his death, meaning that the love story between the two men would continue to contextualize the work. The friction between an autobiographical impulse and what his dealer Andrea Rosen has described as 'his extreme efforts to liberate himself from concretization'[8] is echoed in the artist's habit of deliberately designating his works as "*Untitled*", but including a descriptor in parenthesis that hints at the work's representational significance and often – as in the case of "*Untitled*" *(Couple)* – allows it to be interpreted within an autobiographical framework.

For art critics writing in the 1990s, Gonzalez-Torres' work seemed inescapably contextualized by his illness. As noted in the previous chapter, Blanchon was convinced that Gonzalez-Torres' awareness of his mortality was the driving force behind his best work. For Nancy Spector, writing in the Guggenheim catalogue in 1995, the 'pleasures of embodiment [in Gonzalez-Torres' work] are tinged with the threat of personal loss . . . the allusions to illness are impossible to ignore'.[9] Even Robert Storr, who stressed that Gonzalez-Torres' art was not solely or even primarily dedicated to the AIDS epidemic, conceded that 'sickness and impending death made this game urgent in ways no one, including Gonzalez-Torres, initially expected'.[10] Like Blanchon, Gonzalez-Torres was particularly wary of allowing his practice to be interpreted in the context of his failing health; according to Rosen, while he was still alive, he made sure that it was not public knowledge that he was ill, as he felt that this information would limit readings of his work.[11] In a conversation between the curators Ann Goldstein and Amanda Cruz, on the occasion of Gonzalez-Torres' posthumous installation in the American Pavilion at the 2007 Venice Biennale, Goldstein notes, 'In retrospect, this is an artist who every day, as a professional artist, made his work with his own imminent mortality in mind. He didn't have the option to think differently. The fact that he knew that his life was most likely extremely limited affected not only the content but the structure of how he made the work.' Amanda Cruz responds, 'He never wanted to be known as the AIDS artist, never wanted to be known by that moniker.'[12] Recent curatorial and academic approaches to Gonzalez-Torres' work have fallen into two broad categories. On the one hand, Gonzalez-Torres' work has been treated as exemplary of a generation of artists making work in response to HIV and AIDS: Jonathan D. Katz, the curator of landmark exhibition *Art AIDS America*, has described Gonzalez-Torres as 'one of the chief theorists of and paradigmatic makers within this moment in American art'.[13] On the other hand, as art critic Darren Jones forcefully argued in a 2017 article published on the website ArtSlant, commercial galleries have repeatedly avoided the invocation of HIV or AIDS in their presentation of the work.[14]

In this chapter, I read selected works by Gonzalez-Torres as pathographic (self)portraits that suggest a distinctive relation to temporality and temporal experience. Since the 1990s, queer and disability scholars have sought to rethink dominant heteronormative, ableist, linear and future-orientated arrangements of time. Elizabeth Freeman's term *chrononormativity* recognizes standard temporal organization as a process of social regulation explicitly linked to capital and its institutions: bodies are coerced into maximum productivity through particular configurations of time, and cultural norms are generated and naturalized through temporal forms including repetitions, rhythms and other ways of marking time that include births, deaths and marriages.[15] For Freeman and others, 'queer' time – understood as asynchronous, multi-temporal and non-linear – offers resistance to repressive heteronormative temporal structures.[16] More recently, disability studies scholar Alison Kafer has extended the concept of queer time to encompass 'crip' time: illness and disability, Kafer suggests, have the capacity to render time 'queer', leading to feelings of asynchrony or temporal dissonance; throughout this chapter, I explore queer, crip and other non-linear time forms through Gonzalez-Torres' work and its critical and curatorial framing.[17]

Developing a (self)-portrait practice

In "*Untitled*" *(Me and My Sister)* (1988) (Figure 27), a little girl of perhaps two years old, wearing a white sundress bleached by bright sunshine, grins up at a figure just outside of the camera's view; seated behind her is a slightly older boy dressed in swimming shorts, his legs crossed with one elbow resting on his

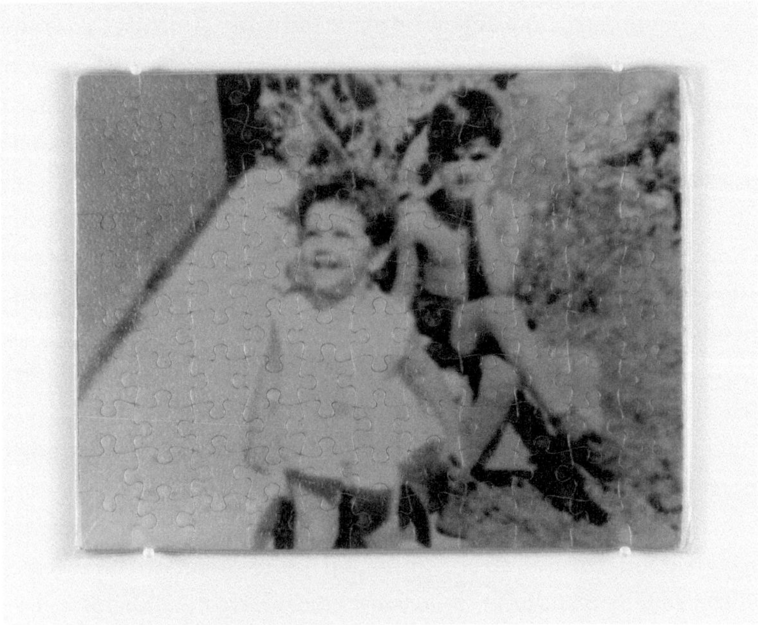

Figure 27 Felix Gonzalez-Torres, *"Untitled" (Me and My Sister)*, 1988. C-print jigsaw puzzle in plastic bag, 7½ × 9½ in. Edition of 3, 1 AP. Photographer: Lance Brewer. © Estate of Felix Gonzalez-Torres. Courtesy Felix Gonzalez-Torres Foundation.

knee as he poses, chin in hands and looking straight at the camera. The image (a re-photographed copy of the original) has been affixed to cardboard, cut to form a small jigsaw puzzle of seven-and-a-half by nine-and-a-half inches, and placed in a clear plastic bag; when exhibited, the bag is fixed to the wall by map pins.[18] Experienced in a gallery setting the work feels intimate, its diminutive size necessitating physical proximity in order to be viewed clearly. Another jigsaw work juxtaposes a photograph of the young artist, an unsmiling teenager with dark hair and a serious gaze, with a photograph of a Spanish civil war memorial topped with the statue of a gun-toting soldier. The text that unites the two pictures – which are gathered together in a single plastic bag – reads 'Madrid 1971' (Figure 28). Like *"Untitled" (Me and Sister)* this work hints at (although never makes explicit) its autobiographical significance.

To what extent can these works be considered as self-portraits? Although they are based on a visual representation of the artist, they also suggest a broader meditation on the operations of memory and personal history, using the artist's own background as source material to build an argument upon. The plastic bags holding together the pieces of puzzle suggest on the one hand forensic enquiry

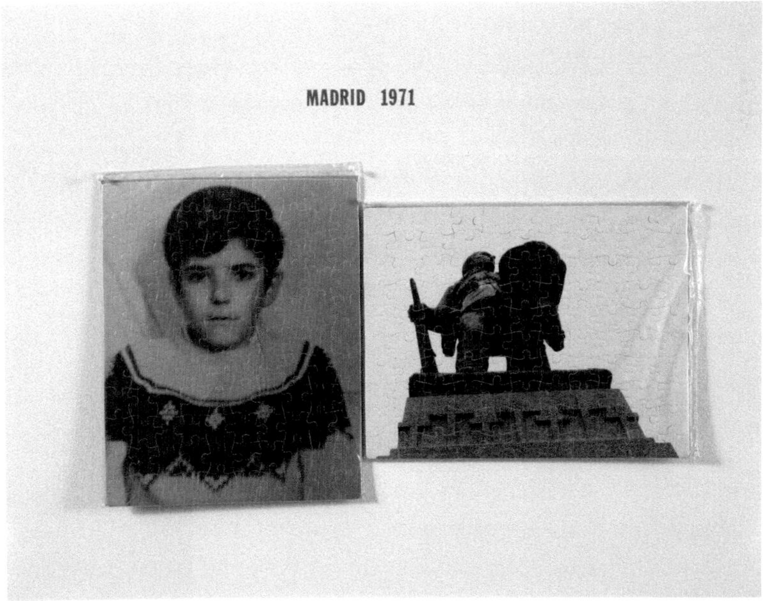

Figure 28 Felix Gonzalez-Torres, *"Untitled" (Madrid 1971)*, 1988. C-print jigsaw puzzle in plastic bag and wall lettering. Three parts; 15 × 18 in. overall. One part: 9½ × 7½ in. One part: 7½ × 9½ in. One part: 1/2 x 3 in. © Estate of Felix Gonzalez-Torres. Courtesy Felix Gonzalez-Torres Foundation.

and the preservation of the photograph as 'evidence', on the other hand, their provisional nature as a mode of display (as opposed to a formal frame, for example) implies a throwaway quality, hinting at the presence of similar images within every family album. This sense of banality is echoed in the process of the works' making, using a standard consumer service that transforms family snapshots into jigsaws and other personal memorabilia. According to Andrea Rosen, Gonzalez-Torres 'was interested in methods that questioned the accepted premise of the photograph, for example, the implication of a reproduction being true, and therefore taken for granted; the desire to stop time, to possess time by capturing a moment'.[19] In *Camera Lucida,* Barthes argues that the photograph does not only immobilize time but 'engorges' it, so that it become 'excessive, monstrous'.[20] The photograph is not, in essence, a memory (in grammatical terms, something to be comprehended in the past perfect tense); instead, the evidentiary force of the photograph actively *blocks* the operations of memory, filling the sight 'by force' and leaving no room for interpretation in the present moment.[21] These 'self-portraits' suggest an attempt to circumvent the totalizing power of the photographic image alluded to by Barthes; by formally enacting the literal break-up of the pictorial field, they bear witness to the irreconcilable distance between the present moment and a past that is continually being remade.

Barthes contrasts the totality of the photographic image ('full, crammed: no room, nothing can be added to it'), to the 'dearth-of-image' that accompanies the reading of a text-based work ('if this novel "takes" me properly, no mental image').[22] In "*Untitled*" (1989), a self-portrait first displayed at the Brooklyn Museum of Art as part of a Visual AIDS curated programme in 1989, Gonzalez-Torres rejected the photographic image altogether in favour of a cryptic series of words and dates of personal significance. In the version installed at the Brooklyn Museum (Figure 29), the work read as follows:

> *Red Canoe* 1987 *Paris* 1985 *Blue Flowers* 1984 *Harry the Dog* 1983 *Blue Lake* 1987 *Interferon* 1989 *Ross* 1983.

The work clearly challenges the traditional precepts of self-portraiture, revealing little about the appearance or 'essence' of the artist, while the refusal to place events in chronological sequence resists the usual conventions of autobiographical writing, suggesting instead the jumbled, frequently non-linear time of personal memory.

The installation of this work at the Brooklyn Museum reveals several things about Gonzalez-Torres' approach to the portrait subject. The work was situated in

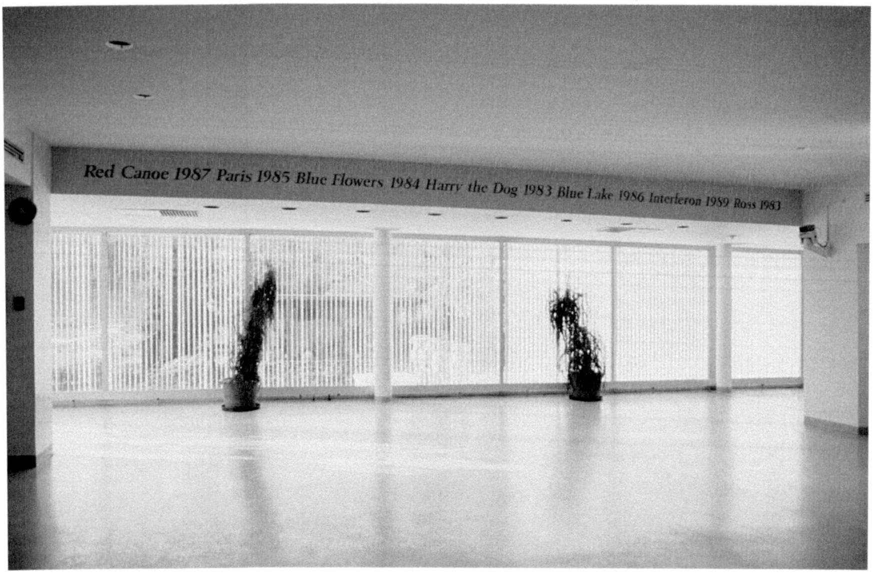

Figure 29 Felix Gonzalez-Torres, "*Untitled*", 1989. Paint on wall. Dimensions vary with installation. Installed in *Untitled: An Installation by Felix Gonzalez-Torres as part of the Visual AIDS Program*. Brooklyn Museum of Art, NY. 1 December 1989–1 January 1990. © Estate of Felix Gonzalez-Torres. Courtesy Felix Gonzalez-Torres Foundation.

a space of the artist's choosing: a low-ceilinged corridor connected to the elevator lobby, on a thin strip of wall between window and ceiling.[23] This marginal space works against the honorific tradition of portraiture, relegating the portrait subject to a barely visible spot in the hallway where he can be literally by-passed. The floor-length window looks out onto Brooklyn's Botanical Gardens; Gonzalez-Torres insisted that the blinds remained open for the duration of the exhibition, placing two pot plants inside the building to make obvious the connection with inside and outside space and, implicitly, between portrait and place, supporting his conviction that a subject is not a discrete entity but is shaped by, and shapes in return, his or her environment. Portraiture, Gonzalez-Torres thus implies, is not simply the representation of an individual but the interrogation of the relationship between that individual and the surrounding world.

The subject of this work is not 'fixed' in a temporal sense in the way that one might expect from a photographic portrait: between the first version shown at the Brooklyn Museum in 1989 and the final version shown during Gonzalez-Torres' lifetime (at the Centro Galego de Arte Contemporaneo, Santiago de Compostella in 1995) the artist added, subtracted and reordered events so that by the time of his death it totalled forty-five entries. This uniquely fluid form of self-portraiture reveals an unfinished subject in a constant state of (self)-production. Its allusions to the passing of time suggest both mortality and re-generation: Lewis Baltz has memorably compared this work to the other 'best-known unexecuted portrait of the last century, that of Dorian Gray'; instead of immortalizing the artist, it embeds him in the flowing passage of time and the associated corruptions of the flesh.[24]

If the photographic image typically signifies coherency and plenitude, this text-based model of subjectivity is understood by the artist to convey instability and flux. Drawing on Jacques Lacan's account of the significance of the 'mirror stage' for the formation of the 'I', Gonzalez-Torres describes the subject as essentially fragmented and temporally unstable:

> When we think of who we are, we usually think of a unified subject. In the present. An immutable entity. This is a mistake that happens, according to Lacan, during our misconception when we at a very tender age discover our image in a mirror ('the mirror stage') and think of ourselves as one a-historical phenomenon. We are not what we think we are, but rather a compilation of texts. A compilation of histories, past, present, and future, always, always shifting, adding, subtracting, gaining.[25]

In a telling slippage between text and subject, Barthes' evocation of the text as a tissue of citations is recalled by Gonzalez-Torres' conceptualization of the subject as a 'compilation of texts'. Just as the text can no longer be regarded as the original expression of a single authorial 'voice', nor can the subject; furthermore, the subject can no longer be comprehended as a straightforward self-representation but must be understood as a construction formed through the response generated in the reader and/or the viewer.

In 2002, six years after Gonzalez-Torres' death, the work was jointly purchased by the Art Institute of Chicago and the San Francisco Museum of Modern Art; the legal agreement between the Felix Gonzalez-Torres Foundation and the two museums stressed the artist's hope that the work would continue to mutate and transform in his absence:

> Not only did Felix know that he would not be able to determine the work's future form, and so was indebted to the owner's involvement, but Felix firmly believed that change was the only way to make the work permanent and relevant. [. . .] In direct relation to his own portrait, the rules and guidelines and intentions of these portrait works create a forum for perpetual life / vitality. The perpetuation of his life without stagnation.[26]

When exhibited at the San Francisco Museum of Modern Art in 2002, Gonzalez-Torres' self-portrait comprised sixty-six entries. The 'self' communicated by this portrait continues to grow and change, no longer at the hands of the artist, but instead at the hands of the two museums (not even individual persons) that currently own it. Miwon Kwon has suggested that it is likely that the work will ultimately become 'a portrait less of Gonzalez-Torres and more a testament to the desire for the artist among the living, either in the form of recollection and memory or as fantasy and projection, or a combination of both'.[27] Kwon's astute observation may equally well be applied to Gonzalez-Torres' practice in a wider sense; the tendency on the part of curators and other commentators to situate the work biographically perhaps reveals as much about a collective desire to claim intimacy with the artist as it does about his own private motivations.

In the early 1990s, Gonzalez-Torres was approached by an art-collecting couple who wanted to commission a puzzle portrait based on photographs from their own childhoods. Gonzalez-Torres refused, suggesting that it would be easy for them to make such a work themselves. Instead, he offered to collaborate with them to create a piece similar to his own text-based self-portrait. Over the next few years, numerous portraits were produced in this way, including those of married couples Karen and Andy Stillpass (1991) and Deane and Lorrin Wong (1991); Gonzalez-Torres' friend and co-member of Group Material, Julie Ault (1991); his dealer Andrea Rosen (1992); the gallery owner Ingvild Goetz (1993); and the collector Robert Vifian (1993).

These works were based on the owner's choice of significant life events; some explained their selection to the artist in long, personal letters, while others preferred to keep their reasons secret and unexplained. Andrea Rosen has described her own experience of having her portrait done in this way:

> It is a very difficult psychological exercise to recount and isolate the experiences, both good and bad, that you imagine influenced the formation of your character. Knowing that it will be installed for others to see whether in your home or on loan to an exhibition, you can't help but think about how you want yourself to be presented, or *remembered!* Does this potentially influence one's choices?[28]

According to Rosen, Gonzalez-Torres' motives for making these commissions can be related to his own strategy of self-disclosure: he wanted the portrait owners to be able to experience 'what it was like for an artist to expose themselves, to use their own subjectivity as an exemplary gesture'.[29] Once Gonzalez-Torres received the material, he decided upon the order of events, which he felt should appear non-chronologically. Since most people were inclined to choose personally meaningful dates and occasions – weddings, births and deaths – Gonzalez-Torres 'completed' the portraits by adding in significant public events, indicating the way in which the subject is formed by external social and historical forces as much as by internal, private ones. In a letter sent to the collector Robert Vifian, Gonzalez-Torres explained his thoughts on the relationship between the public and private realms. The 'private' individual is a social construction, as private activity cannot be separated from public policy; citing his own right to love whom he chooses, Gonzalez-Torres concludes: 'Public life is private life. [. . .] In our culture, everything is related to everything.'[30] Far from merely representing a discrete and unique individual, the portrait thus always exceeds itself, constituting an intricate network of personal, social and political signifiers.

In the same letter, Gonzalez-Torres describes his portraits as 'an attempt at dealing with the theoretical and limited aspects of portraiture' and tries to define his 'subjective idea of what a portrait is, or can be'.[31] Elaborating on the notion of the denoted content versus connoted context of a portrait, Gonzalez-Torres describes the denoted as the most easily identifiable elements of a portrait: the gender of the portrayed subject, his or her clothing, the background detail and so forth. However, it is the connoted context that Gonzalez-Torres finds the most exciting: the viewer's own gendered, cultural, social and economic background means that they will be led to read a portrait in specific, individual ways. (Here Gonzalez-Torres' theoretical perspective diverges from Barthes': if for Barthes the reader 'is a man without history, without biography, without psychology',[32] then for Gonzalez-Torres the 'reader' will always bring their own history, biography and psychology to the work.) Thus a portrait is not, as in the traditional formation, a meeting between the portrayed and the portrayer but is instead an ongoing three-way interaction between artist, subject and viewer.

Significantly, the owners of these works have the right to add or subtract from the text at will. The portrait's 'subjects' become its authors; thus, all commissioned portraits effectively convert into self-portraits over time. Kwon has described these works as the most extreme example of the artist's 'masochistic' logic, in that they allow for a complete erasure of the artist's contribution as portraitist.[33] This is also the case with his own self-portrait: as the work waxes and wanes according to the desires of the two museums that share ownership, the artist is over a period of time expunged from the work. For Kwon, the impulse to relate Gonzalez-Torres' formal working strategy to the real-life circumstances of his illness and death proves irresistible; the artist's obliteration of self paradoxically provides the means to endure after his death. Instead of trying to leave a concrete record of his existence that insists, 'I was here', Gonzalez-Torres opts to become absorbed into the world as 'a form of becoming, to become part of other's being limitlessly, forever'.[34] Facing death, he fashions his own dispersal, giving a new meaning to the concept of the 'death of the author'.[35] This strategy of self-dispersal is echoed by Gonzalez-Torres' work in a wider sense: in the physical form of the jigsaws (in which the pictorial self can be literally separated into pieces) as well as in the works for which he is best known, the glistening fields of cellophane-wrapped sweets and angular stacks of pristine paper sheets, both designed to be taken away piece by piece by the viewing public. While Robert Blanchon's practice merely *suggests* the disappearance of the artist, Gonzalez-Torres' 'giveaway' works actively *perform* that dissipation through time and implicate the participating viewer in it.

The works discussed in this section reveal the 'self' as fluid and changeable, constructed predominantly by outside forces rather than through any deliberate strategy of individual self-fashioning. Despite the use of autobiographical material, works such as the text-based self-portrait, "*Untitled*", are arguably as much a reflection on the abstract operations of subjectivity as they are a personal expression of the artist's self, and in this they undoubtedly challenge conventional understandings of self-portraiture. By performing the metaphorical death of the author, these works hand interpretative power over to their viewer; while this strategy ensures the endurance of the work beyond the artist's 'real' death, it also means that the sexual politics and AIDS-related contexts of the work are frequently under-acknowledged.

Falling out of time

One of Gonzalez-Torres' most poignant paired works, "*Untitled*" *(Perfect Lovers)* (1991) (Figure 30), comprises two mass-produced analogue clocks arranged side by side on a blue wall, their plastic casings just touching. The hands of the two clocks are synchronized, and the owner of the work is tasked with the responsibility for maintaining their unity: because the clocks can be perpetually reset, the work is, in effect, infinite.[36] The identical nature of the two timepieces is commonly understood to signal a same-sex relationship, and the work is often read as a double portrait. The paired form accounts for a large proportion of Gonzalez-Torres' self-referential or autobiographical works, which typically invoke a nameless, featureless couple through disembodied yet insistently physical configurations that include entangled strings of lights ("*Untitled*" *(Couple)*, 1993); glistening piles of wrapped sweets ("*Untitled*" *(Lover Boys)*, 1991); angular stacks of paper ("*Untitled*" *(Double Portrait)*, 1991); blue curtains installed in the windows of a chosen room ("*Untitled*" *(Loverboy)*, 1989); two

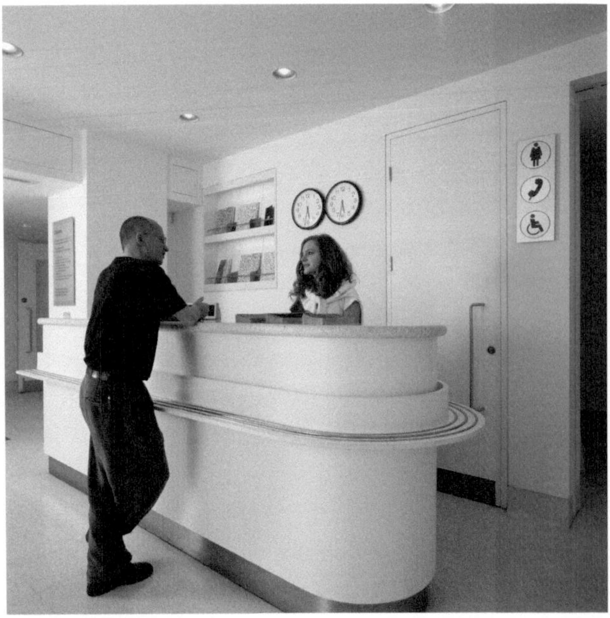

Figure 30 Felix Gonzalez-Torres, *"Untitled" (Perfect Lovers)*, 1987–90. Wall clocks. Original clock size: 13½ in. diameter each. Edition of 3, 1 AP. Installed in *Felix Gonzalez-Torres*, Serpentine Gallery, London, England, UK. 1 June–16 July 2000. Cur. Lisa G. Corrin. (With satellite venues: Camden Arts Centre, Chelsea and Westminster Hospital, Royal College of Art, Victoria and Albert Museum, and Royal Geographical Society, London, England, UK.) Photographer: Stephen White. © Estate of Felix Gonzalez-Torres. Courtesy Felix Gonzalez-Torres Foundation.

floor-length mirrors (*"Untitled" (Orpheus, Twice)*, 1991); or, displayed on a giant public billboard, two white pillows on a rumpled empty bed (*"Untitled"*, 1991).

Gonzalez-Torres was emphatic about the influence of his relationship with Laycock on his practice, stating in an interview: 'I think at times my only public has been my boyfriend, Ross',[37] and 'When people ask me, "Who is your public?" I say honestly, without skipping a beat, "Ross". The public was Ross. The rest of the people just come to the work'.[38] Although the recurrent paired forms are never conclusively tied to the bodies of Gonzalez-Torres and his partner, the barest snippet of biographical knowledge allows a viewer to interpret them in these terms. As Robert Storr notes, in these projected 'portraits' the two men appear as 'evanescent rather than substantial [. . .] Gonzalez-Torres and his partner appear – and disappear – as unique but intangible personas, whilst simultaneously playing the role of the floating signifiers of the viewers' desire and mortality'.[39]

Gonzalez-Torres' own comments on this piece both underplay its suggestively homoerotic nature and indicate that the sublimation of the sexed or gendered body might constitute a deliberate move to facilitate the 'presence' of the gay male body in conservative cultural institutions at a time when that presence was seriously restricted. Referring to the news that the Republican Senator Ted Stevens (one of the most homophobic anti-art congressmen) was planning to visit his show at the Hirshhorn, Gonzalez-Torres reflected: 'he's going to have a really hard time trying to explain to his constituency how pornographic and how homoerotic two clocks side by side are. He came there looking for dicks and asses. There was nothing like that. Now you try to see the homoeroticism in the clock piece, "*Untitled*" *(Perfect Lovers)*.'[40] For Jan Avgikos, writing in *Artforum* in 1991, "*Untitled*" *(Perfect Lovers)* suggests a politics of sexual identity, rather than a personal narrative of love and loss.[41] Speaking about Gonzalez-Torres' wider practice, Avgikos labels the work 'personal in nature [but] not constituted in terms of individual expression', and concludes that Gonzalez-Torres' practice 'works against the expressionist model, based on an expressive self and an empathetic viewer who receives pre-constituted meanings, by proposing a collective social and psychic space in which the holder actively participates in the construction of meaning'.[42]

Avgikos' essay anticipates curator Nicholas Bourriaud's treatment of Gonzalez-Torres' practice in his influential book *Relational Aesthetics* (2002). Bourriaud rejects a biographical reading of Gonzalez-Torres' coupled forms and manages to almost entirely avoid any discussion of sexuality, sickness and death. Bourriaud opens his analysis by noting that the 'basic unit of Gonzalez-Torres' aesthetic is two-fold, and dual';[43] he observes that 'overall, Gonzalez-Torres' work is well and truly organised around an autobiographical project, but a two headed, shared autobiography'; and suggests that 'from start to finish, Gonzalez-Torres told the tale not of an individual, but of a couple'.[44] Yet ultimately Bourriaud is disinterested in biography or queer politics (he openly sneers at the 'widespread trend' of reducing the work to 'an agenda for gay activism'),[45] and instead uses the figure of the couple as a starting point for expounding his theory of 'relational' art. 'Relational aesthetics' denotes a range of art practices that, rather than asserting an independent 'private' aesthetic space, operate in the sphere of social interaction.[46] Art, Bourriaud argues, is inherently social; unlike television or literature, which are defined by acts of private consumption, or even theatre and cinema, in which no live comment is made about what is seen, an art exhibition involves shared perception and analysis in a specific space and time. In the 1990s, many artists choose to foreground the social relations that are latent in all visual art, by creating convivial, interactive encounters. Watching visitors interact with one of Gonzalez-Torres' 'candy spill' installations,

Bourriaud observes people 'grabbing as many candies as their hands and pockets could hold; in doing so, they were being referred to their social behaviour, their fetishism and their cumulative concept of the world'.[47] The significance of such works, based on a physical encounter, is not to be found in the private life of the artist, nor in the historical conditions of the work's inception, but in the collective and cumulative experience of beholders in front of it.

Bourriaud suggests that the antecedent to relational art can be found in minimalist sculpture, which similarly requires the presence of the viewer as an integral part of the work. In 'Art and Objecthood' (1967), Michael Fried described the relationship between viewer and minimalist object principally in spatial terms, with the viewer being treated as an abstract ocular presence. For Bourriaud, 'relational' art such as Gonzalez-Torres' goes significantly beyond this, foregrounding the beholder's physicality as an embodied being. If the experience of minimalist art is, as Bourriaud argues, 'constructed in the distance separating eye and work', then an encounter with one of Gonzalez-Torres' installations is 'worked out in inter-subjectivity', and is thus defined less by a physical space than by its time span: 'Time of manipulation, understanding, decision-making, going beyond the act of "rounding off" the work by looking at it'.[48] For Bourriaud, 'time' is primarily significant in that it delineates the contemporary viewer's encounter with the work; no thought is spared for the temporal specificity of the work's background of AIDS and queer politics, or for the ways in which time might be queered, cripped or experienced in other ways.

An intimate interpretation of "*Untitled*" *(Perfect Lovers)* is offered by Gonzalez-Torres in the form of a love letter to Laycock, archived by the artist before his death and now published in Julie Ault's collected volume of essays on the artist's practice. The letter pairs a rough sketch of the two timepieces with a text celebrating the relationship between the two men:

> Lovers 1988
> Don't be afraid of the clocks, they are our time, time has been generous to us. We imprinted time with the sweet taste of victory. We conquered fate by meeting at a certain TIME in a certain space. We are a product of the time, therefore we give back credit were [*sic*] it is due: time.
> We are synchronized, now and forever.
> I love you.[49]

In *The Phenomenology of Perception*, Maurice Merleau-Ponty draws a distinction between 'constituted time' and 'time itself'.[50] Constituted time signifies recorded, objective time, understood as a linear series of relational moments designated 'before' and 'after'. Time itself – what might be described as phenomenological time – is generated by the subject, or more accurately, through the ongoing inter-relationship between the subject and the world. *"Untitled" (Perfect Lovers)* reveals time as both empirical *and* phenomenological; indeed, the work's affective potential depends both on a recognition of the conventions of constituted time and on an understanding of time as individual and experiential. The time of love, Gonzalez-Torres suggests, has a tempo of its own: the endlessly circular motion of the two sets of hands simultaneously suggests futurity (two lives entwined together for eternity) and a privileging of the present moment (time stands still when you are with the one you love). Initially positing time as a threat (by alluding to temporal finitude), the text ends by claiming the couple's synchronicity with it, 'victorious', having claimed it as their own.

As well as an exposition on the twisted temporalities of love, *"Untitled" (Perfect Lovers)* might also be considered as an opportunity for conceptualizing the peculiar rhythms and cadences of the time of illness and the temporalities of care. María Puig de la Bellacasa has described 'care time' as something that 'suspends the future and distends the present'.[51] Often installed above gallery reception desks peculiarly reminiscent of hospital waiting rooms (e.g. at the Serpentine Gallery in 2000) or in office spaces (The Renaissance Society at the University of Chicago, 1994), the clocks operate as a reminder that (health) care is frequently shaped both by bureaucracies of waiting (for clinical care or treatment) and by sustained temporal practices of maintenance, attentiveness and shared endurance.[52]

In a 1991 interview, Gonzalez-Torres further contextualized the clock piece in terms of his and Laycock's shared mortality:

> Time is something that scares me . . . or used to do. The piece I made with the two clocks was the scariest thing I have ever done. I wanted to face it. I wanted those two clocks right in front of me, ticking.[53]

In their paper on cancer survivorship and temporality, Jackie Stacey and Mary Bryson demonstrate how the experience of critical illness can affect the sufferer's relationship with time. In contrast to the linearity of normal life narratives, Stacey and Bryson argue, cancer survivorship (for example) introduces a troubled sense of time that can be characterized as random and fragmented, with an increased emphasis on the present. Through a reading of artists' films that reflect on the experience of cancer, the authors suggest that the works' formal structures echo the temporal disorientation that is often a feature of critical ill health, and 'undo any conventional sense of time's linear, causal dynamics, offering instead the perceptual disturbances that mark a body returned to its present through the physical and emotional demands of life-threatening illness'.[54] For example, Barbara Hammer's film, *A Horse Is Not a Metaphor* (2008), tracks the filmmaker's diagnosis with and treatment for ovarian cancer. The film encourages the viewer's disorientation by interweaving two types of time frame: narrative progression (described as a prerequisite of cancer survivorship) and a warping of conventional linear time through repetition, slow motion, superimposition and extreme close-ups. Stacey and Bryson's description of the film's dominant aesthetic project as 'a desire to dwell in the present, and to generate a spectatorship that is also of this present'[55] resonates with the privileging of present time in Gonzalez-Torres' *"Untitled" (Perfect Lovers)*; more broadly, Hammer's film and Gonzalez-Torres' artworks both communicate a sense of time as individual, warped or distorted and decidedly non-normative.

Drawing on a wealth of scholarship, Stacey and Bryson label this non-normative time 'queer' time. They are careful to qualify the usage of this term, suggesting that the extent to which the 'warped' time of cancer belongs to queer temporality depends upon whether this 'queerness' refers only to the odd, the uncanny or the indeterminate, or if cancer's time warp in *Horse* 'is queer in the sense that sexuality is already present in this disturbance to temporality'.[56] If Hammer's *Horse* is read in the context of her previous work as a lesbian filmmaker, it becomes 'impossible not to read the temporality of her body's agony and ecstasy as defined by its battle against its sexual disqualifications'.[57] The authors conclude that, in the case of Hammer's film, 'cancer [. . .] warps a time already unsettled by sexual illegitimacies'.[58] Similarly, if Gonzalez-Torres' practice is contextualized in terms of the fragile health of himself and his partner, and, in wider terms against the background of the AIDS crisis as a social, political and cultural phenomenon, we might productively read his works through the concept of queer time, using the term to bring together issues of illness, eroticism, sexuality and embodiment.

The development of the concept of 'queer time' can be usefully traced to the period in which Gonzalez-Torres was working: Jack Halberstam writes that queer time 'emerges most spectacularly, at the end of the twentieth century, from within those gay communities whose horizons of possibility have been severely diminished by the AIDS epidemic' and Elizabeth Freeman notes that the dominant cultural rhetoric of the AIDS epidemic configured gays and lesbians as having no past: 'no childhood, no origin or precedent in nature, no family traditions or legends, and, crucially, no history as a distinct people'.[59] Simon Watney's essay 'In Purgatory' (1994) defines the 1990s in terms of a strange co-habitation between the dead and the still-living, implying a kind of 'split' time that might equally well be described as 'queer'. Watney argues that Gonzalez-Torres' work must be understood in the context of a 'culture of dying', in which memorializing creative practices play an important role. Watney opens by describing a cartoon in *The New Yorker* that for him typifies 'a certain distinct sensibility of the '90s'.[60] The cartoon depicts a balding man seated at a table and pouring over an obituary page; the man is depicted from behind, and so, peering over his shoulder, the reader of *The New Yorker* is able to peruse the epitaphs with him: 'Two Years Younger Than You', 'Exactly Your Age', 'Three Years Your Junior', 'Twelve Years Older Than You', 'Five Years Your Senior' and 'Your Age On the Dot'. For Watney, this drawing evokes the way in which 'many hundreds of thousands of American gay men start their everyday, reminded of their survivor status – so far. The endless routine of sickness, dying and death also ages the survivors prematurely, as entire networks of friends vanish, and with them the wealth of accumulated memory, taste, and hard-won practical wisdom they shared'.[61] Watney describes the world that he inhabits, surrounded by friends that he knows to be dead but nonetheless 'sees' constantly, as 'Purgatory', a place where the living must continue to fight on behalf of the deceased.

Watney's essay makes a clear case for reading Gonzalez-Torres' practice through a politics of autobiography. For Watney, Gonzalez-Torres' work is politically significant in its exposure of homophobic discourse and the way in which it draws attention to 'the discursive formations which frame policy and practice in relation to the everyday lives of gay men in the AIDS epidemic'.[62] This type of political art, Watney implies, is also inescapably personal. In support of his argument, Watney compares the reception of two pieces, both posters intended for display on public billboards. The first consists of a matt black background with two low-set lines of white text that read as follows: *People With AIDS Coalition 1985 Police Harassment 1969 Oscar Wilde 1895 Supreme / Court 1986 Harvey Milk 1977 March On Washington 1987 Stonewall Rebellion 1969.* This work was conceived as time- and site-specific and was first displayed in 1989, on the twenty-year anniversary of the 1969 Stonewall riots, on a billboard above Sheridan Square in Greenwich Village, just around the corner from where the riots took place. The second consists of a single image of a double bed, the sheets slept-in and the pillows bearing the imprint of two heads. Watney criticizes an interpretation of these two works offered by British artist and critic Terry Atkinson, who describes the former as 'remembering the gains acquired from a tradition of political culture', and the latter as an image of 'pathos [. . .] personally rich and formally bleak'. Atkinson's opposition of the political and the personal, Watney suggests, constitutes a crude oversimplification of these two works, which both speak of the *lack* of definite boundaries between 'public' and 'private'. The privacy of the bedroom invades public space, just as the 1986 Supreme Court Ruling judged that American gay men had no constitutional right to privacy in their own homes.[63] Watney cites the artist to support his case: 'There is no private space anymore. Our intimate desires, fantasies, dreams, are intercepted by the public sphere.'[64] In a climate of AIDS-related homophobia, the personal is clearly also profoundly political. Gonzalez-Torres' creative practice can thus be understood as the distillation of personal experience – as a gay man and as a person with AIDS – into an aesthetic, and implicitly political, position.[65] Extending Watney's argument, one might suggest that to ignore the autobiographical elements of Gonzalez-Torres' work (as Bourriaud does, and as – following Jones' argument – a number of commercial galleries also do) is to repress its significance as a creative response to the sexual politics of the AIDS epidemic.

In recent years, the work has been re-marketed for contemporary audiences, leading to accusations that it has been 'de-queered', de-historicized or de-politicized. In her perceptive essay 'Split Witness' (2010), Adair Rounthwaite suggests that the 'elegant, minimalist' vocabulary employed by Gonzalez-Torres lends his work a 'timeless' air; because of this, 'the propensity on the part of curators to draw the work out of its historical context and into the present has been far more marked for the work of Gonzalez-Torres than for the work of any other artist of his generation who dealt with the AIDS crisis'.[66] This is evidenced by the choice of Gonzalez-Torres as the representative of the United States at the Venice Biennale in 2007, a contemporary art event that more usually focusses on the work of living artists. Many commentators expressed surprise that an openly gay HIV-positive artist had been chosen, and it was optimistically suggested that the decision might represent a progressive liberal break with conservative cultural politics. Through a close analysis of the discourse surrounding Gonzalez-Torres' work at the Biennale, Rounthwaite reveals that what might initially be seen as a radical nomination is actually anything but.[67] The selection of works exhibited in the American pavilion had been edited to remove any references to queer sexuality; gone were almost all the doubled pieces, all the works with 'Loverboy' in the title, the empty double bed, the queer history datelines and all specific mentions of Laycock.[68] By carefully deconstructing the language of the nomination tender (written by Nancy Spector, the curator of the 1995 Guggenheim retrospective and a close acquaintance of Gonzalez-Torres), Rounthwaite notes how the proposal's insistence on the ability of the work to 'defy simple categorization' shrewdly emphasizes its flexibility for use in different ideological contexts. Concluding that the pavilion represented 'a sadly dequeered presentation of Gonzalez-Torres' art',[69] Rounthwaite reflects that Gonzalez-Torres proved a savvy political choice on the part of the American State Department's Bureau of Educational and Cultural Affairs: although his aesthetic influence on younger artists is well known and his reputation as a politically engaged artist is secure, his work is totally flexible in its meaning and thus available for appropriation for conservative ends.

Rounthwaite initially reads "*Untitled*" *(Perfect Lovers)* as a meditation on mortality and survivorship. The twinned clocks are destined to ultimately lose time and break their perfect union: inevitably, the battery of one clock will start to fail before the other, so that as a pair they 'carry out a mechanical performance, losing synch, slowing down, and stopping, one ahead of the other'.[70] Drawing on Ross Chamber's description of 'dual autobiography' as a genre that substitutes 'the dual subjectivity of aftermath, a "haunted" self, for the supposedly self-sufficient personal self of the genre's tradition',[71] Rounthwaite reads the work as expressive of a subjective and temporal split. Quoting directly from Chambers, Rounthwaite notes that "*Untitled*" *(Perfect Lovers)* haunts us as the living 'because it enacts an intimacy of measured and unmeasured time';[72] the instrument that we normally employ to measure time becomes a metaphor for the crossover between the time of the living and the non-time of the dead:

> The time measured in "*Untitled*" *(Perfect Lovers)* represents life, and the fact that time is measured as the almost co-ordination of two different acts of measuring depicts life itself as something that occurs in this space of approximate co-ordination. This poses the painful question of what happens to [. . .] the last in the pair to die, who lives on in a state of aftermath in which life is still defined as collective, but the shared space of temporal overlap has run out.[73]

Gonzalez-Torres frequently described his work as a dialogue with Laycock; speaking to Robert Nickas soon after Laycock's death, he admitted, 'Not having a dialogue with Ross is a real handicap. Now the dialogue is just one person.'[74] A two-way conversation continues to inform the work, however, as Laycock becomes a ghost who contributes to the creative process through his present absence. For Rounthwaite, the 'haunting' effect of "*Untitled*" *(Perfect Lovers)* evokes not only the personal relationship between Gonzalez-Torres and Laycock but also the disjunction between the circumstances of the work's inception (in Watney's words, a 'culture of dying') and the rather different conditions of its present-day presentation. Building on Watney, Rounthwaite argues that the 'timeless' quality of

Gonzalez-Torres' work is an effect of a 'haunting', where the traces of the original process of bearing witness to AIDS begin to take on a life of their own.[75]

A synecdoche for "*Untitled*" *(Perfect Lovers)* appears in Vincent Chevalier and Ian Bradley-Perrin's poster *Your Nostalgia Is Killing Me* (2013), where two black-and-white clocks are camouflaged against the Keith Haring-inspired wallpaper in a glitchy, computer-generated image of a young person's bedroom packed with campy AIDS nostalgia. In this work, Chevalier and Perrin deploy camp as what Elizabeth Freeman has called a 'mode of archiving'; Freeman draws attention to the 'temporally hybrid aspect of camp', which as an aesthetic strategy depends on resuscitating 'obsolete' cultural signals.[76] *Your Nostalgia Is Killing Me* plays with a form of temporal drag: associated with 'retrogression, delay and the pull of the past on the present', drag can be a usefully distorting obstacle to linear narratives of generational 'progress'.[77] Suggesting 'the movement time of collective political fantasy',[78] temporal drag offers a way of connecting to disavowed political histories, opening up a tactile relationship to a collective past, one not simply performative or citational but physical and erotic. We experience temporal drag at play in Gonzalez-Torres' work, in the slowing, stopping and eventual resetting of the clocks, which move in and out of synchrony with each other; in the flux of the candy spill installations, which shrink and replenish over of a period of time according to the intentions of the owner or curator; and in the refusal of 'progress' suggested by the immobile pencil lines of the serialized 'bloodwork' charts. Simultaneously in and out of time, this work is not so much 'timeless' as the occasion of a complex folding of different historical moments and temporal experiences that are both individual and collective.[79] While 'haunting' implies an ethical injunction to attend to the ghosts of the past, temporal drag has a different set of connotations, suggesting campy playfulness as well as, perhaps, the tedious 'drag' associated with some forms of overt identity politics.[80] A kind of 'stuck' time, temporal drag is structured by reiteration and repetition: in Judith Butler's ground-breaking work on drag, repetition is both the condition for the production of (heteronormative) subjectivity and a technique for subverting or resisting those norms.[81] As a key stratagem for subjectivity and survival in Gonzalez-Torres' work, repetition and its temporal rhythms will be explored in the next two sections of this chapter.

Remembering, repeating and resisting

Gonzalez-Torres' best-known works are the installations of brightly wrapped candies of varying colours, brands, weights and configurations. Spector refers to the confectionary installations as 'pushing the limits of the [portrait] genre', claiming that 'Gonzalez-Torres has also utilized "portraiture" to reference the body as a physical entity'.[82] Of a total of nineteen confectionary-based works, six can be classified as portraits. The first five of these were made in 1991, the year that Laycock passed away; this was also the year of the death of Gonzalez-Torres' father, although this is less often commented upon. These include three of Laycock alone: "*Untitled*" *(Portrait of Ross in L.A.)*, "*Untitled*" *(Rossmore)* and "*Untitled*" *(Ross)*; one of himself and Laycock combined, "*Untitled*" *(Lover Boys)*; and one of his father, "*Untitled*" *(Dad)*; the sixth portrait was made in 1992, for the collector Marcel Brient, "*Untitled*" *(Portrait of Marcel Brient)*.

"*Untitled*" *(Portrait of Ross in L.A.)* (Figure 31) consists of a large stack of sweets in brightly hued wrappers; Gonzalez-Torres initially used 'Fruit Flashers' (allegedly Laycock's favourite brand of confectionary), although specified that if this brand was not available, similar could be used. The parenthetical title of the work hints at the autobiographical context: Gonzalez-Torres and Laycock resided in different cities for much of their relationship, Gonzalez-Torres in New

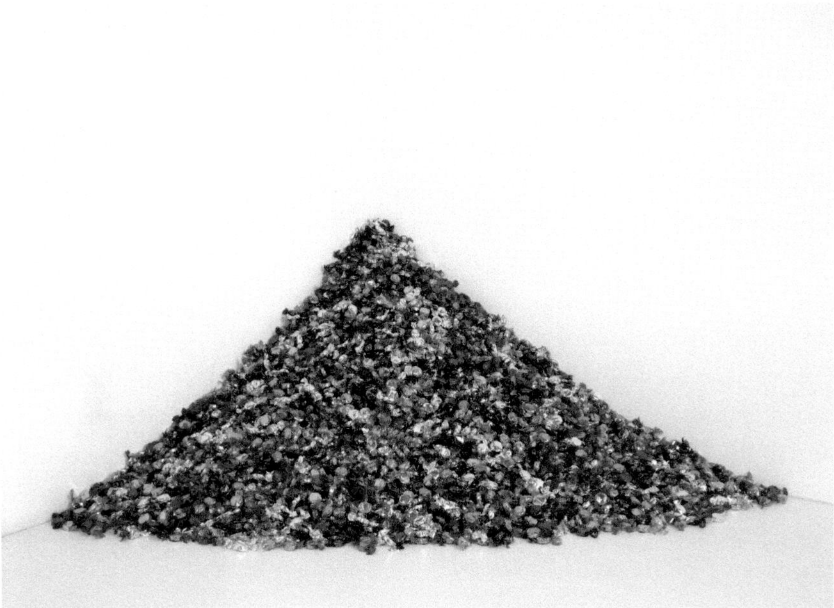

Figure 31 Felix Gonzalez-Torres, *"Untitled" (Portrait of Ross in L.A.)*, 1991. Candies in variously coloured wrappers, endless supply. Overall dimensions vary with installation. Ideal weight: 175 lb. Installed in *Felix Gonzalez-Torres*, Luhring Augustine Hetzler Gallery, Los Angeles. 19 October–16 November 1991. Photographer: James Franklin. © Estate of Felix Gonzalez-Torres. Courtesy Felix Gonzalez-Torres Foundation.

York and Laycock in Toronto, but in the autumn of 1990 Gonzalez-Torres spent a term teaching at CalArts in Los Angeles, and for this period of time he and Ross were able to live together.[83] By this point, Laycock was already quite ill, but despite this, it appears to have been an immensely happy time, memorialized in a number of works. The sweets can in theory be arranged in any configuration but, in practice, have most often been displayed piled generously into a corner. The ideal weight of the stack of sweets is 175 pounds; this is usually understood as corresponding to Laycock's 'ideal' body mass at the start of his illness but may also be interpreted as the generalized weight of a healthy male (the same ideal weight is used in "*Untitled*" *(Portrait of Dad)*, 1991). The intention is that each person who experiences the work will take away a sweet from the pile, which they are free to consume or keep as they wish. The sweets are replenished at intervals determined by the work's owner or the museum's curator: in some exhibitions they have been replenished on a daily basis, while in others the pile has been allowed to completely disappear before being replaced. At its most literal, this process echoes the wasting of Laycock's body, and his eventual death, as well as articulating a fantasy of renewal and eternal life.

As well as being moving for its autobiographical content, it is also subversive on a political level. David Wojnarowicz (with whom Gonzalez-Torres is frequently contrasted) said that upon his death he wanted his corpse to be thrown onto the steps of the White House as an indictment against Reagan's lack of action on the epidemic. "*Untitled*" *(Portrait of Ross in L.A.)* is a subtle variation on this: laying the 'body' of the person with AIDS out upon the floor of the museum, inviting the audience to touch this infected form, even to put a part of it into their mouths and to make it a part of their own bodies; the work ultimately makes the audience become complicit in its disappearance. The erotic valences of the installation are unmistakable. In the words of Robert Storr, 'mouthing the candy' is essential to experiencing the work and making its meaning: 'It is no accident that one must actively suck the hard shelled morsel to release its flavor, nor that the shell is soft and clotted. All these performative requirements and sensations mimic oral sex. Still more specifically, in cases where the candies used in the artist's corner are lollipops, the act of sucking mimics fellatio.'[84] Playing with notions of sex and contamination, Gonzalez-Torres' work seduces the viewer (conventionally assumed to be heterosexual and HIV negative) into a direct physical encounter with the stigmatized body of the person with AIDS.[85]

Spector sees 'pliant savory bodies languorously waiting to be plucked and consumed'[86] and connects this eroticism to Bataille's description of the transgression of corporeal boundaries, and thus to the endangerment of the integrity of selfhood: 'Eroticism is, in essence, a form of bodily excess (to borrow a key term from Bataille), in which the integrity of selfhood is inherently endangered.'[87] In these works, the self is consistently spilling over into otherness: most evidently into the bodies of the consuming participants but also in the uncertainty as to exactly who the referent of these 'portraits' might be. Most critical commentary implies that these works can refer to both Laycock and to Gonzalez-Torres himself (this holds true even when a work is parenthetically labelled as a portrait of Laycock); Gonzalez-Torres' efforts to come to terms with the demise of Laycock are effectively inseparable from his attempts to deal with his own illness and mortality.

The same processes of disappearance and renewal that structures the sweet spills also informs a second set of giveaway pieces that consist of precisely arranged stacks of printed posters intended to be taken by gallery visitors. Like the sweet spills, these paper piles each have an ideal configuration, which varies with each individual work (each sheet of paper usually measures somewhere between 8½ × 11 in. and 33 × 45 in.). The printed matter falls into three dominant categories: typeset fonts, usually in black or white on a contrasting background; minimal photographic compositions of sea or sky; or geometric formations. Some posters extend the theme of double portraiture: for example, the touching gold circles of "*Untitled*" *(Double Portrait)* (1991), which mimic the clocks of "*Untitled*" *(Perfect Lovers)*. Another reworks Gonzalez-Torres' text-based self-portrait strategy (*Red Canoe* 1987 *Paris* 1985 *Harry the Dog* 1983 *Blue Lake* 1987 *Interferon* 1989 *Ross* 1984), reprinting the words in black typeface across the bottom of white sheets of paper.[88]

That Gonzalez-Torres felt an intimate personal connection with such works, and even regarded them as a stand-in for his own embodied subjecthood, is evident from a number of comments made by the artist. Towards the end of his life, in a 1995 interview with Robert Storr, the artist reflected:

> I've become burnt out with trying to have some kind of personal presence in the work. Because I'm not my art. It's not the form and not the shape, not the way these things function that's being put into question. What is being put into question is me.[89]

This contradictory statement reveals not only a desire for personal presence but also the realization that this must always be elusive. The assertion 'I'm not my art' is challenged by the claim that the work problematizes his existence as a subject. On one level this is a self-conscious reworking of Barthes' theory of the death of the author: what is being put into question (by a corpus of work that privileges the active engagement of the viewer) is Gonzalez-Torres' role as an author figure, rather than his individual identity or embodied actuality. Yet on another level, the deep personal connection that Gonzalez-Torres repeatedly claimed to have felt with his work suggests that he experienced the process of 'being put into question' as emotionally and physically painful.[90]

In 1989, Gonzalez-Torres had been invited to participate in the inaugural exhibition of an un-named gallery, in a show of works that addressed issues of politics and sexuality. For the opening night the gallery had hired a team of muscular men dressed in leather trousers and Barbara Kruger T-shirts, tasked with greeting guests, serving drinks, and rolling up and putting elastic bands around sheets of paper from Gonzalez-Torres' stack and handing out as souvenirs. Unsure of what to do with the sheets they had been handed and not having had the chance to directly experience the work themselves, many recipients simply discarded their sheets on the way out of the exhibition. When Gonzalez-Torres arrived at the opening, he was horrified to find them abandoned. His reaction was not simply because giving away the sheets undermined the potential effect of the work that comes with the participants' active choice to take a sheet. As he later confided to Rosen, he hated to be present when people were taking the sheets of paper from the stacks or candies from the pile, as 'he felt it was an invasion of the self, a demise of his own body'. As Rosen reflects, 'Metaphysically, there was an obvious physical corollary between himself and his work. I never realized how tangible it actually became to him.'[91]

More so than any of Gonzalez-Torres' other works, the sweet spills and paper stacks make palpable the weighty physicality of the embodied subject. In interviews Gonzalez-Torres was absolutely explicit about the paper stacks being a metaphor for the body (although the question of exactly *whose* body was at stake always remained ambiguous):

> when I'm dealing with the body, it is more exciting to have a stack of blue paper than a sculpture that is just a body; this is because in our culture the body is constructed through language [. . .] When you take these pieces of paper out of the stack and the stack disappears, I think that is a very beautiful and poignant metaphor for the body, which is always decaying and disappearing.[92]

In a similar way to that in which the text-based portraits insist on the historical changeability of the subject, the sweet spills and paper stacks both perform the temporal nature of embodiment. In a roundtable on queer temporalities, Carla Freccero (a scholar of queer early modernism) notes that 'it's so hard to think the body's temporality as anything other than linear and homogenous,' and attributes this linearity to 'the brutal hegemony of the visual's conceptualization of the body'.[93] In heteronormative terms, the body follows a typically undeviating narrative of maturation, adulthood, the infirmities of old age, death and, finally, decay. As I suggested earlier in this chapter in relation to *"Untitled" (Perfect Lovers)*, life-threatening illnesses disrupt these norms, replacing them with a sense of time that is repetitive, circular, retrogressive or otherwise distorted. As an alternative to the temporality of the straight and standardized body, Freccero raises the possibility of 'a far queerer experience of the body's persistence in time,' and suggests that this experience might be sought in the realms of fantasy and the unconscious and accessed through the language of psychoanalysis.[94] Gonzalez-Torres' sweet spills and poster stacks are particularly suggestive of the 'queer' temporality of the body, evoking a mutable human form that by turns diminishes and expands in an infinite cycle.

Gonzalez-Torres described his motivation for these works in psychoanalytic terms, terms, as a pre-emptive strike against the possibility of loss:

> I wanted to make an artwork that could disappear, that never existed, and it was a metaphor for when Ross was dying. So it was a metaphor that I would abandon this work before the work abandoned me. I'm going to destroy it before it destroys me.[95]

Gonzalez-Torres' explanation recalls Freud's account of the child's game 'fort-da' in 'Beyond the Pleasure Principal' (1920).[96] A young boy in a family with which Freud was staying had a habit of taking a wooden reel on a piece of string and throwing it under his cot so that it disappeared, before reeling it in again by its string. As he did so, he would say '*fort*' (the German for 'gone'), hailing the toy's reappearance with the joyful announcement '*da*' ('there'). Freud connects this with the child's efforts to master and understand the disappearance and return of his mother via the repetition of a distressing experience. Freud offers a number of interpretations of this. Initially he suggests that the going away of the mother/toy might be thought of as a necessary preliminary to her departure. Freud then rejects this explanation, pointing out that the first act of departure was often staged without its pleasurable ending. Instead, Freud suggests that by throwing away the toy, the child is revenging himself on the mother that went away. The action takes on a defiant meaning: 'All right then, go away! I don't need you. I'm sending you away myself.'[97]

Gonzalez-Torres was familiar with Freud's writing on loss and repetition, observing:

> Freud said that we rehearse our fears in order to lessen them. In a way, this 'letting go' of the work, this refusal to make a static form, a monolithic sculpture, in favor of a disappearing, changing, unstable, and fragile form was an attempt on my part to rehearse my fears of having Ross disappear day by day right in front of my eyes.[98]

In 'Remembering, Repeating and Working Through' (1914), Freud describes repetition as an analytical technique; the purpose of analysis is to remember something that has been repressed and to work through it in order to discharge it.[99] Prior to treatment, the patient will 'repeat' instead of remember: for example, he will not remember that he used to be critical of his parents' authority but will instead consistently assume a fault-finding attitude towards the psychoanalyst. The 'repetition compulsion' involves a kind of 'stuck' time: the patient knows that he is repeating *something*, but because he doesn't know that he is repeating something from the past, he unwittingly repeats the present as though it was in the past. The task of the analyst is to recover that which the patient has failed to remember, 'to fill in the gaps in memory' and 'to overcome resistance due to repression'[100] and thus to move through the 'stuck' time of the past and into the fullness of the present moment.

As memorials to a lost love, the sweet spills have their own peculiar temporality, looking back at a happier time, while simultaneously existing only in the present. One might be tempted to describe them as 'melancholic', since their repetitive structure appears to suggest an unwillingness to 'complete' the work of mourning.[101] Selected critics have used these works to challenge Freudian notions of mourning and melancholia and move beyond them. For example, Emily Boone Hagenmaier uses Gonzalez-Torres' work to contest Freud's pathologizing definition of melancholia as 'stuck' mourning, proposing that it offers the possibility of a 'dynamic, collective and celebratory process of queer mourning'.[102] Against Freud, Giorgio Agamben defines 'the ambiguous melancholic project' as the transformation 'into an object of amorous embrace what should have remained only an object of contemplation'.[103] This passionate (rather than cerebral) connection with the lost object opens up a space for the existence of the *unreal*; in Hagenmaier's words 'a hopeful place for imagining alternative ties between past and present, loss and what remains'.[104] Everyone who takes and eats the candy is implicated in this process of amorous, queer, collective mourning. As Hagenmaier approvingly concludes:

> participatory spectators of one of Gonzalez-Torres' candy sculptures transgress the boundary between the dead and the living and ensure an active, social

> memorial to the dead. [. . .] This suggests a vision of mourning as creative and unifying, rather than destructive and alienating. By sharing his loss and joy, Felix Gonzalez-Torres moves us to consider our own.[105]

Hagenmaier's rather idealistic reading echoes medievalist Carolyn Dinshaw's suggestion that queer time might offer a means of connecting affectively with the past, by offering 'the possibility of touching across time, collapsing time through affective contact between marginalized people now and then'.[106] With queer historical touches, Dinshaw argues, we can 'form communities across time'. To what extent might Gonzalez-Torres' work truly constitute a dialogue with the past, given that they are so frequently exhibited outside of their historical contexts? There is often a disjunction between how the artist spoke about his works (and how those in the art world accordingly perceive them) and the way in which the average gallery visitor experiences the work. Jonathan Katz has expressed concern that the giveaway works in particular are most often encountered simply in terms of their playfulness and are thus evacuated of their political significance.[107]

The operations of 'remembering, repeating and working through' reflect on contemporary framings of the work. In Freud's texts repetition is the sign of a repressed trauma: people repeat traumatic events over and over again in an attempt to regain mastery and control. This repetition has a physical dimension, belonging in the realm of actions rather than thoughts or ideas: 'The patient does not *remember* anything of what he has forgotten and repressed, but *acts* it out. He reproduces it not as a memory but as an action; he *repeats* it without, of course, knowing that he is repeating it.'[108] Thus, reproduction actually takes the form of, or blocks, remembering. The aim of analysis is to curb the patient's compulsion to repeat and turn it into a motive for remembering. Turning his attention to the artistic play of adults, Freud notes the contradiction that genres such as tragedy do not spare the spectators the most painful of experiences and yet can be experienced pleasurably. Gonzalez-Torres' works are about play and pleasure: the satisfaction of taking away a small gift, of owning a work of art, of consuming sugary foodstuffs or simply of feasting visually on the rainbow colours of a field of cellophane wrappings. Read through the pleasure principle, these works might be read as the collective repression of a difficult subject, a repressed trauma that can only be 'worked through' by resorting to enjoyable actions. The current curatorial emphasis on the unmitigated pleasure afforded by these works (often implicit in the term 'generosity') constitutes a social resistance to remembering AIDS, as the repressed material is *repeated* as a contemporary experience instead of being *remembered* as something belonging to the past.[109]

Crip time, care work and maintenance time

"*Untitled*" *(Perfect Lovers)* is typical of Gonzalez-Torres' treatment of the body: de-sublimated into incorporeal forms, the body is, as Nancy Spector has astutely remarked, present everywhere in Gonzalez-Torres' work, yet rarely visible as such.[110] Simon Watney reads this corporeal absence in directly political terms, in the context of the AIDS crisis. Noting the widespread media tendency to either demonize or heroize people with AIDS, Watney observes how Gonzalez-Torres 'has stepped away from contestation which is grounded on the bodies of people with AIDS and their representations'.[111]

Gonzalez-Torres was well aware of the problems inherent in many media depictions of AIDS. He rejected the stereotype of the debilitated AIDS victim, claiming that this, as well as 'garish' medical images, was inadequate:

> When people think about AIDS, they think of images of hospital beds, medicine, needles, and all such garish things. That's not AIDS. That's part of it, but AIDS also, unfortunately, includes discrimination, fear, shame, desperation, and political repression. The fact that gays still cannot serve openly in the military, because people still want to believe it's just a gay disease – that's AIDS too. I don't need to see an image of someone dying in a hospital bed to understand AIDS. No one needs to see that; we've seen it before, and we'll see more.[112]

I read Gonzalez-Torres' multiple sequences of hand-painted graphs charting his and Laycock's 'bloodwork' as an attempt to offer an alternative representation to the over-determined AIDS victim.[113] "*Untitled*" *(31 Days of Bloodwork – Steady Decline)* (1994), to take just one example, comprises thirty-one sheets of graph paper each with a straight line pencilled diagonally from upper left to lower right. As the parenthetical title indicates, the work denotes the results of a cycle of blood tests, with the number of pages corresponding to the time period across which tests were carried out. The certificate of authentication for (*31 Days*) provides detailed instructions for installation – 'The canvases are marked with an order. Ideally they may be installed in order, on one wall, in one line, with 1½ in. (4 cm) between each canvas' – but also offers other options: 'Alternatively, the canvases may be configured to the owner's liking. All canvases may be installed together as one piece, or may be installed individually or in groups of any number of canvases.'[114] In practice, the work not only has most often been installed horizontally along a wall, suggesting a narrative (if a static, unchanging one), but has also on occasion been displayed as a grid.

Gonzalez-Torres reused this motif in an almost obsessive manner. The *catalogue raisonné* published by the Sprengl Museum (1997) indicates that twenty-one separate bloodwork sequences were produced between 1988 and 1994: "*Untitled*" *(7 Days of Bloodworks)* (1988); a diptych "*Untitled*" *(Bloodworks)* (1989); a five-part series "*Untitled*" *(Bloodworks)* (1989); five individual works catalogued as "*Untitled*" *(t-Cell Count)* (1990), each comprising a single page of graphite, coloured pencil and gouache; "*Untitled*" *(14 Days of Bloodworks)* (1991); two versions of "*Untitled*" *(7 Days of Bloodworks)* (1991); "*Untitled*" *(31 Days of Bloodworks)* (1991); a four-part work "*Untitled*" *(Bloodworks)* (1992); a single-page "*Untitled*" *(False Hope – Bloodwork)* (1992); in 1993, a thirteen-part work "*Untitled*" *(Steady Decline)* (1993); "*Untitled*" *(9 Days of Bloodwork – Steady Decline and False Hope)* (1993); "*Untitled*" *(7 Days of Bloodwork – Steady Decline)* (1993); "*Untitled*" *(19 Days of Bloodwork – Steady Decline)* (1994); "*Untitled*" *(21 Days of Bloodwork – Steady Decline)* (1994); and two single-page works both called "*Untitled*" *Bloodwork – Steady Decline)* (1994) (Figure 32).[115]

The graphs map the primary medical signifier of AIDS, a declining T-cell count. Several critics have read these charts as affective narratives of declining health: Robert Storr describes them as 'a chillingly contemporary vanitas';[116] in Nancy Spector's analysis the body is 'stricken', and the line is 'plunging [. . .] marking the reality of AIDS' destructive force in the most graphic of terms'.[117] For Spector they also signify 'the scopic regime of the medical system', a system which must transform the patient into an abstracted object in order to function efficiently,[118] and indicate the dehumanising nature of medical language: 'the translation of the life spirit of the body into numerical sequences'.[119]

This reading is partly supported by Gonzalez-Torres' own commentary:

> It was this that struck me when I first saw an extensive bloodwork done on Ross in the form of numbers and codes. I said to him, 'Honey, this is your blood. Right here. This is it.' There was not a drop of blood there. There wasn't anything red. And it was even more frightening because all the numbers could easily be reversed. It is a total abstraction; it is the body. It is your life.[120]

As well as a kind of fascinated horror at the reduction of his lover's body to numeric code, Gonzalez-Torres' statement communicates a sense of wonderment similar to that expressed by Mark Morrisroe – ('THAT'S A MASTERPIECE!') – on looking at his own X-rays for the first time.[121] Like Morrisroe's creatively re-appropriated X-rays, Gonzalez-Torres' bloodwork charts act as intimate (if unconventional) medical portraits. What could be more a precise signifier of a subject's essential identity than their own blood?[122]

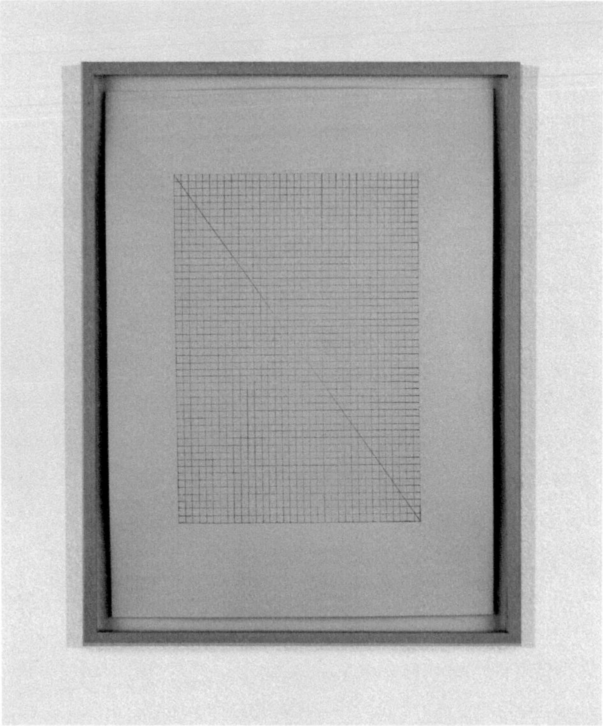

Figure 32 Felix Gonzalez-Torres, "*Untitled*" *(Bloodwork – Steady Decline)*, 1994. Graphite and gouache on paper. Framed. 16½ × 12 3/8 in. (41.9 × 31.4 cm). Photographer: Peter Muscato. © Estate of Felix Gonzalez-Torres. Courtesy Felix Gonzalez-Torres Foundation.

Although initially the graphs appear to be a mechanical series of faint lines swiftly pencilled onto sheets of squared paper, they are in fact painstakingly produced, with each individual square meticulously painted in delicately coloured tempura or gouache; the work is completed by the addition of the pencil line. This hand-crafted quality imbues them with a tactile sensuality echoing that found in Mark Morrisroe's X-ray prints and confers on the two-dimensional drawings a sense of the body's physicality that is more usually associated with three-dimensional works. The carefully hand-crafted nature of each page challenges Spector's claim that the graphs present the empirical evidence of an illness (by recording the depletion of T-cells, each sheet of graph paper 'indexes a present state that will soon no longer be; it maps a topos of life on the verge of death').[123]

In Roland Barthes' unconventional autobiography, *Roland Barthes by Roland Barthes*, the author includes, by way of self-representation, a reproduction of one of the medical charts kept at the end of his bed when he was a young boy in a tubercular sanatorium. Every month, a new sheet was pasted onto the old one, so that, by the end, there were yards of them; Barthes describes this as 'a farcical way of writing one's body within time'.[124] Tuberculosis, Barthes writes, had 'its own interminable time', condemned to spend months confined to bed, one was sick or cured 'abstractly, purely by the doctor's decree'.[125] Gonzalez-Torres' bloodwork charts echo the 'interminable time' of Barthes' tubercular sanatorium; in their sheer number they mark the minutes, hours and days devoted to medical appointments. But rather than writing the body 'through time' (as Barthes puts it) Gonzalez-Torres' graphs appear to suggest stasis and endurance: the line never moves but remains stuck or suspended on its customary diagonal.

Barthes' words and Gonzalez-Torres' graphs invoke a peculiar form of temporality that disability scholar Alison Kafer has termed 'crip time'.[126] Crip time and queer time overlap: as I noted earlier in this chapter, and as Kafer also recognizes, queer time is often defined through reference to illness and disability, with the implication that illness and disability renders time 'queer'. Illness might cause time to slow and may also cause 'feelings of asynchrony or temporal dissonance'.[127] Kafer observes that familiar categories and experiences of illness and disability are already temporally conceived, involving (re)orientations in and to time, and notes that futurity is often framed in curative terms and used to support compulsory able-bodiedness (sick and disabled people cannot be part of a narrative of forward progress unless 'cured'). The bloodwork charts recognize the queer temporal experience of crip time: the line does not shift, time does not move forward as expected, and the future (normatively curative) is refused in favour of the here and now.

Gonzalez-Torres' compulsive diagramming of the sick body can be read as a practice of care. In her book *Enduring Time*, Lisa Baraister theorizes stuck or suspended time as characteristic of the repetitive temporal structure of care or maintenance work.[128] Drawing on Joan Tronto's definition of care as an 'activity that includes everything we do to maintain, continue, and repair our "world" so that we can live in it as well as possible', Baraister posits maintenance practices (which might include cooking, cleaning, washing and other tasks traditionally associated with female labour) as care work.[129] To maintain or to care, Baraitser argues, is 'repetitive, time consuming, arduous, boring and tedious', but it is also necessary for making and maintaining social relations, accomplished primarily through processes of touching.[130] The meticulous, handmade and careful nature of Gonzalez-Torres' 'bloodwork' charts makes visible the tactile and repetitive nature of caring for an ill lover. What is more, these micro-repetitions do not only index the work of care or maintenance work within a personal relationship but might also recall the repetition involved in the work of activism: as Monica Pearl notes, 'ACT UP's successes were built by [. . .] mundane daily repeated but crucial actions.'[131] Read in this register, repetition is not a pathology (e.g. as in a form of melancholia or 'stuck' mourning) but a necessary practice of care and endurance.

* * *

This chapter has explored the nuances of reading Gonzalez-Torres' practice as self-representational and autopathographic. This approach might seem somewhat contentious: even the pieces that make the most overt claim to self-representation (e.g. the text-based "*Untitled*" self-portrait of 1989) appear primarily concerned with probing the workings of subjectivity in general, rather than expressing the artist's unique individuality. Many of his 'portraits' reveal the influence of late twentieth-century thinkers on understandings of subjectivity, including Barthes and Foucault's critique of the subject as a unified and autonomous being, and Lacan's proposal that the coherent subject is a misrecognition, the 'true' subject being instead fragmented and 'in pieces'. Following these thinkers, for Gonzalez-Torres the subject is always unstable, shaped through its relations with others, developing and changing even after its death. One might be tempted to conclude that Gonzalez-Torres' work is about the impossibility of portraiture in its conventional sense.

Yet the practice is underpinned by autobiography: Gonzalez-Torres' love story with Laycock is omnipresent. For those who knew him, Gonzalez-Torres' work was packed with personal references; Rosen suggests that the artist 'relished his identity' and included it within works as an example for others: 'Cuban born, homosexual, a person who went to the Whitney Program, a son, a brother, a lover . . . and so on'.[132] Formally and thematically, the work develops, like Blanchon's, from the specific subject position of being a gay man at a time of extreme homophobia, and from the recognition that producing and circulating one's own representation – even in a form that is coded and oblique – is always a political act. In this sense I concur with Blanchon's opinion that AIDS forms the necessary background to Gonzalez-Torres' strongest work. Selected pieces affectively convey a personal experience of becoming ill and, together with one's partner, facing a dual mortality: the twin clocks evoke the days and weeks spent at medical appointments, and the minutes and hours ticking away as one wonders how much time one might have left; the compulsive repetition of the bloodwork charts evokes the obsessive scrutiny of lab reports in the hope that a T-cell count might begin to ascend; the sweets suggest the anguish of watching one's lover fade away and the pain of surviving his death.

As I noted in the introduction to this book, illness narratives have traditionally been understood as giving form and structure to primarily individual experiences of illness. Challenging this, Stella Bolaki has recently argued that illness narratives are just as frequently characterized by multiplicity: as 'narratives of community' pathographic stories often articulate a collective experience of time and place as much as they do an individual's clinical symptoms.[133] Gonzalez-Torres' work (like Blanchon's) is perhaps most productively understood as articulating a collective and cultural, rather than strictly individual experience of illness. While it alludes to the somatic experiences of a person living with AIDS, it also powerfully invokes the social and political context of the first two decades of the epidemic, when homophobia shaped dominant discourse on the crisis and proscribed the parameters for what was considered representable within the international art world. In this sense, the absence of the concrete physical body in Gonzalez-Torres' practice speaks more powerfully than its visual presence ever could. Illness narratives have typically been assumed to follow a normative progressive linear structure, an assumption that has only relatively recently been explored and critiqued.[134] Gonzalez-Torres' work resists linear, progressive narrative, instead conveying the repetitive rhythms of 'stuck' time: in this chapter I have drawn on queer theory, crip theory and feminist scholarship on temporality and care-giving to explore Gonzalez-Torres' treatment of stuck time as it relates to illness, care and maintenance.

The 'stuck' time articulated by these works also suggests a certain stickiness in the relationship between the crisis years of the epidemic and the historicizing of the epidemic in the present 'post-crisis' moment. In using the term 'stickiness', I am thinking of the work of Sara Ahmed, who describes stickiness as 'an effect of surfacing, as an effect of the histories of contact between bodies, objects, and signs'.[135] Stickiness is a form of relationality: 'a sticky surface is one that will incorporate other elements into the surface such that the surface of a sticky object is in a dynamic process of resurfacing'.[136] Ahmed's sticky surfaces recall Michel Serres' discussion of temporal folding, which he explains via the figure of the baker kneading dough: 'Time enters into the dough, a prisoner of its folds, a shadow of its folding.'[137] Time, for Serres, is sticky: it does not flow in a linear fashion, but rather is a chaotic mix of ruptures, gaps and wells, forking, branching and rolling back on itself. Applied to Gonzalez-Torres' work, stickiness suggests not so much 'timelessness' but an ongoing and unresolved relationality between past and present temporalities of AIDS.

6

Epilogue

In/visible: Picturing HIV in 'endemic time'

This book has focussed on portraits and self-portraits produced between 1987 and 1996, a period commonly understood as the peak of the AIDS epidemic in North America. Since the introduction of effective antiretroviral drugs at the end of the 1990s, HIV has become a manageable chronic condition, at least for those with access to the right pharmaceutical regimes and the living conditions necessary for the successful management of a long-term medical condition. Data from the Center for Disease Control and Prevention shows that the epidemic is far from over: at the end of 2015 over 1.2 million Americans were living with HIV; of these, just over half a million were living with infections classified as stage 3 (AIDS).[1] Moreover, deep-rooted social inequalities mean that the ongoing epidemic does not affect all demographics equally: nearly half of all people living with HIV today in America are black, even though African Americans account for only 12 per cent of the total US population. Nearly 75 per cent of those living with HIV in America are Black males. Black women suffer a prevalence rate only exceeded by black males: Back women's prevalence rates are nearly 50 per cent higher than that of Latino men, which are the next highest group.[2] Changes in the medical management of HIV and new ways of preventing transmission including PrEP and PEP, as well as the growing acknowledgement that HIV does not affect all communities equally, raise new and pressing questions about portraiture and representation in relation to both those living with HIV today and those who experienced the crisis years of the epidemic.

The themes of this book – the interplay between presence and absence, visibility and invisibility – take on new weight and resonance in the light of recent literature that has critiqued the canonization of a predominantly white, male, cis-gendered and middle-class response to the epidemic. The reception of *Art AIDS America* in 2015, discussed in the introduction to this book, intensified existing debates about race, representation and the whitewashing of AIDS, with particular emphasis placed on the very real biopolitical implications of centring white masculinity in cultural conversations about HIV both past and present.[3]

Recent cinematic attempts to dramatize AIDS activism in the 1980s and 1990s – including *How to Survive a Plague* (David France, 2012) and *Dallas Buyer's Club* (Jean-Marc Vallee, 2013) – have been similarly criticized for privileging the stories of 'heroic' individual white males, while relegating women, transgender people and people of colour to the margins of the narrative.[4] As Jih-Fei Cheng notes, relatively little has changed in this respect since the popular AIDS films of the 1990s.[5] Analysing the screenplay of *How to Survive a Plague*, Cheng notes that the absence of women and people of colour is 'marked indelibly and excessively': the sole queer person of colour permitted to speak within the film, the Chicano activist Ray Navarro, disappears from the narrative before the end, rendering him tangential to the history of AIDS activism.[6] Similarly, Nishant Shahani argues that *How to Survive a Plague* and other recent AIDS memory films perform a 'whitewashing' of coalitional histories and a 'visual gentrification of the queer past'.[7] These (re)presentations of AIDS history provide an enduring framework for the relative in/visibility of different populations in relation to HIV and AIDS today and continue to shape epidemiological approaches to the ongoing global epidemic.

Addressing these ongoing structures of in/visibility in relation to historical and contemporary narratives of HIV and AIDS is essential but challenging, often necessitating a shift in normative modes of scholarship. For instance, the collected volume *AIDS and the Distribution of Crises* (2020), edited by Cheng, Juhasz and Shahani, explicitly seeks to decentre cis-gender white gay men as the primary object of academic research, public health initiatives and cultural re-visitations. The editors remark on the structural difficulties that they experienced when attempting to centre the experiences of Black women in particular, who seemed to keep 'sliding off, disappearing from, or moving ever so slightly out of our sight lines'.[8] For the editors, this 'absent presence' became structurally significant, throwing conventional academic practices into crisis.[9]

While acknowledging the necessary limitations of the scope of this present volume, I use this epilogue to explore evolving debates, pointing the reader to significant new scholarship and expanding on the key themes of this book, (self)-portraiture, absence and invisibility, through a reading of self-representational works by the artist Kia LaBeija (b. Kia Michelle Benbow, 1990). LaBeija's multidisciplinary practice – including dance, photography and digital media as well as advocacy – communicates her experience as a young, born-positive queer woman of colour who has grown up with HIV and is driven by a personal and political commitment to make visible the stories of herself and other marginalized positive people, reinserting their narratives into official histories of HIV and AIDS.

LaBeija's best-known work to date is a series of performative photographic self-portraits collectively titled *24* (2014 onwards). One of the most striking pictures in the series, *Eleven* (2015) (Figure 33), shows the young woman being examined by her family physician. Like all her images, the photograph is purposefully and skilfully composed: spot-lit in the centre of the frame, LaBeija is luminous and lustrous in a carmine tulle and sequin prom dress, a single white rose upon her lap. In the shadows to her left, the physician's dark-grey suit blends with the muted blue hues of the clinical space as he wraps a tourniquet around her arm to prepare to draw a blood sample. LaBeija has visited this doctor since she was four years old and, along with her mother, newly diagnosed. At the time, no one expected her to live to maturity: the prom dress, a symbol of the transition from childhood to adulthood, marks and celebrates her survival. The image is a reminder of the importance of consistent, long-term and high-quality healthcare in the management of HIV today and draws attention to the invisible labour of self-maintenance routinely undertaken by people living positive. As the artist notes: 'I go to the doctor all the time, to check my CD4 count, see how my viral load is doing. Am I undetectable? How are my organs doing? It's a method of

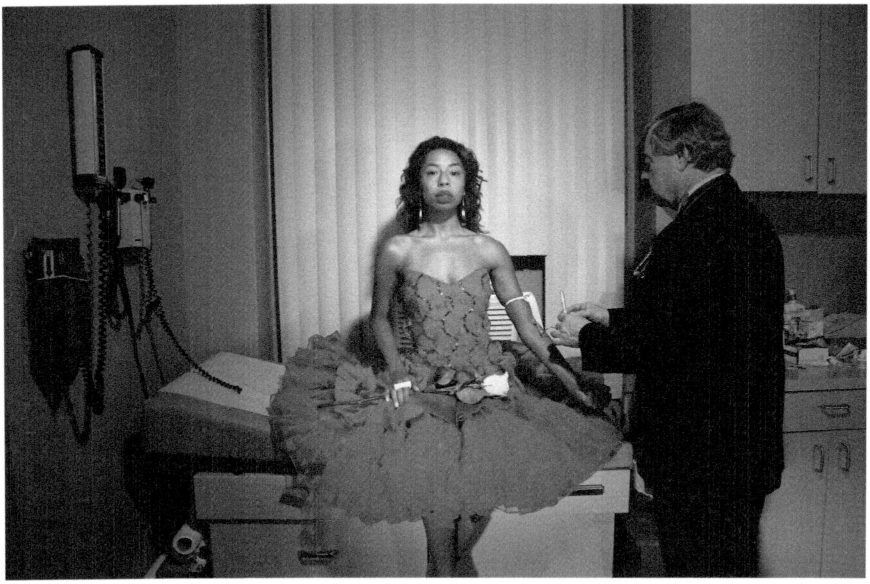

Figure 33 Kia LaBeija, *Eleven*, 2015, from the series 24 (2014 onwards). © Kia LaBeija 2015.

self-care, but one that not many people get to see.'[10] LaBeija draws attention to 'undetectable' as a relatively new serostatus that complicates the previous binary between positive and negative.[11] Effective HIV treatment lowers the viral load in the blood: below a certain level, the viral load is referred to as sufficiently suppressed to be statistically insignificant or 'undetectable' (and thus also non-communicable). As well as making manifest the essential (and often-invisible) personal and professional practices of care necessary for keeping the viral load low, *Eleven* raises critical questions about the role of visual media, including portraiture, in defining health crises: to paraphrase a point made by Julia Jordan-Zachery in her book *Shadow Bodies: Black Women, Ideology, Representation and Politics,* is it a crisis if it is not seen?[12]

LaBeija became a central figure in the conversations about (in)visibility, race, representation and art-world (non)inclusivity that followed the opening of *Art AIDS America.* One of the four (later five) Black-identified artists included in the original show and the only woman of colour, LaBeija was also the only artist representing mother-to-child transmission and the only living positive female artist.[13] As outlined in the introduction to this book, criticism of the exhibition, neatly summarized in the hashtag *#stoperasingblackpeople*, centred on the way in which curatorial decisions had effectively eliminated Black-identified people from past and present histories of HIV and AIDS. This in turn raised fascinating and important questions about how the parameters of what counts as 'art' might need to be redefined in order to present a more inclusive and representative narrative. As the artist and archivist Sur Rodney (Sur) notes, because artists of colour have typically been 'locked out' of the white cube of the art world, to find work that communicates non-white experiences of HIV and AIDS, it is necessary to look beyond the gallery system to other spaces, including (e.g.) clubs, churches, ballrooms and parades.[14]

Shortly after the show's opening and in response to the die-in led by the Tacoma Action Collective, LaBeija released a public statement on her Facebook page. She spoke of the elation that she had felt when selected for the exhibition, and how she had hoped that the inclusion of her work would help to renegotiate the way that people understand what HIV looks like today. On seeing the show's preview in LA, she writes, she was disappointed: 'The images I saw where [*sic*] mostly of gay, white men waisting [*sic*] away [. . .] even the dynamic of the shows patrons was severely disproportioned with those living positive.'[15] In response, LaBeija produced a new work, which she released on her own website in December 2015.[16] Provocatively titled *Your White Walls Can Kiss My Black Ass,* the image depicts the artist naked in a white-walled studio space. Her head is cropped out of the frame and her back is to the camera, drawing the viewer's eye down the camber of her spine, the curve of her body exaggerated by a dancer's pose that transfers her weight onto one foot. A cloud of dark paint stains the floor beneath her. Her body gently brushes the wall; she coalesces with the space and is simultaneously constrained by it, hinting at the complexity of her relationship with art-world institutions.

My own analysis of LaBeija's work does not seek to rehash the debates over *Art AIDS America*. Rather than necessarily locating LaBeija's work within a history of HIV portrait practices, I situate it within contemporary practices of feminist autotheory that take an intersectional approach to illness and disability, drawing on the work of Johanna Hedva and others. I also focus on the still underexplored experiences of women and particularly of children born positive to positive (and often undiagnosed) mothers. While the elegiac work of a generation of male artists focussed on the pain of losing a lover, LaBeija's images express her pain at the loss of her mother, a relatively unmapped experience in artists' responses to the epidemic.[17] Memorializing her mother through an interplay between maternal presence and absence, the work prompts a consideration of the ways in which women and their born-positive babies were 'last served' in early responses to HIV and have since been largely written out of the epidemic by both epidemiological approaches and cultural and art-historical responses.

Sad girls and sick women: Autotheoretical feminist practices

The title of LaBeija's series *24* deliberately conveys a number of autobiographical particularities of time and place, referring to the artist's age when she embarked on the project; the number of years that she had then lived in her childhood home, an apartment block on the westside of midtown Manhattan near Times Square and the theatre district; and the floor number of that apartment. Expanding on my brief reading of *Eleven*, I address three further images from this series, *In My Room*, *Kia and Mommy* and *Mourning Sickness* (all 2014), which were included in the opening Tacoma Art Museum showing of *Art AIDS America*. (*Eleven* was produced after the Tacoma show and was included in the final version of the exhibition at the Alphawood Gallery in Chicago in 2016–17.)[18] The location for all three images is the tightly enclosed domestic space of the apartment referenced in the series' title; the tactic of rendering private spaces publicly visible echoes the approach of an earlier generation of HIV-positive artists, with Felix Gonzalez-Torres' unmade bed billboard (1991) being the most obvious example. But whereas Gonzalez-Torres and his contemporaries experimented with artistic strategies of self-effacement, disembodiment and intentional invisibility, LaBeija's pictures are visual affirmations of a situated and embodied experience. The body as conveyed in these images is not schematized or diagrammatized (as in Gonzalez-Torres' bloodwork charts, for example); it is a particularized body in a specific time and space, connected to other bodies through objects, emotions and relations of care.[19]

In the first image produced for the series, *In My Room*, the artist has placed herself at the centre of the frame, poised on the edge of a faded floral cream couch. Her limbs are folded into a wary, childlike pose, offset by scarlet underwear and matching lipstick; eyeing the camera, she seems hyper-alert, simultaneously vulnerable and self-possessed. The room is a tumbling cacophony of fabrics: the doors of the closet are folded open to reveal garments of silver sequins and white tulle, fuchsia satin and glittering turquoise hung beneath an orderly row of vertiginously heeled shoes. (As Bachelard observes, 'a wardrobe's inner space is also intimate space'.)[20] These textiles are echoed in the faded print of the sofa and bolster, the leopard print cushion, the stuffed horse behind her, the wigs thrown carelessly across the keyboard, the rolls of cloth in the corner of the room and the unidentifiable textiles at the bottom of the image. Objects, as Sara Ahmed recognizes in her critique of the psychologizing and privatization of emotion, can enable (private) emotions to circulate and become social: objects can become 'sticky, or saturated with affect, as sites of personal and social tension'.[21] In Labaija's images, objects are sticky with narrative significance. The tumble of sequinned garments refers to both her participation in New York's ballroom scene and her childhood; many of her neighbours worked in the theatre and would give her clothes left over from performances so that she could play dress-up. Fidelity to these early memories is clearly important to the artist; she reports that her brother's response to the image was one of recollection and evocation: 'Wow – your closet looks just like it did when you were a child.'[22] *Mommy and Me* is shot in the same bedroom: at the centre of the image, illuminated by soft light pooling on the parquet floor, the artist is lying on her back, legs raised and bent against a chest of draws, head turned towards the camera. Her arms are wrapped around a framed photograph of her smiling mother, taken at a family wedding in 1995.[23] Clad in a red sequinned minidress and gold platform stilettoes shoes, LaBeija's pose is simultaneously sultry and semi-foetal, suggesting both adult sexuality and vulnerable child.

The blurred boundaries between adult and child are pushed further still in *Mourning Sickness* (2014), which portrays the artist elegantly and embryonically curled up on her bathroom floor. In interviews LaBeija has described this picture as a performative re-enactment of an adolescence spent being regularly sick before attending high school, with dizziness, tiredness, nausea and vomiting being side effects of the changing regimes of medications necessary to keep her healthy. Sickness means that she was often late for school, resulting in missed classes; feeling unable to discuss her health with her peers, she explained her absenteeism by cultivating a 'cool girl' image of indifference. The bathroom is also a site of mourning: LaBeija recalls locking herself in to cry after her mother's death. Through the pun of the title, which mixes grief with gestational sickness, LaBeija implies a psychic identification with her mother: just as her mother was once pregnant with her, now the daughter is pregnant with grief for the mother. Although sick, she is perfectly made-up, with painted fingernails and jewellery, and wearing an elegant kimono style wrap with a pattern that echoes the baby-blue rug upon which she lies. The artist has described this as a 'glamour shot',[24] the phrase echoing Sur Rodney (Sur)'s description of Mark Morrisroe's final self-portrait, discussed in Chapter 3 of this book. Bathrooms have often offered spaces for artists to articulate social anxieties around 'matter out of place', facilitating the address of bodily functions, fluids and fears of contamination: consider the work of Robert Gober, for example. But LaBeija's bathroom is immaculate, its bleached and gleaming tiles echoing her own impeccable appearance. Whereas male artists of a previous generation, including Mark Morrisroe and Robert Blanchon, used deliberate strategies of abjection, dirt and decay to express the lack of value placed by society on queer men's lives, LaBeija engages a very different aesthetic vocabulary of flawless glamour, acknowledging that this is a deliberate reaction to the phobic images of HIV-positive people that she grew up with in the 1990s. The conscious composition and sumptuous use of texture and colour echo the conventions of fashion photography (David LaChapelle and Cindy Sherman are two obvious influences) as well as contemporary vernacular practices of networked self-imaging. A productive comparison can be made with Leslie Kaliades' black-and-white *Self-Portrait* (1989), shot on a bathroom floor twenty-five years earlier; while Kaliades' gold-sequinned bra top matches LaBeija for glamour, there is something more brutally voyeuristic about Kaliades' picture. The sheer staginess of LaBeija's images serves to deflect any thoughts about voyeurism or visual objectification; she has carefully prepared herself to be looked at and demands that she be at the centre of the camera's gaze.

The gorgeousness of LaBeija's images is always freighted with melancholy, and it is to this affect that I now turn, situating LaBeija's within the context of a rapidly expanding genre of post-internet feminist autotheoretical practices built on women's experiences of mental and physical ill health. Autotheory describes the practices of engaging with theory, life and art from the perspective of one's own lived experience.[25] Lauren Fournier notes that while the term itself is relatively new – it became dominant post-2015, following the publication of Maggie Nelson's *The Argonauts*, which plays on Paul B. Preciado's use of the word in *Testo Junkie* (published in English in 2013) – 'the practice of theorizing from the first person is well established within the genealogies of feminism.'[26] The roots of present-day impulse towards autotheoretical practices can be traced to cross-genre writings by women of colour, including Audre Lorde, Gloria E. Anzaldua, Cherrie Moraga, Sylvia Winter and bell hooks, as well as the work of a number of historical 'sick women' authors including Lorde, Sylvia Plath, Anne Sexton and Charlotte Gilmour Perkins, who used their writing to make visible and theorize experiences of illness, trauma, pain and grief.[27] And although autotheory has often been approached as a predominantly text-based phenomenon, Fournier identifies a substantial lineage of post-1960s feminist autotheoretical visual art practices, including conceptual, video and body and performance art, and 'self-imaging' practices such as performing for the camera or taking selfies.[28]

Two contemporary autotheoretical para-art practices, Audrey Wollen's 'Sad Girl Theory' and Johanna Hedva's 'Sick Woman Theory', are suggestive for reading LaBeija's work, which they are roughly contemporaneous with: 'Sad Girl Theory' was published as a series of Instagram posts between 2015 and 2016, while 'Sick Woman Theory' was originally presented as a lecture in 2015 and published online in 2016.[29] Like LaBeija, both Wollen (b.1992) and Hedva (b.1984) work from positions of chronic illness: Hedva has an autoimmune condition that renders her unable to leave her bed for lengthy periods of time; Wollen's Instagram account alludes to an unspecific chronic disability via a series of selfies taken in hospitals and pain management clinic. Hedva's 'Sick Woman Theory' responds to and critiques Wollen's 'Sad Girl Theory', which proposes that the sadness of young women needs to be understood as a radical act. Rather than always seeing sadness as passive or an admission of personal failure, Wollen argues, it can be re-conceptualized as an active and articulate way of staging resistance: read through Wollen, the sadness exhibited by LaBeija for the camera is not merely personal but also a defiant political gesture. Yet, as Hedva notes, Wollen's autotheoretical posturing centres a model of subjectivity grounded in whiteness, youth, beauty, heteronormativity and well-resourced middle-classness, implicitly raising the question of who gets to (auto) theorize and to what purpose. Asking 'what happens to the sad girl who is poor, queer, and/or not white, when, *if*, she grows up', Hedva places the thinking of Arendt,

Butler, Cvetkovich, Lorde, Southhawk and others alongside their own class- and gender-based experiences of chronic illness.[30] Their text explores the possibility of political protest for sick people: citing Hannah Arendt's belief that to be political one must get one's body into the street, Hedva notes that such a position relies on a public/private binary that has long since broken down and insists that most modes of political protest are (and perhaps always have been) 'internalized, lived, embodied, suffering, and no doubt invisible'.[31] In this context, Hedva writes of '*the trauma of not being seen*' (her italics) as a common experience of (sick) women of colour, who typically have to 'fight for their experience to be not only honoured, but first made visible'.[32]

The text of 'Sick Woman Theory' is accompanied by self-images of the artist, whose markedly performative mode of self-presentation bears noteworthy similarities to LaBeija's own. Posing within the private and domestic space of their own home, Hedva is pictured in their bed and wheelchair, witchy and priestess-like in a full-length long-sleeved scarlet dress with white embroidery at the bodice and cuffs, strings of beads at their neck, their lips painted a glossy black. Sitting in their wheelchair, Hedva's feet resting on a stack of books, the most visible of which are Audrey Lorde's *Sister Outsider* and Alison Kafer's *Feminist, Queer, Crip*: medications pile in their lap, and one hand holds out a pill container while the other grips a Perspex walking cane. Lying on their bed, Hedva points at the books and pharmaceuticals that surround them; wild tendrils of long black hair snake across the green cushion that supports their head.

Hedva and LaBeija's images are part of an emergent genre described by Tamar Tembeck as 'autopathographic selfies' or 'selfies of ill health', which seeks to construct 'a politicised dramaturgy of the lived body, notably by enabling individuals [. . .] to come out as being invisibly ill''.[33] Tembeck's case study is the social media practice of Karolyn Gehrig, instigator of the *#HospitalGlam* movement, which launched in 2014. Gehrig has a chronic connective tissue disorder which makes frequent medical appointments an ordinary part of her life; she documents these visits through her Instagram feed, planning special outfits for the occasion. Like those of LaBeija and Hedva, Gehrig's images draw on the language of fashion photography, engaging a highly deliberate posed and polished aesthetic. The dramaturgical thrust of Gehrig's, Hedva and LaBeija's self-imaging practices is to articulate the centrality of medical experience in their everyday life and to convey their desire to be publicly identified as persons living with illness.[34]

These images are performative (in the Butlerian sense) rather than merely expressive: they bring a particular version of a life into being, rather than illustrating something that already exists prior to photographing it. While autopathographic self-imaging practices are often presumed to offer unmediated access to lived experience, it is more accurate to say that lived experience is given shape and form through the image-making process, rather than constituting a pre-existing actuality.[35] Fournier described contemporary text-based autotheory as 'post-confessional' in that it has been shaped by the performative turn: citing Maggie Nelson's *The Argonauts*, Fournier identifies a shift away from early forms of life writing such as memoir (which is associated with memory) towards the more playful activity of performative writing, which foregrounds instability and self-reflectivity.[36] While LaBeija's images could be read as visual memoir, the (re)enactment of childhood experience and the entangling of remembered past with lived present suggest something more akin to the creative performative process described by Nelson. Memory, both personal and collective, is LaBeija's raw material. Her carefully constructed self-images are not simply about living with a chronic health condition in the present day but about negotiating a relationship with history, forcing a contemporary reckoning with a past from which the presence of women and children has been elided. She recalls watching *United in Anger: A History of ACT UP* and noting the film's absence of archival footage of children at ACT UP meetings. The film's cinematographic memory is at odds with her own: 'I was there, with lots of other children, we did exist.'[37]

A generation of silenced voices

> *I am a child of a generation born to positive mothers, when women were not PWAs. I am a child born of a generation of children who were not built to last, who suckled the breasts of un-tested women, who grew in their wombs and passed through them like rushing waters. I am a child born into a generation where hope came in the form of color-coordinated pills stamped with dates, and times, and schedules. I am a child born into a generation of silenced voices that would not be heard until decades of birthday candles had been blown out.*[38]

In this prose-poem, printed in *TDR* in 2016, LaBeija refers to the historical gendering of the epidemic, recalling an era where women were not counted as people with AIDS. In the early 1990s, when LaBeija was around two years old, her mother began to suffer from a series of medical symptoms that at the time were not recognized as potential indicators of an HIV infection. Cindy Patton has described women as 'last served' by responses to the AIDS epidemic.[39] The Center for Disease Control's 1983 review of the epidemiologic pathways along which HIV was spreading identified homosexual men, haemophiliacs, Haitians, intravenous drug users and the 'female sexual partners of bisexual or intravenous drug using men, and their children' as the groups most at risk of contracting HIV.[40] Yet, subsequent literature abridged the risk groups to the '4Hs' (homosexuals, heroin users, haemophiliacs and Haitians); when women re-entered epidemiological discourse, it was primarily as vectors for (male) infection, generating the fifth alliterative category of 'hookers'. One of the first medical textbooks on AIDS, published in 1984, addressed women only in a chapter on sex workers and their children. It was not until 1993 that the Centers for Disease Control expanded the list of HIV-related illnesses to include the gynaecological abnormalities and cancers by which HIV typically manifests in women.[41]

The failure of epidemiological discourse to adequately account for women is alluded to in Nicholas Nixon's divisive photo-book project *People with AIDS* (1991), explored in Chapter 2 of this book. Nixon's project features four female sitters (out of fifteen sitters in total): Linda Black, Elizabeth Ramos, Laverne Colebut and Sara Paneto. The first- and third-person illness narrative that accompanies the portraits of Ramos tells us that she tested positive in 1985 following a blood donation, and that her physician refused to recognize that this might be the cause of her bronchitis and breathing difficulties, instead treating Ramos for 'stress' and the female malady 'hysteria'.[42] Ramos was eventually admitted to an emergency ward with *pneumocystis* and later won a malpractice suit against her doctor. Nixon photographs Ramos with her young son, Chris: in an image titled 'July 1987', both are dressed in white and both are smiling, Chris gentling pinching his mother's cheeks to force a grin. The image stands out in Nixon's project, where the more usual representation of (non-positive) womanhood is as caregiver or mourner for an adult son. (Therese Frare's pieta-like image of David Kirby (1990), subsequently used in Oliviero Toscani's controversial advertising campaign for the United Colors of Benneton, memorably engaged a similar trope.)[43] The narratives that accompany Nixon's images of HIV-positive women are laden with disapproving allusions to promiscuity and drug use: one of the first things that we learn about Laverne Colebut is that she loved 'tiny lace underpants in hot colors', and Sara Paneto is labelled as a 'recovering addict' raised in the 'Puerto Rican ghettos of New York City and Norwich, Connecticut, [surrounded by] violence, alcohol and drugs'.[44] Only Ramos, who insists 'I never used drugs. I wasn't promiscuous', escapes the camera's judgement, her 'innocence' confirmed pictorially by the presence of her children and her status as devoted mother. Predictably, in Nixon's *People with AIDS*, representations of HIV-positive women swing between the tired tropes of virgin and whore, with women cast as either undeserving victims or promiscuous 'vectors' of transmission.[45]

Writing on the representation of women in mainstream AIDS documentaries in the late 1980s, Alexandra Juhasz recognized the cultural erasure of women (and particularly women of colour), noting that HIV-positive women were only granted a place in public visual culture in the context of heterosexual reproduction and that this conditional visibility tended to be fleeting, with images of HIV-positive mothers swiftly displaced by pictures of their sick but pretty babies.[46] Used as visual stand-ins for their mothers (or alternatively, as Sander Gilman notes, mobilized as affective counter-narratives to phobic images of debilitatingly ill gay men), sick children were afforded a kind of hyper-visibility: writing in 1989, Jan Zita Grover observed that during the period of 1985–9, the number of children with AIDS (which constituted approximately 1% of all AIDS cases in the United States) had received more press attention than the 61 per cent of diagnosed cases among gay men.[47] Read through this historical context of displacement and hyper-visibility, LaBeija's pictures perform a metonymy of their own, wrapping woman and child, mother and daughter, into a single photographic frame. The title of *Mourning Sickness,* for example, implies a psychical identification of daughter with mother: as her mother once carried her, LaBeija is now pregnant with grief for her mother. Posed in her childhood bedroom (*In My Room*), adult Kia in red-hued underwear sits in front of a black-and-white print of herself as a little girl (this photograph appears in the image twice over, once as a print tacked to the folding door and once as a reflection in the mirror; the same photograph featured in LaBeija's video Goodnight, Kia, made for Visual AIDS' Day with(out) Art in 2017). In *Mommy and Me*, adult Kia (in sequinned red mini dress, gold platform heels) cradles a photo of her mother as her mother once cradled her. Images of children typically tried to signal the 'innocence' of the victim and thus the low risk of transmission: children, it was intimated, are not sexually active and therefore cannot pose a threat.[48] In their knowing juxtaposition of childhood innocence with adult sexuality, LaBeija's images directly challenge these cultural tropes, situating the stereotypes of the sick child and sexual woman in nuanced dialogue with each other by playing both roles.

Multiple temporal frames are layered into a single picture: representing herself as both infant and adult, LaBeija's images tangle past and present, mixing the historical moment of crisis with a contemporary state of chronicity, or, to cite Julian Gill-Peterson's formulation, epidemic with endemic time.[49] 'Endemic time' describes a change in the temporality of HIV/AIDS after the introduction of anti-retroviral drugs. Gill-Peterson reworks Foucault's formulation of the historical turn from disciplinary power to bio-power to delineate a shift from an era of epidemics to one of endemics. In an era defined by epidemics, life and death are separate, with death understood as something that 'suddenly swooped down on life'; in an endemic era, however, death is 'something permanent, something that slips into life'.[50] For Gill-Peterson, the contemporary moment is defined by a generational overlapping: an age group who knew epidemic time intersects with one who only know endemic time, generating a sense of 'belatedness' and a present that is out of joint with itself.[51] Foucault's notion of the endemic resonates with Derrida's theory of hauntology, which offers 'a way to come to understand that life and death [. . .] are not opposites'.[52] For Derrida, learning to live with ghosts was a political project of accountability for past and future: a contemporary politics of HIV/AIDS must develop a new politics of 'learning to live with the ghosts produced by the inheritances of the epidemic' as an ethical prerequisite for enduring and indeed thriving in endemic time.[53] LaBeija's images actively perform this project of learning to live with the dead, wrapping mother into child, past into present, and materializing the folds and doublings of non-linear, out-of-joint time.

* * *

Self-representational works by HIV-positive female-identifying artists (especially female artists of colour) have not to date been well represented in the dominant cultural and art history of AIDS in America, although this is changing. When I visited the Visual AIDS archive in 2011 as part of the initial research for this book (the archive had not been digitized at that point), I was keen to explore self-portraits and self-representational work by female artists. I was disappointed: there was at that time relatively little work held by Visual AIDS that met my criteria. In 2022, as I prepare the final version of this manuscript, the now-digitized archive can be sorted by demographic criteria; clicking 'female' returns sixty-five artists, including LaBeija.[54]

The AIDS epidemic of the 1980s and 1990s helped to precipitate a shift in the very nature of visual self-representation. Significantly, this shift did not take place within a vacuum but was equally influenced by new theories of subjectivity and selfhood, and a particularized set of social and political circumstances that created the conditions of in/visibility for certain figurations of personhood.

The tools and techniques of visual self-representation continue to evolve today, as do the social, political and theoretical conditions that shape what can and cannot be seen. By reading selected artworks as creative articulations of lived experiences of critical and chronic illness, this book contributes not only to a rapidly evolving literature on visual and artistic representations of HIV and AIDS but also to developing scholarship at the intersections of art history and medical humanities. The artists' works explored within these pages show how self-representations of illness are never simply unmediated expressions of individual experience, but complex aesthetic and sociocultural entanglements that knowingly engage with art's histories and theories and with wider networks of social and cultural epistemologies and practices.

Notes

Introduction

1 Jonathan D. Katz, 'How AIDS Changed American Art', in *Art AIDS America*, ed. Jonathan D. Katz and Rock Hushka (Tacoma, Seattle and London: Tacoma Art Museum in association with University of Washington Press, 2015), 24–45.
2 Simon Watney, *Policing Desire: Pornography, AIDS and the Media*, 3rd edition (London: Cassell, 1997), 9.
3 Douglas Crimp, 'AIDS: Cultural Analysis / Cultural Activism', *October* 43, no. Winter (1987): 3; Paula Treichler, 'AIDS, Homophobia and Biomedical Discourse: An Epidemic of Signification', *October* 43 (1987): 31.
4 Simon Watney, 'The Spectacle of AIDS', *October* 43 (Winter 1987): 78.
5 PWA Coalition, 'PWA Coalition Portfolio', *October* 43 (1987): 147–68.
6 For example, on activist graphics see Douglas Crimp and Adam Rolston, *AIDS Demographics* (Seattle: Bay Press, 1990); Avram Finkelstein, *After Silence: A History of AIDS through Its Images* (Oakland: University of California Press, 2018); on the AIDS Project Quilt see Marita Sturken, *Tangled Memories: The Vietnam War, the AIDS Epidemic, and the Politics of Remembering* (Berkeley and London: University of California Press, 1997); Gabriele Griffin, *Visibility Blue/s: Representations of HIV and AIDS* (Manchester: Manchester University Press, 2000); Steven Gambardella, 'Absent Bodies: The AIDS Quilt as Social Melancholia', *Journal of American Studies* 45, no. 2 (2011): 213–26; and on public health posters see Roger Cooter and Claudia Stein, 'Coming into Focus: Posters, Power, and Visual Culture in the History of Medicine', *Medizinhistorisches Journal* 42 (2007): 180–209.
7 For examples see Alexandra Juhasz, *AIDS TV: Identity, Community, and Alternative Video* (Durham and London: Duke University Press, 1995); Roger Hallas, *Reframing Bodies: AIDS, Bearing Witness, and the Queer Moving Image* (Durham and London: Duke University Press, 2009); Kylo-Patrick R. Hart, *The AIDS Movie: Representing a Pandemic in Film and Television*, 2nd edition (London and New York: Routledge, 2013).
8 Crimp, 'AIDS', 15.
9 Jan Zita Grover, 'Introduction', in *AIDS: The Artists' Response* (Columbus: Ohio State University, 1989), 2–3.
10 Douglas Crimp, 'Mourning and Militancy', in *Melancholia and Moralism: Essays on AIDS and Queer Politics*, ed. Douglas Crimp (Cambridge, MA: MIT Press, 2002), 129–49.

11 David Deitcher, 'What Does Silence Equal Now?', in *Art Matters: How the Culture Wars Changed America*, ed. Brian Wallis, Marianne Weems, and Philip Yenawine (New York and London: New York University Press, 1999), 108.
12 David Deitcher, 'Death and the Marketplace', *Frieze* 29 (1996): 40–5.
13 Jonathan Katz, 'Hide/Seek: Portraits by Felix Gonzalez-Torres and David Wojnarowicz', accessed 8 April 2014, https://www.youtube.com/watch?v=4iiLMJru7SY.
14 Katz, 'How AIDS Changed American Art'.
15 Alexandra Juhasz and Theodore (Ted) Kerr, 'On Care, Activism, and HIV', in *Health*, ed. Bárbara Rodríguez Muñoz, Whitechapel Documents of Contemporary Art (London and Cambridge MA: Whitechapel Gallery and the MIT Press, 2020), 37–42; see also the use of the term 'silence' in Alexandra Juhasz and Theodore (Ted) Kerr, *We Are Having This Conversation Now: The Times of AIDS Cultural Production* (Durham: Duke University Press, 2022).
16 Deitcher, 'What Does Silence Equal Now?'.
17 Dion Kagan, *Positive Images: Gay Men and HIV/AIDS in the Culture of 'Post-Crisis'* (London and New York: IB Tauris, 2018).
18 Theodore (Ted) Kerr, 'Time Is Not a Line: Conversations, Essays, and Images about HIV/AIDS Now', *We Who Feel Differently*, Fall 2014, http://wewhofeeldifferently.info/journal.php.
19 For a comprehensive account of the culture wars, see Brian Wallis, Marianne Weems, and Philip Yenawine, eds., *Art Matters: How the Culture Wars Changed America* (New York: New York University Press, 1999).
20 Kerr has written about this phenomenon extensively; for selected examples, see Kerr, 'Time Is Not a Line'; Theodore (Ted) Kerr, 'AIDS – Based on a True Story', *Dandelion* 7, no. 1 (2016), https://dandelionjournal.org/article/doi/10.16995/ddl.341/; Alexandra Juhasz and Theodore (Ted) Kerr, 'Who Are the Stewards of the AIDS Archive? Sharing the Political Weight of the Intimate', in *The Unfinished Queer Agenda After Marriage Equality*, ed. Angela Jones, Joseph Nicholas DeFilippis, and Michael W. Yarbrough (London: Routledge, 2018), 88–101; Theodore (Ted) Kerr, 'What You Don't Know About AIDS Could Fill A Museum: Curatorial Ethics and the Ongoing Epidemic in the 21st Century', *On Curating*, no. 42 (2019): 5–17.
21 On The Normal Heart see Griffin, *Visibility Blue/s*, chapter 6; Monica Pearl, *AIDS Literature and Gay Identity: The Literature of Loss* (New York and London: Routledge, 2013), 112–13; For an extensive treatment of HIV in 21st century theatre and performance see Alyson Campbell and Dirk Gindt, eds, *Viral Dramaturgies: HIV and AIDS in Performance in the Twenty-First Century* (London: Palgrave Macmillan, 2018).
22 For a comprehensive oral history of Angels in America, see Isaac Butler and Dan Kois, *The World Only Spins Forward: The Ascent of Angels in America* (New York and London: Bloomsbury, 2018).

23 For a critical study of the 'Patient Zero' myth, see Richard A. McKay, *Patient Zero and the Making of the AIDS Epidemic* (Chicago and London: University of Chicago Press, 2017).

24 Vincent Chevalier and Bradley Perrin, 'Your Nostalgia Is Killing Me', Tumblr, *PosterVirus* (blog), 20 November 2013, https://postervirus.tumblr.com/post/67569099579/your-nostalgia-is-killing-me-vincent-chevalier; quoted in Theodore (Ted) Kerr, 'As We Canonize Certain Producers of Culture We Are Closing Space for a Complication of Narratives', *The Visual AIDS Blog* (blog), 10 December 2013, https://visualaids.org/blog/as-we-canonize-certain-producers-of-culture-we-are-closing-space-for-a-comp; See also Alexander McClelland and Jessica Whitbread, 'PosterVirus: Claiming Sexual Autonomy for People with HIV through Collective Action', in *Mobilizing Metaphor: Art, Culture, and Disability Activism in Canada*, ed. Christine Kelly and Michael Orsini (Vancouver and Toronto: UBC Press, 2016), 76–97; Marika Louise Cifor, '"Your Nostalgia Is Killing Me": Activism, Affect and the Archives of HIV/AIDS' (Doctoral Thesis, Los Angeles, University of California, 2017), https://escholarship.org/uc/item/2312c9bb; Finkelstein, *After Silence*, 201–17.

25 Tomasz Sikora, 'Queer Life-Worlds and the Art of David Wojnarowicz', *Journal of Gender Studies* 29, no. 1 (2020): 76–87.

26 ACT UP New York, 'Drawing Attention to the Modern HIV Epidemic for Act up Artist David Wojnarowicz', n.d., https://actupny.com/drawing-attention-to-the-modern-hiv-epidemic-for-act-up-artist-david-wojnarowicz/.

27 ACT UP New York, 'The Whitney Actions and the Historicization of HIV/AIDS', n.d., https://actupny.com/the-whitney-actions-and-the-historicization-of-hiv-aids/#comment-44.

28 ACT UP New York.

29 Jonathan Katz, 'In/Different America and AIDS', in *Art AIDS America Chicago*, ed. Staci Boris (Chicago: Alphawood Foundation, 2018), 42–3.

30 Jen Graves, 'Tacoma Art Museum's Art AIDS America Is a Messy Masterpeice That Reframes the Past 40 Years of American Art', *The Stranger*, 7 October 2015, https://www.thestranger.com/visual-art/features/2015/10/07/22970740/viral.

31 Tacoma Action Collective, 'Press Release, Die in Protest 12/7 at Tacoma Art Museum', *Tumblr*, 24 December 2015, https://stoperasingblackpeoplenow.tumblr.com.

32 Theodore (Ted) Kerr, 'A History of Erasing Black Artists and Bodies from the AIDS Conversation', *Hyperallergic*, 31 December 2015, https://hyperallergic.com/264934/a-history-of-erasing-black-artists-and-bodies-from-the-aids-conversation/.

33 Katz, 'In/Different America and AIDS', 44.

34 Katz, 'In/Different America and AIDS', 42.

35 Richard Sandell, *Museums, Moralities, and Human Rights* (London and New York: Routledge, 2017), 141–2.

36 Finkelstein, *After Silence*, 217.

37 Thomas E. Yingling, *AIDS and the National Body* (Durham and London: Duke University Press, 1997), 22.

38 Michel Foucault, *The History of Sexuality, Volume 1*, trans. Robert Hurley (London: Penguin, 1990).

39 Fiona Johnstone and Kirstie Imber, 'Introducing the Anti-Portrait', in *Anti-Portraiture: Challenging the Limits of the Portrait*, ed. Fiona Johnstone (London and New York: Bloomsbury, 2020), 1–23.

40 Marcia Pointon, *Portrayal and the Search for Identity* (London: Reaktion Books, 2013), 13.

41 For examples of standard textbook definitions of portraiture, see Richard Brilliant, *Portraiture* (London: Reaktion Books, 1991); Joanna Woodall, 'Introduction: Facing the Subject', in *Portraiture: Facing the Subject*, ed. Joanna Woodall (Manchester: Manchester University Press, 1997), 1–25.

42 Fiona Johnstone, 'Relics, Remains and Other Objects: Non-Mimetic Portraiture in the Age of AIDS', in *Anti-Portraiture: Challenging the Limits of the Portrait*, ed. Fiona Johnstone and Kirstie Imber (London and New York: Bloomsbury, 2020), 195–215.

43 Cindy Patton, 'Heterosexual AIDS Panic: A Queer Paradigm', *Gay Community News*, 9 February 1985; see also Cindy Patton, *Last Served? Gendering the AIDS Pandemic* (London: Taylor and Francis, 1994), 19 and 99–100.

44 Patton, *Last Served? Gendering the AIDS Pandemic*, 19 and 100.

45 Robert Storr, 'Felix Gonzalez-Torres: Être Un Espion', in *Felix Gonzalez-Torres*, ed. Julie Ault (New York and Gottingen: Steidl, 2006), 234.

46 Tamar Tembeck, ed., *Auto/Pathographies* (Alma: Sagamie édition d'art, 2014), 6.

47 Anne Hunsaker Hawkins, *Reconstructing Illness: Studies in Pathography*, 2nd ed. (West Lafayette: Purdue University Press, 1998), 1.

48 Susanna Egan, *Mirror Talk: Genres of Crisis in Contemporary Autobiography* (Chapel Hill and London: University of North Carolina Press, 1999), 28.

49 Ross Chambers, *Facing It: AIDS Diaries and the Death of the Author* (Ann Arbor: University of Michigan Press, 1998), 7.

50 Chambers, *Facing It*, 13.

51 This is particularly true of modern art and mental illness, best exemplified by the mythologizing of Vincent van Gogh's life and art in terms of his self-mutilation and suicide. See Griselda Pollock, 'Artists, Mythologies and Media – Genius, Madness and Art History', *Screen* 21, no. 3 (1980): 57–96 for a critique of this approach.

52 Gemma Blackshaw, 'The Pathological Body: Modernist Strategising in Egon Schiele's Self-Portraiture', *Oxford Art Journal* 30, no. 3 (2007): 379.

53 Tembeck, *Auto/Pathographies*, 8.

54 For examples see Crimp, 'AIDS'; Paula Treichler, *How to Have Theory in an Epidemic: Cultural Chronicles of AIDS* (Durham and London: Duke University Press, 1999); Watney, *Policing Desire*.

55 Lisa Diedrich, *Treatments: Language, Politics, and the Culture of Illness* (Minneapolis: University of Minnesota Press, 2007), xiv.

56 Arlene Croce, 'Discussing the Undiscussable', in *The Crisis of Criticism*, ed. Maurice Berger (New York: The New Press, 1998), 15–29.

57 Alan Radley, *Works of Illness: Narrative, Picturing and the Social Response to Disease* (Ashby-de-la-Zouch: Inkerman Press, 2009), 23.

58 Sander Gilman, *Disease and Representation: Images of Illness from Madness to AIDS* (Ithaca and London: Cornell University Press, 1988).

59 Gilman, *Disease and Representation*; Sander Gilman, *Health and Illness: Images of Difference* (London: Reaktion Books, 1995).

60 Lisa Diedrich locates this emergence around 1980, citing Susan Sontag's Illness as Metaphor (1978) and Audre Lorde's The Cancer Journals (1980) as significant texts. See Lisa Diedrich, *Indirect Action: Schizophrenia, Epilepsy, AIDS, and the Course of Health Activism* (Minneapolis: University of Minnesota Press, 2016), 6–7.

61 Tamar Tembeck, 'Selfies of Ill Health: Online Autopathographic Photography and the Dramaturgy of the Everyday', *Social Media + Society* 2, no. 1 (2016): 3, https://doi.org/10.1177/2056305116641343.

62 Diedrich, *Indirect Action*, 3.

63 Anne Whitehead and Angela Woods, 'Introduction', in *The Edinburgh Companion to the Critical Medical Humanities*, ed. Anne Whitehead and Angela Woods (Edinburgh: Edinburgh University Press, 2016), 1.

64 Arthur Kleinman, *The Illness Narratives: Suffering, Healing, and the Human Condition* (New York: Basic Books, 1988), 3.

65 Further significant texts for narrative medicine include Arthur Frank, *The Wounded Storyteller: Body, Illness, and Ethics* (Chicago and London: University of Chicago Press, 1995); Rita Charon, *Narrative Medicine: Honoring the Stories of Illness* (Oxford: Oxford University Press, 2006).

66 Angela Woods, 'The Limits of Narrative: Provocations for the Medical Humanities', *Med Humanities* 37 (2011): 73–8.

67 Stella Bolaki, *Illness as Many Narratives: Arts, Medicine and Culture* (Edinburgh: Edinburgh University Press, 2016), 6–7.

68 Bolaki, *Illness as Many Narratives*, 11–12.

69 I borrow the term 'erotogenic' from Elisabeth Lebovici, 'In the Darkroom', in *Mark Morrisroe*, ed. Beatrix Ruf and Thomas Seelig (Zurich: JPR Ringier, 2010), 228–39.

70 Roland Barthes, *Camera Lucida: Reflections on Photography*, trans. Richard Howard (London: Vintage, 2000), 81.

71 Gilman, *Health and Illness*, 115.

72 Georges Bataille, *Erotism*, trans. Mary Dalwood (London and New York: Marion Boyars, 1987), 11.

73 Sasha Archibald, 'Robert Blanchon's Archive of Absence', in *Robert Blanchon*, ed. Tania Duvergne and Amy Sadao (New York: Visual AIDS, 2006), 23.

74 Watney, 'The Spectacle of AIDS'.

75 Katz, 'How AIDS Changed American Art'.

76 Darren Jones, 'Galleries Representing Felix Gonzalez-Torres Are Editing HIV/AIDS from His Legacy: It Needs To Stop', *Artslant* (blog), 2017, https://www.poz.com/article/galleries-representing-felix-gonzalez-torres-editing-hiv-aids-from-his-legacy.

77 Robert Storr, 'When This You See Remember Me', in *Felix Gonzalez-Torres*, ed. Julie Ault (New York and Gottingen: Steidl, 2006), 9; Nicolas Bourriaud, *Relational Aesthetics*, trans. Simon Pleasance and Fronza Woods (Dijon: Presses du reel, 2002), 51.

78 Radley, *Works of Illness*; Tembeck, *Auto/Pathographies*.

79 Nancy Spector, *Felix Gonzalez-Torres* (New York: Guggenheim Museum Publications, 1995), 146.

80 For key examples of such talks, see Interview at the Bronx Museum of Art with Sur Rodney (Sur) and Kia Labeija, 12 February 2016, https://youtu.be/AOLShR_Vq48; *Art AIDS America Chicago: Artist Kia Labeija in Conversation with Zac Stafford* (Chicago: Alphawood Foundation, 2017), http://artaidsamericachicago.org/event-videos/; *Living Free: Kia Labeija, from Pathology to Wholeness* (Stanford University, 2017), https://www.youtube.com/watch?v=7jrbUspNXkE.

Chapter 1

1 Center for Disease Control, 'Pneumocystis Pneumonia – Los Angeles', *Morbidity and Mortality Weekly Report*, 30, no. 21 (5 June 1981): 250–2.

2 Lawrence K. Altman, 'Rare Cancer Seen in 41 Homosexuals', *The New York Times*, 3 July 1981.

3 For an account of how prostitutes (and women in general) lost their presence on the AIDS research agenda, see Treichler, *How to Have Theory in an Epidemic*, 42–59.

4 John Langone, 'AIDS: The Latest Scientific Facts', *Discover*, December 1985, 27–52; quoted in Treichler, 'AIDS, Homophobia and Biomedical Discourse', 37.

5 Treichler, *How to Have Theory in an Epidemic*, 74.

6 *Newsweek*, 12 August 1985. For a sustained consideration of the significance of Rock Hudson's illness, see Richard Meyer, 'Rock Hudson's Body', in *The Passionate Camera: Photography and Bodies of Desire*, ed. Deborah Bright (London and New York: Routledge, 1998), 341–60.

7 *Life*, no. 8 (July 1985).

8 Bonnie Johnson, 'A Life Stolen Early', *People* 34, no. 16 (22 October 1990): 70–3 (72).

9 Douglas Crimp, 'How to Have Promiscuity in an Epidemic', *October* 43 (Winter 1987): 270.
10 Crimp, 'How to Have Promiscuity in an Epidemic', 249.
11 Watney, *Policing Desire*, 3.
12 Crimp, 'How to Have Promiscuity in an Epidemic', 250.
13 Randy Shilts, *And the Band Played On* (London and New York: Penguin, 1987), 120.
14 Shilts, *And the Band Played On*, 166.
15 Larry Kramer, *The Normal Heart* (London: Methuen and the Royal Court Theatre, 1986), 115; cited in Shilts, *And the Band Played On*.
16 Crimp, 'How to Have Promiscuity in an Epidemic', 242–4.
17 Crimp, 'How to Have Promiscuity in an Epidemic', 253.
18 Crimp, 'How to Have Promiscuity in an Epidemic', 252.
19 For an account of the setting up of ACT UP, see Deborah Gould, *Moving Politics: Emotion and ACT UP's Fight against AIDS* (Chicago and London: University of Chicago Press, 2009), 4–6.
20 Gould, *Moving Politics*, 4.
21 See for example Chapter Three, 'The Pleasures and Intensities of Activism' in Gould, *Moving Politics*, 181–212.
22 Gregg Bordowitz, 'My Postmodernism', in *The AIDS Crisis Is Ridiculous and Other Writings: 1986-2003*, by Gregg Bordowitz, ed. James Meyer (Cambridge, MA: MIT Press, 2004), 236. 'My Postmodernism' was originally published in *Artforum* 41, no. 7 (2003): 226–9 and 273–4.
23 Douglas Crimp, Interview with Douglas Crimp: ACT UP Oral History Project, interview by Sarah Schulman, 16 May 2007, 17–18, www.actuporalhistory.org/interviews/images/Crimp.pdf.
24 Marek Kohen, 'Ways of Seeing Pornography', *New Statesman* (London), 11 December 1987. Quoted in Watney, *Policing Desire*, x.
25 Crimp, 'AIDS', 3.
26 Bordowitz, 'My Postmodernism', 221.
27 Nancy E. Stoller, 'Foucault in the Streets: New York City Act(s) UP', in *Lessons from the Damned: Queers, Whores, and Junkies Respond to AIDS*, ed. Nancy E. Stoller (New York and London: Routledge, 1988), 114. In addition to those reasons listed by Stoller, we might speculate that Foucault's own death in 1984 from an AIDS-related condition gave his work an additional resonance in the activist context.
28 David Halperin, *Saint Foucault: Towards a Gay Hagiography* (New York and Oxford: Oxford University Press, 1995), 26.
29 Halperin, *Saint Foucault*, 15.
30 Douglas Crimp, 'The Spectacle of Mourning', in *Melancholia and Moralism: Essays on AIDS and Queer Politics* (Cambridge, MA: MIT Press, 2002), 196.

31 Douglas Crimp, 'On the Museum's Ruins', *October* 13 (1980): 41–57.; Douglas Crimp, 'The End of Painting', *October* 16 (n.d.): 69–86.; Michel Foucault, *The Order of Things*, trans. Tavistock / Routledge, 1970 (London and New York: Routledge, 1989).
32 Watney, *Policing Desire*, 18.
33 Watney, *Policing Desire*, 8.
34 Michel Foucault, *Discipline and Punish: The Birth of the Prison*, trans. Alan Sheridan (London: Penguin, 1991), 25. Quoted in Watney, *Policing Desire*, 16.
35 For a detailed history of the Silence=Death project, see Finkelstein, *After Silence*, 27–57.
36 Finkelstein, *After Silence*, 46.
37 For an account of Silence=Death's transformation from poster to placard, see Jack Lowery, *It Was Vulgar and It Was Beautiful: How AIDS Activists Used Art to Fight a Pandemic* (New York: Bold Type Books, 2022), 49–61.
38 William Olander, 'The Window on Broadway by ACT UP/On View at the New Museum, November 20, 1987, to January 24, 1988', 20 November 1987, New Museum Digital Archive, http://archive.newmuseum.org/index.php/Detail/Object/Show/object_id/7910.
39 Simon Leung, quoted in Howard Singerman, 'In Theory and Practice: A History of the Whitney Independent Study Program', *Artforum*, February 2004, 112–17 and 170–1.
40 Crimp, 'AIDS', 3–16.
41 Gran Fury, 'Art and Politics of the 1980s: Language in the Public Sphere: Gran Fury (Tom Kalin and Members) and Helen Molesworth' (panel discussion, Columbia University, NYC, 12 November 2012). See also Alexis Clements, 'We Were Not Making Art, We Were at War', 21 November 2012, http://hyperallergic.com/60650/gran-fury-in-2012/.
42 Robert Rosenblum, 'Life Versus Death: The Art World in Crisis'', in *Art against AIDS* (New York: American Foundation for AIDS Research, 1987), 29–30.
43 Rosenblum, 'Life Versus Death', 32.
44 Crimp, 'AIDS', 7.
45 Crimp, 'AIDS', 6.
46 Crimp, 'AIDS', 7.
47 Deitcher, 'What Does Silence Equal Now?', 99.
48 Deitcher, 'What Does Silence Equal Now?', 99.
49 Hal Foster, 'Postmodernism: A Preface', in *Postmodern Culture*, ed. Hal Foster (London: Pluto Press, 1985), ix–x.
50 Douglas Crimp, 'On the Museum's Ruins', in *Postmodern Culture*, ed. Hal Foster (London: Pluto Press, 1985), 43–56. This essay was originally published in *October* 13 (1980): 41–57; all citations from this point onwards refer to the version in Foster's volume.

51 Crimp, 'On the Museum's Ruins', 53.

52 John Roberts, 'The Museum and the Crisis of Critical Postmodernism', *Third Text* 11, no. 41 (1997): 71.

53 Gran Fury, Gran Fury talks to Douglas Crimp, interview by Douglas Crimp, April 2003, http://www.artforum.com/inprint/id=4466.

54 Cited by Crimp, 'AIDS', 7.

55 Crimp and Rolston, *AIDS Demographics*, 15.

56 For a reasonably balanced account of Reagan's response to AIDS, see Jennifer Brier, *Infectious Ideas: U.S. Political Responses to the AIDS Crisis* (North Carolina: University of North Carolina Press, 2009), 78–121. Also see Carrie C. Sheehan, 'Securitizing the HIV / AIDS Pandemic in U.S. Foreign Policy' (Doctoral Thesis, Washington, DC: American University, 2008). Paula Treichler suggests that Reagan's first public address about AIDS took place on 1 April 1987, where he spoke with approval of mandatory testing (Treichler, *How to Have Theory in an Epidemic*, 57). Other sources suggest that Reagan's first speech devoted exclusively to AIDS was delivered on 1 June 1987, to attendees at a benefit dinner for the Association for AIDS Research; according to reports in *The New York Times* he was booed for his suggestion of mandatory testing. (http://www.nytimes.com/1987/06/01/us/reagan-urges-wide-aids-testing-but-does-not-call-for-compulsion.html?pagewanted=all&src=pm).

57 Lee Edelman, *Homographesis: Essays in Gay Literature and Cultural Theory* (New York and London: Routledge, 1994), 79–92.

58 Cited by Crimp, 'AIDS', 7.

59 Olander, 'The Window on Broadway by ACT UP'.

60 Diane Waldman, 'The Language of Signs', in *Jenny Holzer*, ed. Diane Waldman (New York: Guggenheim Museum Publications, 1989), 9–14.

61 Ann Goldstein, 'Bring in the World', in *Barbara Kruger*, ed. Ann Goldstein (Los Angeles: The Museum of Contemporary Art, Los Angeles, 1999), 31.

62 Goldstein, 'Bring in the World', 35.

63 Interview with AA Bronson, in L'Ecole du Magasin, ed., *AIDS RIOT: Artist Collectives against AIDS, New York, 1987–94*, 12e Session de l'Ecole Du Magasin (Grenoble: Magasin, 2003), 269–74.

64 Gregg Bordowitz, *General Idea: Imagevirus* (London: Afterall, 2010), 12.

65 Deitcher, 'What Does Silence Equal Now?', 105.

66 Deitcher, 'What Does Silence Equal Now?', 104.

67 Elizabeth Hess, 'Safe Combat in the Erogenous Zone', *The Village Voice*, 10 January 1989. Hess would have been thinking of Rosalind Solomon's *Portraits in the Time of AIDS*, at the Grey Art Gallery, New York University, 17 May–2 July, 1988, and Nicholas Nixon's *Pictures of People*, at the Museum of Modern Art, New York, 15 September–15 November, 1988; Solomon and Nixon's photographs of people with AIDS will be examined in detail in Chapter 2 of this book.

68 Hess, 'Safe Combat in the Erogenous Zone'.

69 Kim Levin, 'It's Called Denial', *The Village Voice*, 17 January 1989. Reproduced in Julie Ault, ed., *Show and Tell: A Chronicle of Group Material* (London: Four Corners Books, 2010), 154.

70 Bordowitz, *General Idea*, 94.

71 Roland Barthes, 'The Death of the Author', in *Image, Music, Text*, trans. Stephen Heath (London: Fontana, 1977), 142–8.

72 Michel Foucault, 'What Is an Author?', in *The Foucault Reader: An Introduction to Foucault's Thought*, ed. Paul Rabinow (London and New York: Penguin, 1991), 101–20.

73 Gregg Bordowitz, *The AIDS Crisis Is Ridiculous and Other Writings, 1986-2003*, ed. James Meyer (Cambridge, MA: MIT Press, 2004), 67.

74 Bordowitz, *General Idea*, 94.

75 Deitcher, 'What Does Silence Equal Now?', 99–100.

76 Nan Goldin, *The Ballad of Sexual Dependency*, ed. Marvin Heiferman, Mark Holborn, and Suzanne Fletcher (New York and London: Aperture, 1986); Goldin's own work will be examined in the following chapter.

77 Nan Goldin, 'In the Valley of the Shadow', in *Witnesses: Against Our Vanishing* (New York: Artists Space, 1989), 4–5.

78 Philip-Lorca diCorcia, *Hustlers* (Gottingen: Steidl, 2013).

79 John Russell, 'Images of Grief and Rage in Exhibition on AIDS', *The New York Times*, 16 November 1989.

80 For an in-depth account of Witnesses in relation to the culture wars, see Janet Kraynak, 'Nan Goldin's "Witnesses: Against Our Vanishing"', in *Witness to Her Art: Art and Writings*, ed. Michael Brenson and Rhea Anastas (New York: Bard College, 2006), 34–41.

81 Carol S. Vance, 'The Pleasures of Looking: The Attorney General's Commission on Pornography versus Visual Images', in *The Critical Image: Essays on Contemporary Photography*, ed. Carol Squiers (Seattle: Bay Press, 1990), 38–58; cited by Kraynak, 'Nan Goldin's "Witnesses: Against Our Vanishing"', 36.

82 Vance, 'The Pleasures of Looking', 38.

83 Roger Chapman, 'Andres Serrano', in *Culture Wars: An Encyclopedia of Issues, Viewpoints, and Voices*, ed. Roger Chapman (New York: M.E. Sharpe, 2010).

84 Reverend Donald E. Wildmon, cited in Robert Atkins, 'Stream of Conscience: Andres Serrano's "Piss Christ"', *Village Voice*, 30 May 1989.

85 Senator D'Amato, cited in Chapman, 'Andres Serrano', 507.

86 Kraynak, 'Nan Goldin's "Witnesses: Against Our Vanishing"', 37.

87 Robert Teigrob, 'Robert Mapplethorpe', in *Culture Wars: An Encyclopedia of Issues, Viewpoints, and Voices*, ed. Roger Chapman (New York: M.E. Sharpe, 2010).

88 For a full account of Morrisroe's work in *Witnesses,* see Fiona Johnstone, 'Mark Morrisroe's Self-Portraits and Jacques Derrida's "Ruin"', *Third Text* 25 (2011): 799–809.

The exhibition presents all the works listed previously as Morrisroe's own works; in fact Gail Thacker took the final Polaroid picture, and Morrisroe's estate acknowledges it to be Thacker's work rather than Morrisroe's. The Plexiglass box construction was assembled by his partner Ramsey McPhillips, who also wrote Morrisroe's as yet unpublished biography, excerpts from which were included in the exhibition.

89 Cynthia Carr, *Fire in the Belly: The Life and Times of David Wojnarowicz* (New York: Bloomsbury, 2012), 392.

90 David Wojnarowicz, 'Postcards from America: X-Rays from Hell', in *Witnesses: Against Our Vanishing* (New York: Artists Space, 1989), 6 & 7.

91 Wojnarowicz, 'Postcards from America', 7.

92 Douglas Crimp, 'Mourning and Militancy', *October* 51 (1989): 5.

93 Sigmund Freud, 'Mourning and Melancholia', in *On the History of the Psycho-Analytic Movement, Volume XIV (1914-1916)*, vol. XIV (1914-1916), *The Standard Edition of the Complete Psychological Works of Sigmund Freud* (London: Hogarth Press & The Institute of Psychoanalysis, 1993), 243–58. Freud revised his theory of mourning in 'The Ego and the Id' (1923).

94 Freud; cited in Crimp, 'Mourning and Militancy', 1989, 6. The italics are Crimp's.

95 Freud's treatment of mourning as a solitary activity has been widely criticized by commentators who point out that collective mourning rituals are a common feature of most societies. For example, see Darian Leader, *The New Black: Mourning, Melancholia and Depression* (London: Penguin, 2009), 7–8. Also Sturken, *Tangled Memories*, 201.

96 Watney, *Policing Desire*, 7; quoted in Crimp, 'Mourning and Militancy', 1989, 8.

97 Crimp, 'Mourning and Militancy', 1989, 9.

98 Freud, 'Mourning and Melancholia', 136–7.

99 Crimp, 'Mourning and Militancy', 1989, 9.

100 Freud, 'Mourning and Melancholia', 244.

101 Crimp, 'Mourning and Militancy', 1989, 12.

102 Crimp, 'Mourning and Militancy', 1989, 15–16.

103 Douglas Crimp, 'Melancholia and Moralism: An Introduction', in *Melancholia and Moralism: Essays on AIDS and Queer Politics* (Cambridge, MA: MIT Press, 2002), 17.

104 Roberta Smith, 'Response to AIDS Gains in Subtlety', *The New York Times*, 18 February 1994.

105 *Significant Losses: Artists Who Have Died from AIDS*, College Park, University of Maryland, Art Gallery, 2 November to 23 December, 1994.

106 Deitcher, 'What Does Silence Equal Now?', 93.

107 Gran Fury, 'Good Luck . . . Miss You – Gran Fury', in *AIDS RIOT: Artists Collectives against AIDS, 1987–1994*, ed. 12th Session of the Ecole du Magasin (Caroline Engel, Nicholas Fenouillat, Aurélie Guitton, Benedetta di Loreto, Flora Loyau, Ivana Mestrov, Anna Olszewska) (Grenoble: Magasin, 2003), 301–6.

108 Kagan, *Positive Images*.

Chapter 2

1 Nixon, *Pictures of People*; Rosalind Solomon, *Portraits in the Time of AIDS* (Grey Art Gallery, New York University, 17 May–2 July 1988).

2 Douglas Crimp, 'Portraits of People with AIDS', in *Melancholia and Moralism: Essays on AIDS and Queer Politics* (Cambridge, MA: MIT Press, 2002), 83–107; Jan Zita Grover, 'Visible Lesions: Images of the PWA', in *Out in Culture: Gay, Lesbian and Queer Essays on Popular Culture*, ed. Corey K. Creekmur and Alexander Doty (Durham and London: Duke University Press, 1995), 354–81.

3 Grover, 'Visible Lesions', 361.

4 Grover, 'Visible Lesions', 361.

5 'Filme en Direct Quatre Jours Avant Sa Mort'.

6 Sander Gilman, 'AIDS and Syphilis: The Iconography of Disease', *October* 43 (1987): 3. Also Gilman, *Disease and Representation*, 1–3.

7 Gilman, *Disease and Representation*, 1.

8 Grover, 'Visible Lesions', 362; Grover's emphasis.

9 Grover, 'Visible Lesions', 366.

10 Watney, 'The Spectacle of AIDS'.

11 Watney, 'The Spectacle of AIDS', 78.

12 Watney, 'The Spectacle of AIDS', 78; Watney's emphasis.

13 *Bright Eyes* was aired on Channel Four in December 1984 in the late night timeslot *The Eleventh Hour*, a series that showcased independent work. In 1987 it was shown in exhibitions at the New Museum of Contemporary Art, the Museum of Modern Art, and the Kitchen in New York City; and in the programmes of the San Francisco Lesbian and Gay Film Festival, and the Los Angeles Lesbian and Gay Film and Video Festival. For an extended analysis of *Bright Eyes*, see Martha Gever, 'Pictures of Sickness: Stuart Marshall's "Bright Eyes"', *October* 43 (1987): 108–26.

14 See Cesare Lombroso, *Criminal Man*, trans. Mary Gibson and Nicole Hahn Rafter (Durham, NC: Duke University Press, 2006); Lombroso's text was first published in Italian in 1876, and underwent five editions in his lifetime, the final edition being published in 1896–7.

15 Havelock Ellis, *The Criminal*, 4th edition (London: The Walter Scott Publishing Company, 1910).

16 Grover, 'Visible Lesions', 366.

17 A slightly different approach to the relationship between the sick and erotic body is set out in Sander Gilman's analysis of public health posters. Gilman suggests that AIDS awareness posters subvert the cultural assumption that the ill body will be visually marked as ugly, and argues that such images become eroticized precisely to counter the historical associations between homosexuality and deviancy and disease. See 'The Body Beautiful and AIDS' in Gilman, *Health and Illness*, 115–72.

The uncomfortable relationship between illness and eroticism will be taken up in Chapter 3 of this book in relation to Mark Morrisroe's late self-portraits.

18 Crimp, 'Portraits of People with AIDS', 106; Crimp's emphasis. The notion of the PWA as killer is taken up by Leo Bersani in his essay 'Is the Rectum a Grave?', *October* 43 (1987): 197–222; Bersani's text will be explored in Chapter 4 of this book in relation to the work of Robert Blanchon.

19 Shilts, *And the Band Played On*, 198; See also Steven Capsuto's startling observation that 'television usually sexualized GLBT characters only if they were serial killers'; Steven Capsuto, *Alternate Channels: The Uncensored Story of Gay and Lesbian Images on Radio and Television* (New York: Ballantine Books, 2000), 222.

20 Grover, 'Visible Lesions', 357; Grover's emphasis.

21 Several of Rosett's photographs are reproduced in PWA Coalition, 'PWA Coalition Portfolio'.

22 Gregg Bordowitz and David Deitcher, 'Art, Activism, and Everyday Life', *Documents* 11 (1998): 36.

23 Crimp, 'Portraits of People with AIDS', 100.

24 Nicholas Nixon and Bébé Nixon, *People with AIDS* (Boston: David R. Godine, 1991), vii.

25 Peter Galassi, 'Introduction', in *Pictures of People*, ed. Nicholas Nixon (New York: The Museum of Modern Art, New York, 1988), 26.

26 Grover, 'Visible Lesions', 355.

27 'No More Pictures without Context', reproduced in Crimp, 'Portraits of People with AIDS', 87.

28 Crimp, 'Portraits of People with AIDS', 86.

29 Crimp, 'Portraits of People with AIDS', 87.

30 Crimp, 'Portraits of People with AIDS', 87.

31 See 'Artist's Statement', in Rosalind Solomon, *Portraits in the Time of AIDS* (New York: Grey Art Gallery & Study Center, 1988), unpaginated.

32 Grover, 'Visible Lesions', 373 and 374.

33 Crimp, 'Portraits of People with AIDS', 86.

34 Galassi, 'Introduction', 9.

35 Thomas Sokolowski, 'Preface', in *Portraits in the Time of AIDS*, ed. Rosalind Solomon (New York: Grey Art Gallery & Study Center, 1988), unpaginated; my italics.

36 Gary Indiana, untitled interview, *Artforum* 26, no. 6 (February 1988): 77; quoted by Galassi, 'Introduction', 27.

37 Galassi, 'Introduction', 27.

38 Crimp, 'Portraits of People with AIDS', 88.

39 Sokolowski, 'Preface', unpaginated. Despite the liberal rhetoric of this passage, a close reading reveals one of the most important ethical difficulties presented by Nixon and Solomon's exhibitions, which do not constitute portrait galleries of *individuals* with AIDS, so much as a collective portrait *of the disease itself*.

40 Emmanuel Levinas and Richard Kearney, 'Dialogue with Emmanuel Levinas', in *Face to Face with Levinas*, ed. Richard A. Cohen (Albany: State University of New York Press, 1986), 23–4.

41 See for example George Piggford, '"In Time of Plague": AIDS and Its Significations in Hervé Guibert, Tony Kushner and Thom Gunn', *Cultural Critique* 44 (2000): 169–96.; and Ranen Omer-Sherman, 'The Fate of the Other in Tony Kushner's "Angels in America"', *Melus* 32, no. 2 (2007): 7–30.

42 Emmanuel Levinas, *Ethics and Infinity: Conversations with Philippe Nemo*, trans. Richard A. Cohen (Pittsburgh: Duquesne University Press, 1985), 85–6.

43 Levinas, *Ethics and Infinity*, 85–6.

44 Levinas, *Ethics and Infinity*, 87.

45 Judith Butler, *Precarious Life: The Powers of Mourning and Violence* (London and New York: Verso, 2006), 142. Butler does not entirely dismiss the ethical potential of photography. Instead, she proposes the 'critical image' as a means of ensuring humanization through the image. The critical image must work the difference that prevents identification from collapsing into identity. (I can identify with someone only in so far as they are different to me.) It thus must 'not only fail to capture its referent, but *show* this failing' (Butler, *Precarious Life*, 146).

46 Butler, *Precarious Life*, 141 and 143.

47 Judith Butler, *Bodies That Matter* (London and New York: Routledge, 1993), 146.

48 Quoted in Susie Linfield, *The Cruel Radiance: Photography and Political Violence* (Chicago: Chicago University Press, 2011), 5.

49 Susan Sontag, *On Photography* (Harmondsworth: Penguin, 1979), 4.

50 Sontag, *On Photography*, 4.

51 Sontag, *On Photography*, 12.

52 Allan Sekula, *Photography against the Grain: Essays and Photo Works, 1973–83* (Halifax: Press of the Nova Scotia College of Art and Design, 1984). Quoted in Linfield, *The Cruel Radiance*, 7.

53 Allan Sekula, 'The Body and the Archive', *October* 39 (1986): 6.

54 Sekula, 'The Body and the Archive', 10.

55 Galton first proposed his procedure for composite photography in 1877, and its use proliferated over the following three decades. See Sekula, 'The Body and the Archive', 40–54; and Francis Galton, 'Composite Portraits, Made by Combining Those of Many Different Persons into a Single Figure', *The Journal of the Anthropological Institute of Great Britain and Ireland* 8 (1879): 132–44.

56 Sekula, 'The Body and the Archive', 62.

57 Craig Owens, 'The Discourse of Others: Feminists and Postmodernism', in *Postmodern Culture*, ed. Hal Foster (London: Pluto Press, 1985), 69. For a useful overview of the work and its critical reception, see Steve Edwards, *Martha Rosler: The Bowery in Two Inadequate Descriptive Systems* (London: Afterall, 2012).

58 Allan Sekula, 'Dismantling Modernism, Reinventing Documentary (Notes on the Politics of Representation)', *The Massachusetts Review* 19, no. 4 (1978): 867.
59 Sekula, 'Dismantling Modernism, Reinventing Documentary', 867.
60 Martha Rosler, 'In, around, and Afterthoughts (on Documentary Photography)', in *3 Works* (Halifax: The Press of Nova Scotia College of Art and Design, 1981), 59–86.
61 Rosler, 'In, around, and Afterthoughts', 77–8.
62 Rosler, 'In, around, and Afterthoughts', 73. Rosler is not entirely negative about the future of documentary photography; she notes that 'we do not yet have a real documentary' and ponders the possibility that a 'radical' version of the genre might still be brought into existence (p. 80).
63 Crimp, 'Portraits of People with AIDS', 98.
64 Sekula, 'Dismantling Modernism, Reinventing Documentary', 865. Quoted in Crimp, 'Portraits of People with AIDS', 98.
65 Galassi, 'Introduction', 26.
66 Galassi, 'Introduction', 10.
67 Galassi, 'Introduction', 12.
68 Andy Grundberg, 'Nicholas Nixon Seeks a Path to the Heart', *The New York Times*, 11 September 1988, H37.
69 Sontag, *On Photography*, 23.
70 Galassi, 'Introduction', 26; quoted in Crimp, 'Portraits of People with AIDS', 85.
71 Grundberg, 'Nicholas Nixon Seeks a Path to the Heart', 38; quoted in Crimp, 'Portraits of People with AIDS', 84.
72 Galassi, 'Introduction', 27.
73 Grover, 'Visible Lesions', 372.
74 Grover, 'Visible Lesions', 371.
75 Sekula, 'Dismantling Modernism, Reinventing Documentary', 860.
76 Sekula, 'Dismantling Modernism, Reinventing Documentary', 883.
77 Chris Townsend, *Art and Death* (London and New York: I.B. Tauris, 2008), 69.
78 Townsend, *Art and Death*, 76.
79 Townsend, *Art and Death*, 75.
80 Emmanuel Levinas, *God, Death and Time*, trans. B. Bergo (Stanford, CA: Stanford University Press, 2000), 105; quoted in Townsend, *Art and Death*, 75.
81 Townsend, *Art and Death*, 75.
82 Cf. Luc Sante's description of Goldin as a 'portraitist of souls' in Luc Sante, 'All Yesterday's Parties', in *Nan Goldin: I'll Be Your Mirror*, ed. Nan Goldin, David Armstrong and Hans Werner Holzworth (New York: Whitney Museum of American Art, 1996), 103. Also Goldin's comment: 'That whole thing of African tribes having this theory that their soul would be stolen by photography: I think the wrong people had the camera. I always say if you're photographing your own tribe, then there's not actually that danger of the soul being stolen. I think that you

can actually give people access to their own soul.' Nan Goldin, 'On Acceptance: A Conversation. Nan Goldin Talking with David Armstrong and Walter Keller', in *Nan Goldin: I'll Be Your Mirror*, ed. Nan Goldin, David Armstrong and Hans Werner Holzworth (New York: Whitney Museum of American Art, 1996), 103.

83 Marvin Heiferman, 'Pictures of Life and Loss', in *Nan Goldin: I'll Be Your Mirror*, ed. Nan Goldin, David Armstrong and Hans Werner Holzworth (New York: Whitney Museum of American Art, 1996), 277.

84 Jonathan Weinberg, *Fantastic Tales: The Photography of Nan Goldin* (London: Tate Publishing / The Pennsylvania State University Press, 2005), 1.

85 E. Coulthard and Nan Goldin, *I'll Be Your Mirror* (Blast! Films, 1995).

86 Goldin, 'On Acceptance', 454.

87 Goldin, *The Ballad of Sexual Dependency*, 6. We might take as a mild challenge to Goldin's assertion Luc Sante's recollection of attending the slide shows: 'Her pictures sometimes made people uncomfortable. They might be agreeable voyeurs of the splendours and miseries of others, but then there would suddenly flash a shot of them weeping or pissing or listing hard to the lee, and you could feel them stiffen on the folding chair next to yours . . .' Sante, 'All Yesterday's Parties', 101.

88 For an assessment of responses to Goldin's work, see Liz Kotz, 'Aesthetics of "Intimacy"', in *The Passionate Camera: Photography and Bodies of Desire*, ed. Deborah Bright (London and New York: Routledge, 1998), 204.

89 Catherine Lampert, 'Family of Own Gender', in *The Devil's Playground*, ed. Nan Goldin (London: Phaidon, 2003), 56.

90 Deitcher, 'Death and the Marketplace', 44.

91 Goldin, *The Ballad of Sexual Dependency*, 6.

92 Nan Goldin, 'Nan Goldin on Cookie Mueller', *The Digital Journalist. 20 Years: AIDS and Photography* (blog), 2001, http://digitaljournalist.org/issue0106/voices_goldin.htm.

93 Nan Goldin, *Cookie Mueller: Photographs* (New York: Pace/MacGill, 1991).

94 'Nan Goldin: I'll Be Your Mirror', The Whitney Museum of American Art, 3 October 1996–5 January 1997; 'Nan Goldin: Devil's Playground', The Whitechapel Gallery, 26 January–1 April 2002.

95 Elisabeth Sussman, *Nan Goldin: I'll Be Your Mirror* (New York: Whitney Museum of American Art, 1996), 256.

96 Goldin, *Cookie Mueller*, 1. Goldin's text is also reproduced in Sussman, *Nan Goldin*, 256. Goldin's observation in *The Cookie Portfolio* echoes one made almost thirteen years earlier, where Goldin connects her photography practice to the suicide of her older sister: 'recently, I've realized my motivation [to photograph] has deeper roots. I don't really remember my sister. [. . .] I remember my version of her, of the things she said, of the things she meant to me. But I don't remember the tangible sense of who she was, her presence, what her eyes looked like, what her voice sounded like. I don't ever want to be susceptible to anyone else's version of my history. I don't

ever want to lose the real memory of anyone again.' Goldin, *The Ballad of Sexual Dependency*, 9.

97 Barthes, *Camera Lucida*, 77.

98 Barthes, *Camera Lucida*, 76.

99 Nan Goldin, '20 Years: AIDS and Photography', *The Digital Journalist* (blog), June 2001, http://digitaljournalist.org/issue0106/voices_goldin.htm.

100 Kotz, 'Aesthetics of "Intimacy"', 212.

101 Kotz, 'Aesthetics of "Intimacy"', 212.

102 Lukas Engelmann, *Mapping AIDS: Visual Histories of an Enduring Epidemic* (Cambridge: Cambridge University Press, 2018), 92; see also Lukas Engelmann, 'Photographing AIDS: Capturing AIDS in Pictures of People with AIDS', *Bulletin of the History of Medicine* 90, no. 2 (2016): 250–78.

103 Engelmann, *Mapping AIDS*, 48.

104 Bruce Silverstein Gallery, 'Rosalind Solomon. Portraits in the Time of AIDS, 1988. 6 June–2 August 2013' (Press Release, June 2013), https://www.brucesilverstein.com/exhibitions/rosalind-solomon3/press-release; Theodore (Ted) Kerr and Rosalind Solomon, 'People Didn't Want to Look at the Work. Perhaps People Are More Willing to Look at It Now', *The Visual AIDS Blog* (blog), 24 July 2013, https://visualaids.org/blog/people-didnt-want-to-look-at-the-work.-perhaps-people-are-more-willing-to-l; Theodore (Ted) Kerr and Rosalind Solomon, 'I Didn't Know What to Do after the AIDS Project. It Was so Intense', *The Visual AIDS Blog* (blog), 24 July 2013, https://visualaids.org/blog/i-didnt-know-what-to-do-after-the-aids-project.-it-was-so-intense#.UfBFw1Od778.

105 Holland Cotter, 'Rosalind Solomon: Portraits in the Time of AIDS, 1988 [Review]', *New York Times*, 19 July 2013, Late Edition (East Coast) edition, https://www.proquest.com/newspapers/rosalind-solomon-portraits-time-aids-1988/docview/1400944549/se-2.

106 Rosalind Solomon, Oral history interview with Rosalind Fox Solomon, interview by Linda Yablonsky, October 2016, Smithsonian Archives of American Art, https://www.aaa.si.edu/download_pdf_transcript/ajax?record_id=edanmdm-AAADCD_oh_384311.

Chapter 3

1 Bataille, *Erotism*, 11.

2 Jane Hudson, in Teresa Gruber, *'There Was a Sense of Family . . .' The Friends of Mark Morrisroe* (Nurnberg: Verlag fur Moderne Kunst, 2012), 78.

3 Grover, 'Visible Lesions'; Crimp, 'Portraits of People with AIDS'.

4 Grover, 'Visible Lesions', 369.

5 Teresa Gruber, 'Biography', in *Mark Morrisroe*, ed. Beatrix Ruf and Thomas Seelig (Zurich: Ringier Collection, 2010), 442–7.
6 Uncatalogued documentation in the Mark Morrisroe Archive, Fotomuseum Winterthur.
7 Pat Hearn, 'Mark Morrisroe: A Survey from the Estate', in *Boston School: Mark Morrisroe (1959-1980), A Survey from the Estate*, ed. Lia Gangitano (Boston: Institute of Contemporary Art, 1995), 59.
8 Jane Hudon, in Gruber, *'There Was a Sense of Family . . .' The Friends of Mark Morrisroe*, 78.
9 Lia Gangitano, ed., *Boston School: Mark Morrisroe (1969-1989): A Survey from the Estate* (Boston: Institute of Contemporary Art, 1995), 13.
10 Jane Hudson, 'Comments on Mark Morrisroe: The Punk Years at the Museum School', in *Boston School: Mark Morrisroe (1959–80), A Survey from the Estate*, ed. Lia Gangitano (Boston: Institute of Contemporary Art, 1995), 64; Hudson speaking in Gruber, *'There Was a Sense of Family . . .' The Friends of Mark Morrisroe*, 78.
11 Barry Schwabsky, 'Irresponsible Images: The Photographs of Mark Morrisroe', *The Print Collector's Newsletter* 25, no. 2 (June 1994): 49.
12 Linda Yablonsky, 'Mark Morrisroe in New York', in *Mark Morrisroe*, ed. Beatrix Ruf and Thomas Seelig (Zurich: JRP Ringier, 2010), 298.
13 Fionn Meade, 'At the Eleventh Hour', in *Mark Morrisroe*, ed. Beatrix Ruf and Thomas Seelig (Zurich: JRP Ringier, 2010), 134.
14 José Esteban Muñoz, 'Morrisroe's Melodramatics' (presentation, Artists Space, New York, 23 April 2011), http://artistsspace.org/programs/mark-morrisroe-neo-romantic-iconography-and-the-performance-of-self/.
15 David Joselit, 'Mark Morrisroe's Photographic Masquerade', in *Boston School: Mark Morrisroe (1959-1980), A Survey from the Estate*, ed. Lia Gangitano (Boston: Institute of Contemporary Art, 1995), 66–80.
16 Barthes, *Camera Lucida*, 103, 14.
17 Barthes, *Camera Lucida*, 14, 12.
18 Barthes, *Camera Lucida*, 9.
19 Hervé Guibert, *Ghost Image*, trans. Robert Bononno (Los Angeles: Sun & Moon Press, 1996).
20 Hervé Guibert, *To The Friend Who Did Not Save My Life*, trans. by Linda Coverdale (London: Quartet, 1995); *The Compassionate Protocol*, trans. James Kirkup (London: Quartet, 1993); *Cytomegalovirus: A Hospitalization Diary*, trans. Clara Orban and Elliot Weisenberg (Lanham and London: University Press of America, 1996).
21 Guibert, *Ghost Image*, 83.
22 Guibert, *Ghost Image*, 153.
23 The 'spectral turn' also represents a strand of cultural theory in France, Britain and America that embrace the language of ghosts and spectrality, taking its cue

from Jacques Derrida, *Specters of Marx: The State of Debt, the Work of Mourning, and the New International*, trans. Peggy Kamuf (New York and London: Routledge, 1994). See Martin Jay, 'The Uncanny Nineties', in *Cultural Semantics: Keywords of Our Time* (Cambridge, MA: University of Massachusetts Press, 1998), 157–64.

24 Lebovici, 'In the Darkroom', 231.

25 Lebovici, 'In the Darkroom', 232.

26 Lebovici arrives at Freud by way of Leo Bersani's essay 'Foucault, Freud, Fantasy and Power', *GLQ: A Journal of Lesbian and Gay Studies* 2, no. 1–2 (1995): 11–33; I shall return to Bersani's text later in the chapter.

27 Sigmund Freud, *Three Essays on the Theory of Sexuality*, ed. James Strachey (London: Hogarth Press & The Institute of Psychoanalysis, 1962), 49.

28 Elizabeth Grosz, *Space, Time, and Perversion* (New York and London: Routledge, 1995), 196.

29 David Joselit and Collier Schorr, 'Mark Morrisroe: Photographic Process and Psychic Structure' (panel discussion, Artists Space, New York, 16 April 2011).

30 Alphonso Lingis, *Libido* (Albany: SUNY Press, 1985).

31 Grosz, *Space, Time, and Perversion*, 197.

32 Hervé Guibert, 'The Cancerous Image', in *Ghost Image*, trans. Robert Bononno (Los Angeles: Sun & Moon Press, 1996), 154–8.

33 Guibert, 'The Cancerous Image', 155–6.

34 Guibert, 'The Cancerous Image', 156.

35 Guibert, 'The Cancerous Image', 157.

36 Guibert, 'The Cancerous Image', 157.

37 Guibert, 'The Cancerous Image', 158.

38 Laura U. Marks, *The Skin of the Film: Intercultural Cinema, Embodiment, and the Senses* (Durham and London: Duke University Press, 2000).

39 Marks, *The Skin of the Film*, vii.

40 Didier Anzieu, *The Skin Ego*, trans. Chris Turner (New Haven: Yale University Press, 1989), 210.

41 Anzieu, *The Skin Ego*, 17.

42 Quoted in Joselit, 'Mark Morrisroe's Photographic Masquerade', 69.

43 Joan Riviere, 'Womanliness as Masquerade', in *Psychoanalysis and Female Sexuality*, ed. Henrik M Ruitenbeck (New Haven: College and University Press, 1966), 209–20; Mary Ann Doane, 'Film and the Masquerade: Theorising the Female Spectator', *Screen* 23, no. 3–4 (1982): 74–88; Judith Butler, *Gender Trouble* (London and New York: Routledge, 1990). Joselit is careful to distinguish 'performativity' from either 'performance' or 'theatricality', although many accounts of Morrisroe's work treat the terms as if they are interchangeable.

44 Joselit, 'Mark Morrisroe's Photographic Masquerade', 74; Joselit's emphasis.

45 Joselit, 'Mark Morrisroe's Photographic Masquerade', 79; Joselit's emphasis.

46 Ramsey McPhillips, 'Who Turned Out the Limelight? The Tragi-Comedy of Mark Morrisroe', in *Loss Within Loss: Artists in the Age of AIDS*, ed. Edmund White (Madison: University of Wisconsin Press, 2001), 109.
47 Stephen Kern, *The Culture of Time and Space, 1880-1918* (Cambridge, MA: Harvard University Press, 1983), 147.
48 Bettyann Kevles, *Naked to the Bone: Medical Imaging in the Twentieth Century* (New Brunswick: Rutgers University Press, 1997), 130.
49 Robert Mattison, *Robert Rauschenberg: Breaking Boundaries* (New Haven: Yale University Press, 2003), 136.
50 Bice Curiger, *Meret Oppenheim: Defiance in the Face of Freedom* (Cambridge, MA: MIT Press, 1989), 66; see also Renée Riese Hubert, 'From Déjeuner En Fourrure to Caroline: Meret Oppenheim's Chronicle of Surrealism', in *Surrealism and Women*, ed. Mary Ann Caws, Rudolf Kuenzli and Gwen Raaberg (Cambridge, MA: MIT Press, 1991), 46–7.
51 Akira Mizuta Lippit, *Atomic Light (Shadow Optics)* (Minneapolis: University of Minnesota Press, 2005), 52.
52 Lippit, *Atomic Light*, 29–30.
53 Rosalind Krauss, 'Notes on the Index: Part 1', *October* 3 (Spring 1977): 75.
54 Krauss, 'Notes on the Index', 75.
55 Jane Livingston, 'Man Ray and Surrealist Photography', in *L'Amour Fou: Photography & Surrealism*, ed. Rosalind Krauss and Jane Livingston (New York: Abbeville Press, 1985), 128.
56 Livingston, 'Man Ray and Surrealist Photography', 128.
57 Michel Foucault, *The Birth of the Clinic*, trans. A.M. Sheridan (London: Routledge, 1989), 65.
58 Foucault, *The Birth of the Clinic*, 65.
59 Foucault, *The Birth of the Clinic*, 105.
60 See Kevles, *Naked to the Bone*, 265.
61 For a discussion of humoral theory see Gail Kern Paster, *The Body Embarrased: Drama and the Discipline of Shame in Early Modern England* (New York: Cornell University Press, 1993), 1–22; and Nancy Sirasi, *Medieval and Early Renaissance Medicine* (Chicago: University of Chicago Press, 1990), 104–5.
62 Devan Stahl, 'Living into the Imagined Body: How the Diagnostic Image Confronts the Lived Body', *Medical Humanities* 39, no. 1 (2013): 54.
63 Lawrence Chau, 'Mark Morrisroe', *Flash Art*, October 1988.
64 Kevles, *Naked to the Bone*, 120.
65 Linda Dalrymple Henderson, 'X Rays and the Quest for Invisible Reality in the Art of Kupka, Duchamp, and the Cubists', *Art Journal* 47 (Winter 1988): 330.
66 Akira Mizuta Lippit, 'Reflections on Spectral Life', *Discourse* 30, no. 1–2 (2008): 40.

67 Lisa Cartwright, *Screening the Body: Tracing Medicine's Visual Culture* (Minneapolis: University of Minnesota Press, 1995), 117.
68 Cartwright, *Screening the Body*, 115.
69 Cartwright, *Screening the Body*, 115.
70 Thomas Mann, *The Magic Mountain*, trans. H. T. Lowe-Porter (London: Secker and Warburg, 1946), 241.
71 Mann, *The Magic Mountain*, 348.
72 Mann, *The Magic Mountain*, 218–19.
73 Mann, *The Magic Mountain*, 215.
74 Mann, *The Magic Mountain*, 215.
75 Cartwright, *Screening the Body*, 157.
76 Kevles, *Naked to the Bone*, 266.
77 Guibert, *Ghost Image*, 65.
78 Guibert, *Ghost Image*, 110.
79 Rafael Sanchez and Sur Rodney Sur, *The Architecture of Loss: Mark Morrisroe, 1959–89*, April 2011, http://www.thebody.com/visualaids/web_gallery/2011/sanchez/statement_full.html.
80 Sanchez and Sur, *The Architecture of Loss*.
81 Gilman, *Health and Illness*, 66.
82 Kenneth Clark, *The Nude: A Study of Ideal Art* (London: John Murray, 1956), 1.
83 Clark, *The Nude*, 23.
84 For a considered account of art-historical distinctions between nakedness and nudity, see Lynda Nead, *The Female Nude: Art, Obscenity and Sexuality* (London and New York: Routledge, 1992), 12–16.
85 John Berger, *Ways of Seeing* (London and Harmondsworth: BBC and Penguin, 1972), 54.
86 T. J. Clark, *The Painting of Modern Life: Paris in the Art of Manet and His Followers* (London: Thames & Hudson, 1985), 146.
87 Michael Callen, 'Remarks of Michael Callen, American Public Health Association Annual Meeting, Las Vegas, Nevada, 1986', *Surviving and Thriving with AIDS: Hints for the Newly Diagnosed*, March 1987, 40.
88 Laura Mulvey, 'Visual Pleasure and Narrative Cinema', *Screen* 16, no. 3 (1975): 6–18.
89 Mulvey, 'Visual Pleasure and Narrative Cinema', 12; cited in Kenneth MacKinnon, 'After Mulvey: Male Erotic Objectification', in *The Body's Perilous Pleasures: Dangerous Desires and Contemporary Culture*, ed. Michele Aaron (Edinburgh: Edinburgh University Press, 1999), 13. Since the publication of Mulvey's article, counter-claims have been made exploring the existence of a specifically female or homoerotic gaze; nonetheless, much of this work is, as MacKinnon demonstrates, couched in terms that betray a degree of discomfort about regarding the male as passive object rather than active subject.

90 Craig Owens, 'Posing', in *Beyond Recognition: Representation, Power, and Culture*, ed. Scott Bryson, Barbara Kruger, Lynne Tillman and Jane Weinstock (Berkeley: University of California Press, 1992), 201.
91 Dick Hebdige, 'Posing. . . Threats, Striking. . . Poses: Youth, Surveillance, and Display', *SubStance* 37–8 (1983): 86; quoted by Owens, 'Posing', 202.
92 Amelia Jones has explored the 'rhetoric of the pose' at length in relation to the practice of feminist body artist Hannah Wilke.
93 Mapplethorpe died on 9 March 1989, and Morrisroe died four months later on 24 July, suggesting that Mapplethorpe's final self-portrait is likely to have preceded Morrisroe's by several months.
94 Vince Aletti, 'Shot Through the Heart', *Village Voice*, 8 February 2000.
95 Aletti, 'Shot Through the Heart', 67.
96 Peggy Phelan, *Unmarked: The Politics of Performance* (London and New York: Routledge, 1993), 40.
97 Phelan, *Unmarked*, 53.
98 Phelan, *Unmarked*, 40.
99 Richard Meyer, 'Imagining Sadomasochism: Robert Mapplethorpe and the Masquerade of Photography', *Qui Parle* 4, no. 1 (Fall 1990): 76.
100 Meyer, 'Imagining Sadomasochism', 75.
101 Richard Marshall, ed., *Robert Mapplethorpe: Autoportrait* (Santa Fe: Arena Editions, 2001).
102 Meyer, 'Imagining Sadomasochism', 65.
103 Meyer, 'Imagining Sadomasochism', 67.
104 Carrie Sandahl, 'Bob Flanagan: Taking It Like a Man', *Journal of Dramatic Theory and Criticism* XV, no. 1 (2000): 97.
105 Andrea Juno and V. Vale, *Bob Flanagan: Supermasochist* (San Francisco: Research Publications, 1993), 11; cited in Sandahl, 'Bob Flanagan', 101.
106 Sandahl, 'Bob Flanagan', 101.
107 Kirby Dick, *Sick: The Life and Death of Bob Flanagan, Supermasochist* (Lexicon Home Entertainment, 1997); cited in Sandahl, 'Bob Flanagan', 101.
108 Chambers, *Facing It*, 44.
109 Emily Apter, 'Fantom Images: Hervé Guibert and the Writing of "Sida" in France', in *Writing AIDS: Gay Literature, Language, and Analysis*, ed. Timothy F. Murphy and Suzanne Poirier (New York: Columbia University Press, 1993), 87.
110 Owens, 'Posing', 214.
111 Owens, 'Posing', 214; Owens' emphasis.
112 Bersani, 'Foucault, Freud, Fantasy and Power', 23.
113 Bersani, 'Foucault, Freud, Fantasy and Power', 23.
114 Bataille, *Erotism*, 11.
115 Pascal de Duve, *Cargo Vie* (Paris: J.C. Lattes, 1993); trans. and cited in Chambers, *Facing It*, 13–14.

Chapter 4

1 Michel Beaujour, *Poetics of the Literary Self-Portrait*, trans. Yara Milos (New York and London: New York University Press, 1991), 4.
2 Archibald, 'Robert Blanchon's Archive of Absence', 28.
3 Amy Sadao, 'Foreword', in *Robert Blanchon*, ed. Tania Duvergne and Amy Sadao (New York: Visual AIDS, 2006), 9.
4 Freud, 'Mourning and Melancholia', 244.
5 Crimp, 'Melancholia and Moralism', 8.
6 Andrew Sullivan, 'When Plagues End', *The New York Times Magazine*, 10 November 1996, 52–62; 76–7; 84.
7 Crimp, 'Melancholia and Moralism', 4–5.
8 Crimp, 'Melancholia and Moralism', 8.
9 Crimp, 'Melancholia and Moralism', 9.
10 Crimp, 'Melancholia and Moralism', 9.
11 Deitcher, 'Death and the Marketplace', 44.
12 Gran Fury, 'Good Luck . . . Miss You – Gran Fury'.
13 Robert Blanchon Archive, Fales, Box 5, Folder 9.
14 Archibald, 'Robert Blanchon's Archive of Absence', 26.
15 Archibald, 'Robert Blanchon's Archive of Absence', 26.
16 Crimp, 'Mourning and Militancy', 2002, 140.
17 bell hooks, 'Is Paris Burning?', in *Black Looks: Race and Representation* (London: South End Press, 1992), 145–56.
18 Sherrie Levine, 'Five Comments', in *Blasted Allegories: An Anthology of Writing by Contemporary Artists*, ed. Brian Wallis (New York: The New Museum, 1987), 92–3.
19 Foucault, *The History of Sexuality, Volume 1*, 58–73.
20 Julia Kristeva, *Powers of Horror: An Essay on Abjection*, trans. Leon S. Roudiez (New York: Columbia University Press, 1982); Julia Kristeva, *Black Sun: Depression and Melancholia*, trans. Leon S. Roudiez (New York: Columbia University Press, 1989).
21 Watney, 'The Spectacle of AIDS'.
22 Bersani, 'Is the Rectum a Grave?'.
23 Archibald, 'Robert Blanchon's Archive of Absence', 23.
24 Archibald, 'Robert Blanchon's Archive of Absence', 31.
25 Fred Camper, 'Writing on the Wall/Robert Blanchon: Gum, Waste, Indentations, Stains, and Envelopes', *Chicago Reader*, 2 February 1996.
26 Fred Camper, 'Shooting Star', *Chicago Reader*, 26 January 2001.
27 Robert Blanchon Archive, Fales, Box 4, Folder 9.
28 Roberta Smith, 'Felix Gonzalez-Torres, 38, A Sculptor of Love and Loss', *The New York Times*, 11 January 1996.
29 Robert Blanchon Archive, Fales, Box 2, Folder 19.

30 Archibald, 'Robert Blanchon's Archive of Absence', 23.
31 'Disappearing Act', 1998; Leslie Tonkonow Artworks and Projects, and Bound and Unbound, NYC; curated by Kirby Gookin and Robin Kahn.
32 Robert Blanchon Archive, Fales. Box 4, Folder 16.
33 Crimp, 'Mourning and Militancy', 2002, 140.
34 Quoted in Archibald, 'Robert Blanchon's Archive of Absence', 26.
35 Archibald, 'Robert Blanchon's Archive of Absence', 26.
36 Artist's Statement, Fall 1991, Robert Blanchon Archive, Fales, Box 4, Folder 17.
37 Archibald, 'Robert Blanchon's Archive of Absence', 29.
38 The Robert Blanchon Estate Project use parentheses to denote titles used by the artist, and square brackets to denote those added by the Estate; I have chosen to follow the same convention here.
39 See Carr, *Fire in the Belly*, 544.
40 Richard Brilliant, *Portraiture* (London: Reaktion Books, 1991), 62–6.
41 Archibald, 'Robert Blanchon's Archive of Absence', 29.
42 Stephen Spender, 'Confessions and Autobiography', in *Autobiography: Essays Theoretical and Critical*, ed. James Olney (Princeton: Princeton University Press, 1980), 115–21 (p. 116).
43 *Public/ Private*, Betty Rymer Gallery, The School of the Art Institute of Chicago, Chicago, IL, (1992).
44 *Family Affair: Gay and Lesbian Issues of Domestic Life*, Atlanta College of Art, Atlanta, GA (1995).
45 Robert Blanchon Archive, Fales, Box 4, Folder 9.
46 Robert Blanchon, '[never realized]: 4 Opportunistic Infections for Public Viewing and Consumption', in *Robert Blanchon*, ed. Tania Duvergne and Amy Sadao (New York: Visual AIDS, 2006), 109–15 (p. 112).
47 Blanchon, '[never realized]: 4 Opportunistic Infections for Public Viewing and Consumption', 111.
48 Blanchon, '[never realized]: 4 Opportunistic Infections for Public Viewing and Consumption', 111.
49 Blanchon, '[never realized]: 4 Opportunistic Infections for Public Viewing and Consumption', 115.
50 Blanchon, '[never realized]: 4 Opportunistic Infections for Public Viewing and Consumption', 115.
51 Blanchon, '[never realized]: 4 Opportunistic Infections for Public Viewing and Consumption', 115.
52 Sidonie Smith and Julia Watson, *Reading Autobiography: A Guide for Interpreting Life Narratives* (Minneapolis: University of Minnesota Press, 2001), 3.
53 Smith and Watson, *Reading Autobiography*, 3.
54 Barthes, 'The Death of the Author', 142.
55 Chambers, *Facing It*, 7.

56 Chambers, *Facing It*, 8.

57 Robert Blanchon Archive, Fales, Box 5, Folder 9.

58 Camper, 'Writing on the Wall/Robert Blanchon'.

59 Tania Duvergne and Amy Sadao, eds., *Robert Blanchon* (New York: Visual AIDS, 2006), 160.

60 Beaujour, *Poetics of the Literary Self-Portrait*, 4.

61 Smith and Watson, *Reading Autobiography*, 70.

62 Michel Leiris, *Scratches*, trans. Lydia Davis, The Rules of the Game (Baltimore and London: Johns Hopkins University Press, 1991), i, 14.

63 Kristeva, *Powers of Horror*.

64 Melissa E. Feldman, 'The Portrait: From Somebody to Nobody', in *Face-Off: The Portrait in Recent Art*, ed. Melissa E. Feldman (Philadelphia: Institute of Contemporary Art, University of Pennsylvania, 1994), 10.

65 Feldman, 'The Portrait', 10.

66 Christine Fanthome, 'The Influence and Treatment of Autobiography in Confessional Art: Observations on Tracey Emin's Feature Film Top Spot', *Biography* 29 (2006): 30–42. Born in the same year as Blanchon, Emin's most famous confessional works, *Everyone I Have Ever Slept With* (1995) and *My Bed* (1999) were produced, respectively, one year before and three years after Blanchon's installation.

67 Sidonie Smith and Julia Watson, 'The Rumpled Bed of Autobiography: Extravagant Lives, Extravagant Questions', *Biography* 24, no. 1 (Winter 2001): 5.

68 Hallas, *Reframing Bodies*, 113.

69 Foucault, *The History of Sexuality, Vol. 1*, 59.

70 Kristeva, *Powers of Horror*, 3.

71 Jack Ben-Levi et al., 'Introduction', in *Abject Art: Repulsion and Desire in American Art* (New York: Whitney Museum of American Art, 1993), 7.

72 Ben-Levi et al., 'Introduction', 7.

73 Simon Taylor, 'The Phobic Object: Abjection in Contemporary Art', in *Abject Art: Repulsion and Desire in American Art* (New York: Whitney Museum of American Art, 1993), 59–83.

74 Kristeva, *Black Sun*, 4.

75 Kristeva, *Black Sun*, 12.

76 Sigmund Freud, *The Interpretation of Dreams*, trans. James Strachey, The Penguin Freud Library, eighth edition (London and New York: Penguin, 1976), IV, 507.

77 Sigmund Freud, 'Fragment of an Analysis of a Case Study of Hysteria (1905 [1901])', in *A Case of Hysteria: Three Essays on Sexuality and Other Works, Vol. VII (1901-1905)*, The Standard Edition of the Complete Psychological Works of Sigmund Freud (London: Hogarth Press & The Institute of Psychoanalysis, 1953), 1–122.

78 Camper, 'Writing on the Wall/Robert Blanchon'.
79 Robert Blanchon Archive, Fales, Box 5, Folder 9.
80 Freud, 'Mourning and Melancholia', 243.
81 Kristeva, *Black Sun*, 7.
82 Watney, 'The Spectacle of AIDS', 80.
83 Watney, 'The Spectacle of AIDS', 77.
84 Watney, 'The Spectacle of AIDS', 77.
85 Watney, 'The Spectacle of AIDS', 73.
86 Watney, 'The Spectacle of AIDS', 79.
87 Laura Mulvey, 'A Phantasmagoria of the Female Body: The Work of Cindy Sherman', *New Left Review* 1, no. 188 (August 1991): 138.
88 Mulvey, 'A Phantasmagoria of the Female Body', 145.
89 Mulvey, 'A Phantasmagoria of the Female Body', 148.
90 Watney, 'The Spectacle of AIDS', 83.
91 Crimp, 'How to Have Promiscuity in an Epidemic', 253.
92 Grover, 'Visible Lesions', 357.
93 Peter Stallybrass and Allon White, 'The Sewer, the Gaze and the Contaminating Touch', in *The Politics and Poetics of Transgression* (London: Methuen, 1986), 125–48.
94 Georges Bataille, *Visions of Excess: Selected Writings, 1927-1939*, ed. and trans. Allan Stoekl (Minneapolis: University of Minnesota Press, 1985), 31.
95 Bataille, *Visions of Excess*, 31.
96 In the context of abstract expressionism the most frequent use of the phrase 'stain' occurs in relation to a female artist, Helen Frankenthaler; Lisa Saltzmann proposes that the stain is culturally associated with femininity (Lisa Saltzmann, 'Reconsidering the Stain: On Gender, Identity, and the New York School Painting', in *Reading Abstract Expressionism: Context and Critique*, ed. Ellen Landau (New Haven: Yale University Press, 2005), 560–80.) Pollock is typically constructed in virile, masculine American terms, with his pored and dripped paintings seen as explicitly sexual, 'casting paint like seed . . . It was, demonstrably, the real thing . . . painting composed of . . . ejaculatory splat' (William Feaver, 'The Kid from Cody', (1979), as quoted in Anna C. Chave, 'Pollock and Krasner: Script and Postscript', in *Pollock and After: The Critical Debate*, 2nd Edition (London and New York: Routledge, 2000, 329–47.) Blanchon's sad, spent little stains provide a striking counterpart and convey a visceral bodily negativity that might be more easily associated with the female body.
97 Rosalind Krauss, *The Optical Unconscious* (Cambridge, MA: MIT Press, 1993).
98 Krauss, *The Optical Unconscious*, 245.
99 Krauss, *The Optical Unconscious*, 276.

100 Rosalind Krauss, 'The Crisis of the Easel Picture', in *Jackson Pollock: New Approaches*, ed. Kirk Varnedoe and Pepe Karmel (New York: The Museum of Modern Art & Harry Abrams, 1999), 155–79.

101 Camper, 'Writing on the Wall/Robert Blanchon'.

102 Steve Knezevich, 'Robert Blanchon at LACPS', *LA Weekly*, 26 December 1996.

103 For an account of the sinks, urinals and drains, see Richard Flood, 'The Law of Indirections', in *Robert Gober: Sculpture and Drawing*, ed. Richard Flood, Gary Garrels, and Ann Temkin (Minneapolis: Walker Arts Center, 1999), 22.

104 Robert Gober, 'Interview: Richard Flood and Robert Gober', in *Robert Gober: Sculpture and Drawing*, ed. Richard Flood, Gary Garrels and Ann Temkin (Minneapolis: Walker Arts Center, 1999), 123.

105 See Elisabeth Sussman on the multiple interpretations of the drain: Elisabeth Sussman, 'Robert Gober: Installation and Sculpture', in *Robert Gober: Sculptures and Installations, 1979-2007*, ed. Theodora Vischer (Basel: Schaulager Basel, 2007), 24.

106 Helen Molesworth, 'Stops and Starts', *October* 92 (2000): 161.

107 Flood, 'The Law of Indirections', 12.

108 Flood, 'The Law of Indirections', 12.

109 Gober, 'Interview', 128.

110 In response to Craig Gholson's question about Duchamp's urinal, Gober states: 'They [the critics] say it preoccupies me, but to me what's interesting is that it seems to be preoccupying them. They're the ones who are always writing about it, not me. It's not a piece that particularly lives in my soul. It's an interesting piece, it's a great piece, but it seems to be on their minds, not mind.' Robert Gober, in Robert Gober by Craig Gholson, 1989, http://bombmagazine.org/article/1252/robert-gober (accessed 28 April 2014).

111 Sussman, 'Robert Gober', 19.

112 Flood, 'The Law of Indirections', 11.

113 Some important examples of this include Anna C. Chave, 'Minimalism and Biography', *The Art Bulletin* 82, no. 1 (2000): 149–63; and Susan Best, *Visualizing Feeling: Affect and the Feminine Avant-Garde* (London and New York: I.B. Tauris, 2011).

114 Hal Foster, 'The Crux of Minimalism', in *The Return of the Real: Art and Theory at the End of the Century* (Cambridge, MA: MIT Press, 1996), 59.

115 Foster, 'The Crux of Minimalism', 59.

116 Foster, 'The Crux of Minimalism', 50.

117 Michael Fried, 'Art and Objecthood', in *Art in Theory, 1900-2000*, ed. Charles Harrison and Paul Wood (Oxford: Blackwell, 1992), 840; Fried's emphasis.

118 Freud, *The Interpretation of Dreams*, 474.

119 Knezevich, 'Robert Blanchon at LACPS', 41.

120 Butler, *Bodies That Matter*, 61.

121 Robert Blanchon Archive, Fales, Box 4, Folder 7.
122 Bersani, 'Is the Rectum a Grave?'.
123 Bersani, 'Is the Rectum a Grave?', 211–12; Bersani's emphasis.
124 Bersani, 'Is the Rectum a Grave?', 212.
125 Bersani, 'Is the Rectum a Grave?', 217.
126 Lee Edelman, *No Future: Queer Theory and the Death Drive* (Durham and London: Duke University Press, 2004), 2.
127 Edelman, *No Future*, 3.
128 Edelman, *No Future*, 3.
129 Edelman, *No Future*, 5.
130 For an account of the gains to be made by gay men and women from deliberately adopting an abject subject position, see Craig Houser, 'I, Abject', in *Abject Art: Repulsion and Desire in American Art*, ed. Jack Ben-Levi et al. (New York: Whitney Museum of American Art, 1993), 85–100.

Chapter 5

1 Gunhild Hagestad, 'On-Time, off-Time, out of Time? Reflections of Continuity and Discontinuity from an Illness Perspective', in *Adulthood and Aging: Research on Continuities and Discontinuities*, ed. V. L. Bengston (New York: Springer, 1996), 204–22; quoted in Jackie Stacey and Mary Bryson, 'Queering the Temporality of Cancer Survivorship', *Aporia* 4 (2012): 5–17; emphasis in original.
2 Crimp, Interview with Douglas Crimp: ACT UP Oral History Project, 44.
3 Douglas Crimp, *Melancholia and Moralism: Essays on AIDS and Queer Politics* (Cambridge, MA: MIT Press, 2002).
4 Douglas Crimp, 'AIDS: Cultural Analysis / Cultural Activism', *October* 43, no. Winter (1987): 16; Crimp's essay is addressed in detail in chapter one of this book.
5 Crimp, Interview with Douglas Crimp: ACT UP Oral History Project, 46.
6 Robert Nickas, 'Felix Gonzalez-Torres: All the Time in the World', in *Felix Gonzalez-Torres*, ed. Julie Ault (New York and Gottingen: Steidl, 2006), 40. This interview was originally published in *Flash Art*, 161 (1991), 86-89; all citations in this book refer to the 2006 version.
7 Andrea Rosen, '*"Untitled" (The Neverending Portrait)*', in *Felix Gonzalez-Torres*, ed. Dietmar Elger (Stuttgart: Cantz Verlag, 1997), 54.
8 Rosen, '*"Untitled" (The Neverending Portrait)*', 56.
9 Spector, *Felix Gonzalez-Torres*, 171.
10 Storr, 'When This You See Remember Me', 9.

11 Rosen, '"*Untitled" (The Neverending Portrait)*', 44.
12 Amanda Cruz, Suzanne Ghez, and Ann Goldstein, 'Reflections on a Proposal for 1995', in *Felix Gonzalez-Torres: America*, ed. Nancy Spector (New York: Guggenheim Museum Publications, 2007), 57.
13 Katz, 'How AIDS Changed American Art'.
14 Jones, 'Galleries Representing Felix Gonzalez-Torres Are Editing HIV/AIDS from His Legacy'.
15 Elizabeth Freeman, *Time Binds: Queer Temporalities, Queer Histories* (Durham and London: Duke University Press, 2010), 3.
16 For example, see Carolyn Dinshaw et al., 'Theorizing Queer Temporalities: A Roundtable Discussion', *GLQ: A Journal of Lesbian and Gay Studies* 13, no. 2–3 (2007): 177–95.
17 Alison Kafer, *Feminist, Queer, Crip* (Bloomington and Indianapolis: Indiana University Press, 2013).
18 Gonzalez-Torres created approximately fifty-six jigsaw puzzles in this way. See Deborah Cullen, 'Felix Gonzalez-Torres: The Jigsaw Puzzles', in *Searching for Sebald: Photography as W.G. Sebald*, ed. Lise Patt and Christel Dillbohner (Los Angeles: ICI Press, 2007), 350–9 for more information on the jigsaw works.
19 Rosen, '"*Untitled" (The Neverending Portrait)*', 51.
20 Barthes, *Camera Lucida*, 91.
21 Barthes, *Camera Lucida*, 91.
22 Barthes, *Camera Lucida*, 89.
23 Rosen, '"*Untitled" (The Neverending Portrait)*', 50.
24 Lewis Baltz, '(Sans Titre), Felix Gonzalez-Torres', in *Felix Gonzalez-Torres*, ed. Julie Ault (New York and Gottingen: Steidl, 2006), 214.
25 Julie Ault, ed., *Felix Gonzalez-Torres* (New York and Gottingen: Steidl, 2006), 170.
26 Co-ownership agreement accompanying the certificate for *'Untitled'*, 1989. Quoted in Miwon Kwon, 'The Becoming of a Work of Art: FGT and a Possibility of Renewal, a Chance to Share, a Fragile Truce', in *Felix Gonzalez-Torres*, ed. Julie Ault (New York and Gottingen: Steidl, 2006), 308.
27 Kwon, 'The Becoming of a Work of Art', 308.
28 Rosen, '"*Untitled" (The Neverending Portrait)*', 51; Rosen's emphasis.
29 Rosen, '"*Untitled" (The Neverending Portrait)*', 52.
30 Ault, *Felix Gonzalez-Torres*, 171.
31 Letter to Robert Vifian, dated 3 December 1994, in Ault, 170–1.
32 Barthes, 'The Death of the Author', 148.
33 Kwon, 'The Becoming of a Work of Art', 305.
34 Kwon, 'The Becoming of a Work of Art', 309.
35 Kwon, 'The Becoming of a Work of Art', 309.
36 A rule around the work is that the clocks can fall out of synchrony, but if one of the clocks stops, they should be fixed or replaced, as the case may be.

37 Nickas, 'Felix Gonzalez-Torres', 40.
38 Storr, 'Être Un Espion', 233. This interview was originally published in *Art Press* 198 (1995): 24–32; all citations refer to the 2006 version.
39 Storr, 'When This You See Remember Me', 9.
40 Storr, 'Être Un Espion', 238.
41 On Gonzalez-Torres and Minimalism, see also Spector, *Felix Gonzalez-Torres*, 156–7.
42 Jan Avgikos, 'This Is My Body: Felix Gonzalez-Torres', *Artforum* 29, no. 6 (February 1991): 81 and 82.
43 Bourriaud, *Relational Aesthetics*, 50.
44 Bourriaud, *Relational Aesthetics*, 51.
45 Bourriaud, *Relational Aesthetics*, 50.
46 Bourriaud, *Relational Aesthetics*, 14.
47 Bourriaud, *Relational Aesthetics*, 56.
48 Bourriaud, *Relational Aesthetics*, 59. Bourriaud's account of the time span of relational art can be compared to Fried's critique of the 'temporal' aspect of the Minimalist object. A sensation of endlessness is central to the experience of minimal art, and Fried understands this indefinite duration is paradigmatically theatrical: 'as though theatre confronts the beholder, and thereby isolates him, with the endlessness not just of objecthood but of time both passing and to come, simultaneously approaching and receding, as if apprehended in an infinite perspective.' In modernist painting and sculpture, the experience of it has no duration, because such works are timeless and eternal, and entirely present within themselves. Fried concludes: 'presentness is grace'. Minimalist art is thus by inference non-present: it exists only in time, not in itself. See Fried, 'Art and Objecthood', 843–4. When Bourriaud claims that the experience of the Minimalist object is spatial rather than temporal, my suspicion is that he is wilfully misreading Fried.
49 Reproduced in Ault, *Felix Gonzalez-Torres*, 155.
50 Maurice Merleau-Ponty, *The Phenomenology of Perception*, trans. Colin Smith (London and New York: Routledge, 2002), 482.
51 María Puig de la Bellacasa, *Matters of Care: Speculative Ethics in More than Human Worlds* (Minneapolis: University of Minnesota Press, 2017), 206.
52 On temporal practices and healthcare, see Lisa Baraister and William Brook, 'Watchful Waiting: Temporalities of Crisis and Care in the UK National Health Service', in *Vulnerability and the Politics of Care*, ed. Victoria Browne et al., vol. 235, Proceedings of the British Academy (Oxford: Oxford University Press, n.d.), 230–47.
53 Nickas, 'Felix Gonzalez-Torres', 45.
54 Stacey and Bryson, 'Queering the Temporality of Cancer Survivorship', 6.
55 Stacey and Bryson, 'Queering the Temporality of Cancer Survivorship', 11.

56 Stacey and Bryson, 'Queering the Temporality of Cancer Survivorship', 15.
57 Stacey and Bryson, 'Queering the Temporality of Cancer Survivorship', 15.
58 Stacey and Bryson, 'Queering the Temporality of Cancer Survivorship', 15.
59 Judith Halberstam, *In a Queer Time and Place: Transgender Bodies, Subcultural Lives* (New York and London: New York University Press, 2005), 2; Elizabeth Freeman, 'Introduction', *GLQ: A Journal of Lesbian and Gay Studies* 13, no. 2–3 (2007): 162.
60 Simon Watney, 'In Purgatory: The Work of Felix Gonzalez-Torres', *Parkett* 39 (1994): 38.
61 Watney, 'In Purgatory', 38.
62 Watney, 'In Purgatory', 40.
63 'Supreme Court 1986' refers to the Supreme Court's decision on *Bowers v Hardwick*, which effectively criminalized certain sexual activities when carried out by two (consenting) male adults; gay men thus had no protection from state jurisdiction, even in the supposed 'privacy' of their own bedrooms. See Spector, *Felix Gonzalez-Torres*, 23–5.
64 Watney, 'In Purgatory', 41. Watney is quoting from Robert Nickas' interview, 'Felix Gonzalez-Torres: All the Time in the World', *Flash Art* 161 (1911): 86-89.
65 As Gonzalez-Torres insisted, 'aesthetics are politics. They're not even *about* politics, they *are* politics'. Storr, 'Être Un Espion', 234.
66 Adair Rounthwaite, 'Split Witness: Metaphorical Extensions of Life in the Art of Felix Gonzalez-Torres', *Representations* 109 (Winter 2010): 36.
67 Rounthwaite, 'Split Witness', 49.
68 The only exception to this was a new work, consisting of two white Carrara marble pools, and described in terms totally different from those usually used to describe the other paired works, as 'two adjoining reflecting pools that form a figure of eight, the sign of infinity, as both a silent mirror on our collective culture and a beacon of hope'. Rounthwaite, 'Split Witness', 50.
69 Rounthwaite, 'Split Witness', 51.
70 Rounthwaite, 'Split Witness', 40.
71 Ross Chambers, *Untimely Interventions: AIDS Writing, Testimonial, and the Rhetoric of Haunting* (Ann Arbor: University of Michigan Press, 2004), 260; cited in Rounthwaite, 'Split Witness', 40.
72 Chambers, *Untimely Interventions*, 227–8; cited in Rounthwaite, 'Split Witness', 42.
73 Rounthwaite, 'Split Witness', 42.
74 Nickas, 'Felix Gonzalez-Torres', 51.
75 Rounthwaite, 'Split Witness', 36.
76 Freeman, *Time Binds*, 68.
77 Freeman, *Time Binds*, 62.
78 Freeman, *Time Binds*, 65.

79 On temporal folding, see Michel Serres' discussion of baker's dough in Michel Serres, *Rome: The Book of Foundations* (Stanford: Stanford University Press, 1991), 81; see also Lisa Baraitser's discussion of Serres in Lisa Baraister, *Enduring Time* (London and New York: Bloomsbury, 2017), 32–45.
80 I am thinking here of Freeman's ironic reference to the anachronistic lesbian feminist as the 'big drag': see Freeman, *Time Binds*, 59–65.
81 Butler, *Gender Trouble*, 198–9.
82 Spector, *Felix Gonzalez-Torres*, 146.
83 Rosen, '*"Untitled" (The Neverending Portrait)*', 56.
84 Storr, 'When This You See Remember Me', 8.
85 Katz, 'Hide/Seek'.
86 Spector, *Felix Gonzalez-Torres*, 147.
87 Spector, *Felix Gonzalez-Torres*, 150.
88 Kwon, 'The Becoming of a Work of Art', 287.
89 Storr, 'Être Un Espion', 239.
90 In the interview with Storr, Gonzalez-Torres directly refers to that pain, and his desire to control it: 'I'm going to destroy it [the work] before it destroys me. That was my little amount of power when it came to this work. I didn't want it to last, because then it couldn't hurt me. [. . .] I control that pain. That's really what it is'. Storr, 'Être Un Espion', 239.
91 Rosen, '*"Untitled" (The Neverending Portrait)*', 47.
92 Tim Rollins, 'Felix Gonzalez-Torres: Interview', in *Felix Gonzalez-Torres*, ed. William S. Bartman (New York: ART Press, 1993), 28.
93 Freccero, speaking in Dinshaw et al., 'Theorizing Queer Temporalities', 193.
94 Freccero, speaking in Dinshaw et al., 'Theorizing Queer Temporalities', 193.
95 Storr, 'Être Un Espion', 239.
96 Sigmund Freud, 'Beyond the Pleasure Principle (1920)', in *Beyond the Pleasure Principle, Group Psychology and Other Works, Vol. XVIII (1920-1922)*, vol. XVIII, The Standard Edition of the Complete Psychological Works of Sigmund Freud (London: Hogarth Press & The Institute of Psychoanalysis, 1955), 7–64.
97 Freud, 'Beyond the Pleasure Principle (1920)', 16.
98 Rollins, 'Felix Gonzalez-Torres', 13.
99 Sigmund Freud, 'Remembering, Repeating and Working Through (Further Recommendations on the Technique of Psycho-Analysis) (1914)', in *The Case of Schreber, Papers on Technique, and Other Works, Vol. XII (1911-1913)*, vol. XII, The Standard Edition of the Complete Psychological Works of Sigmund Freud (London: The Hogarth Press and the Institute of Psychoanalysis, 1958), 145–56.
100 Freud, 'Remembering, Repeating and Working Through', 148.
101 Freud considered melancholia a pathological form of 'incomplete' mourning, see Sigmund Freud, 'Mourning and Melancholia', in *On the History of the Psycho-*

Analytic Movement, Volume XIV (1914-1916), The Standard Edition of the Complete Psychological Works of Sigmund Freud (London: Hogarth Press & The Institute of Psychoanalysis, 1993), 243–58 (p. 244).

102 Emily Boone Hagenmaier, 'Untitled (Queer Mourning and the Art of Felix Gonzalez-Torres)', in *Dying, Assisted Death and Mourning*, ed. Asa Kasher (Amsterdam and New York: Editions Rodolphi BV, 2009), 157–68.

103 Hagenmaier, 'Untitled (Queer Mourning and the Art of Felix Gonzalez-Torres)', 161.

104 Hagenmaier, 'Untitled (Queer Mourning and the Art of Felix Gonzalez-Torres)', 161.

105 Hagenmaier, 'Untitled (Queer Mourning and the Art of Felix Gonzalez-Torres)', 165.

106 Dinshaw et al., 'Theorizing Queer Temporalities', 178.

107 Katz, 'Hide/Seek'.

108 Freud, 'Remembering, Repeating and Working Through', 150.

109 Freud, 'Beyond the Pleasure Principle', 18.

110 Spector, *Felix Gonzalez-Torres*, 140.

111 Watney, 'In Purgatory', 40.

112 Spector, *Felix Gonzalez-Torres*, 166.

113 While this is a widely shared interpretation, the Felix Gonzalez-Torres Foundation note that this does not necessarily reflect the specific intentions of the artist.

114 Kwon, 'The Becoming of a Work of Art', 299; Kwon is quoting directly from the back of a certificate.

115 Dietmar Elger, ed., *Felix Gonzalez-Torres: Catalogue Raisonné* (Stuttgart: Cantz Verlag, 1997).

116 Storr, 'When This You See Remember Me', 25.

117 Spector, *Felix Gonzalez-Torres*, 120.

118 Spector, *Felix Gonzalez-Torres*, 166–7.

119 Spector, *Felix Gonzalez-Torres*, 167.

120 Spector, *Felix Gonzalez-Torres*, 176.

121 Ramsey McPhillips, 'Who Turned out the Limelight? The Tragi-Comedy of Mark Morrisroe', in *Loss Within Loss: Artists in the Age of AIDS*, ed. Edmund White (Madison: University of Wisconsin Press, 2001), 109.

122 Although produced in a very different context, Marc Quinn's DNA-based 'portrait', *Sir John Edward Sulston* (2001), operates according to a similar logic; Sulston was a central figure in the development of DNA analysis. See Sarah Howgate and Sandy Nairne, *A Guide to Contemporary Portraits* (London: National Portrait Gallery, 2009), 13.

123 Spector, *Felix Gonzalez-Torres*, 120.

124 Roland Barthes, *Roland Barthes by Roland Barthes*, trans. Richard Howard (New York: Hill and Wang, 1977), 35.

125 Barthes, *Roland Barthes by Roland Barthes*, 35.

126 Kafer, *Feminist, Queer, Crip*.

127 Kafer, *Feminist, Queer, Crip*, 34.

128 Lee Edelman, 'Tearooms and Sympathy; or, The Epistemology of the Water Closet', in *Homographesis: Essays in Gay Literary and Cultural Theory* (New York and London: Routledge, 1994), 148–72; Baraister, *Enduring Time*.

129 Joan Tronto, *Moral Boundaries: A Political Arguement for an Ethics of Care* (London: Routledge, 1993), 14 cited Baraister, *Enduring Time*, 14.

130 Baraister, *Enduring Time*, 70.

131 Monica Pearl, '"A Thousand Kindred Spirits" Reflections on AIDS Activism and Representations of AIDS in US Culture and Conversation', *Radical History Review* 140 (2021): 223.

132 Rosen'*"Untitled" (The Neverending Portrait)*', 58.

133 Bolaki, *Illness as Many Narratives*, 1–2.

134 Woods, 'The Limits of Narrative'; Angela Woods, 'Beyond the Wounded Storyteller: Rethinking Narrativity, Illness and Embodied Self-Experience', in *Health, Illness and Disease: Philosophical Essays*, ed. Havi Carel and Rachel Cooper (Newcastle: Acumen, 2013).

135 Sara Ahmed, *The Cultural Politics of Emotion* (Edinburgh: Edinburgh University Press, 2014), 91.

136 Ahmed, *The Cultural Politics of Emotion*, 91.

137 Serres, *Rome*, 81; for a discussion of Serres and temporal folding, see Baraister, *Enduring Time*, 32–4.

Chapter 6

1 Centres for Disease Control and Prevention, 'HIV Surveillance Report, 2016; Vol. 28', November 2017, https://www.cdc.gov/hiv/pdf/library/reports/surveillance/cdc-hiv-surveillance-report-2016-vol-28.pdf.

2 Adam Geary, *Antiblack Racism and the AIDS Epidemic: State Intimacies* (New York: Palgrave Macmillan, 2014). See also Julia S. Jordan-Zachery, *Shadow Bodies: Black Women, Ideology, Representation, and Politics* (New Brunswick: Rutgers University Press, 2017). Cathy J. Cohen, *The Boundaries of Blackness: AIDS and the Breakdown of Black Politics* (Chicago and London: Chicago University Press, 1999).

3 On the erasure of Black people in *Art AIDS America*, see also Kerr, 'A History of Erasing Black Artists'; Theodore (Ted) Kerr, 'AIDS 1969: HIV, History, and Race', *Drain*, 2016, http://drainmag.com/aids-1969-hiv-history-and-race/; Tyrone Palmer, 'Under the Rainbow', *The New Inquiry*, 28 July 2015, https://thenewinquiry.com/under-the-rainbow/.

4 On how to survive a plague, see Jih-Fei Cheng, 'How to Survive: AIDS and Its Afterlives in Popular Media', *Women's Studies Quarterly* 44, no. 1/2 (2016): 73–92; Nishant Shahani, 'How to Survive the Whitewashing of AIDS: Global Pasts, Transnational Futures', *QED: A Journal in GLBTQ Worldmaking* 3, no. 1 (2016): 1–33. On Dallas Buyers' Club, see Akkadia Ford, 'The Dallas Buyers Club: Who's Buying It?', *TSQ: Transgender Studies Quarterly* 4, no. 1 (2017): 135–40; Laura Copier and Eliza Steinbock, 'On Not Really Being There: Trans* Presence/Absence in Dallas Buyers Club', *Feminist Media Studies* 18, no. 5 (2018): 923–41.

5 Cheng, 'How to Survive', 73.

6 Cheng, 'How to Survive', 78.

7 Shahani, 'How to Survive the Whitewashing of AIDS', 4.

8 Jih-Fei Cheng, Alexandra Juhasz, and Nishant Shahani, 'Foreword', in *AIDS and the Distribution of Crises* (Durham: Duke University Press, 2020), xxiii.

9 Cheng, Juhasz, and Shahani, 'Foreword', xxiii–xxiv.

10 Kia Labeija, quoted in Amelia Abraham, 'Photographing Black, Female, HIV Positive Power', *Refinery 29* (blog), 30 December 2016, https://www.refinery29.com/en-us/kia-labeija-on-photographing-black-queer-femme-power.

11 See Maria Cifor and Cait McKinney, 'Reclaiming HIV/AIDS in Digital Media Studies', *First Monday* 25, no. 10 (2020) for an analysis of LaBeija's digital work for PosterVirus, #undetectable (2016).

12 Julia S. Jordan-Zachery, 'Safe, Soulful Sex: HIV/AIDS Talk', in *AIDS and the Distribution of Crises*, ed. Jih-Fei Cheng, Alexandra Juhasz, and Nishant Shahani (Durham: Duke University Press, 2020), 93; see also Jordan-Zachery, *Shadow Bodies*.

13 Interview at the Bronx Museum of Art with Sur Rodney (Sur) and Kia LaBeija), 12 February 2016, https://youtu.be/AOLShR_Vq48. 'I identify as being a black artist, but I'm also a mixed artist too. I'm Filipino, and African-American, and Polynesian, all different types of things.' Kia LaBeija quoted in Annabel Graham, 'The Underside of Glamour: An Interview of Kia LaBeija', *Autre.Love* (blog), 18 January 2018, https://autre.love/interviewsmain/2018/1/18/the-underside-of-glamour-an-interview-of-kia-labeija. The exhibition threw up several problems about categorizing art around racialized categories. For Labeija, being 'Black-identified' is a strategic identification.

14 Interview at the Bronx Museum of Art with Sur Rodney (Sur) and Kia LaBeija).

15 Kia LaBeija, 20 December 2015. Cited on the Tacoma Action Collective's Facebook page, https://www.facebook.com/TacomaActionCollective. Accessed 14 October 2021.

16 The image was released December 2015. It has since been removed from the web.

17 On artists' responses to the loss of a parent to HIV and AIDS, see Emily Colucci, 'Touch across Time: Familial Loss And Its Remains in Art during the Ongoing HIV/AIDS Pandemic', ed. Theodore (Ted) Kerr, *On Curating*, What You Don't Know About AIDS Could Fill a Museum, no. 42 (2019): 272–82; and 'Visual AIDS'

Panel, The Personal and the Political: Losing Parents to AIDS, with Alysia Abbott, Kia Benbow, Mathew Rodrigues, and Sarah Shulman, Hosted by the New York Public Library', https://www.youtube.com/watch?v=BnZsMDEZV98; for a novel that memorializes a father lost to AIDS, see Alysia Abbott, *Fairyland: A Memoir of My Father* (New York and London: W. W. Norton, 2013).

18 The individual images are untitled in the initial catalogue *Art AIDS America*, with all three appearing under the series title *24*. The images are titled in the exhibition checklist for the catalogue for *Art AIDS America Chicago*.

19 LaBeija describes these images as exploring 'lived experience in space' in 'Interview at the Bronx Museum of Art with Sur Rodney (Sur) and Kia LaBeija)'.

20 Gaston Bachelard, *The Poetics of Space* (New York: Penguin, 2014), 99.

21 Ahmed, *The Cultural Politics of Emotion*.

22 Kia LaBeija and Alex Fialho, 'Living Free: Kia LaBeija, From Pathology to Wholeness' (Lecture and conversation, IDA Stanford, 17 May 2017), https://www.youtube.com/watch?v=7jrbUspNXkE.

23 LaBeija and Fialho, 'Living Free'.

24 Theodore (Ted) Kerr, Amy Sadao, and Nelson Santos, 'Love Happened Here: Art, Archives, and a Living History', in *Art AIDS America*, ed. Jonathan Katz and Rock Hushka (Tacoma, Seattle and London: Tacoma Art Museum in association with University of Washington Press, 2016), 68.

25 Lauren Fournier, 'Sick Women, Sad Girls, and Selfie Theory: Autotheory as Contemporary Feminist Practice', *Auto/Biography Studies* 33, no. 3 (2018): 643; see also Lauren Fournier, *Autotheory as Feminist Practice in Art, Writing, and Criticism* (Cambridge, MA: MIT Press, 2021).

26 Fournier, *Autotheory as Feminist Practice in Art, Writing, and Criticism*, 8.

27 Fournier, 'Sick Women, Sad Girls, and Selfie Theory', 647–9.

28 Fournier, 'Sick Women, Sad Girls, and Selfie Theory', 644; Fournier, *Autotheory as Feminist Practice in Art, Writing, and Criticism*; Amelia Jones, *Self/Image: Technology, Representation, and the Contemporary Subject* (New York: Routledge, 2006), 134.

29 Audrey Wollen, 'Tell Me about Sad Girl Theory', Instagram photo, *@tragicqueen* (blog), 22 June 2014; Johanna Hedva, 'Sick Woman Theory', 2016, http://johannahedva.com/SickWomanTheory_Hedva_2020.pdf.

30 Hedva, 'Sick Woman Theory', 8.

31 Hedva, 'Sick Woman Theory', 9.

32 Hedva, 'Sick Woman Theory', 4 and 8.

33 Tembeck, 'Selfies of Ill Health', 1.

34 Similar self-imaging practices include artist Carolyn Lazard's In Sickness and Study (2015 onwards), an Instagram-based project that depicts the artist's arm, mid blood-transfusion, holding up a series of books. On Lazard and Wollen, see Fournier, 'Sick Women, Sad Girls, and Selfie Theory', 649–50; On Carolyn Lazard,

see Giulia Smith, 'Carolyn Lazard', *Art Monthly*, 2019; and Giulia Smith, 'Chronic Illness as Critique: Crip Aesthetics across the Atlantic', *Art History* 44, no. 2 (2021): 286–310.

35 As Stuart Hall recognized, there is no 'true' representation of people or events in an art work; for Hall, culture is not a direct transcription of lived experience but the means through which subjects seek to order and make sense of that lived experience. Stuart Hall, 'The Work of Representation', in *Representation: Cultural Representations and Signifying Practices*, ed. Stuart Hall (London: Sage and Open University Press, 1997), 44–51; Kobena Mercer, 'Stuart Hall and the Visual Arts', *Small Axe* 19, no. 1 (2015): 78–87.

36 Fournier, *Autotheory as Feminist Practice in Art, Writing, and Criticism*, 16.

37 Kia LaBeija, Interview at the Bronx Museum of Art with Sur Rodney (Sur) and Kia LaBeija).

38 Kia LaBeija, 'Rebirth', *TDR: The Drama Review* 60, no. 4 (2016): 2–3.

39 Cindy Patton, *Last Served? Gendering the AIDS Pandemic* (London: Taylor and Francis, 1994).

40 Bill Rodriguez, 'Biomedical Models of HIV and Women', in *The Gender Politics of HIV/AIDS in Women*, ed. Nancy Goldstein and Jennifer L. Manlowe, Perspectives on the Pandemic in the United States (New York and London: New York University Press, 1997), 34.

41 Patton, *Last Served? Gendering the AIDS Pandemic*, 13.

42 Nixon and Nixon, *People with AIDS*, 90.

43 See Henry A. Giroux, 'Consuming Social Change: The "United Colors of Benetton"', *Cultural Critique* 26 (1993–94): 5–32.

44 Nixon and Nixon, *People with AIDS*, 134 and 146.

45 Nan Goldin's *Cookie Portfolio*, explored in detail in Chapter 2 of this book, arguably offers a more complex portrayal of an HIV-positive woman as a mother. In the first image of the portfolio, *Cookie with Max at My Birthday Party, Provincetown*, 1977, Max rests on Cookie's lap: he is around five or six years old and presumably tired by the party, although he manages to return Goldin's photographic gaze with gentle curiosity. Cookie's hands – bejewelled, tattooed and golden-fingernailed – are tenderly folded across his little tummy. Max's black superhero mask echoes his mother's trademark thick black eyeliner. Later in the *Portfolio* we meet Max again, now a young man: this time the roles are reversed and it is he who holds his mother, one arm wrapped protectively around her as they sit together on the humbug-stripped sofa in the New York apartment that they share.

46 Alexandra Juhasz, 'The Contained Threat: Women in Mainstream AIDS Documentary', *Journal of Sex Research* 21, no. 1 (1990): 25–46.

47 Gilman, 'AIDS and Syphilis', 105; Grover, 'Visible Lesions', 356.

48 Gilman, 'AIDS and Syphilis', 105.

49 Julian Gill-Peterson, 'Haunting the Queer Spaces of AIDS: Remembering ACT UP/ New York and an Ethics for an Endemic', *GLQ: A Journal of Lesbian and Gay Studies* 19, no. 3 (2013): 279–300.

50 Michel Foucault, *Society Must Be Defended: Lectures at the College de France, 1975–76*, trans. David Macey (London and New York: Penguin, 2003), 244.

51 Gill-Peterson, 'Haunting the Queer Spaces of AIDS', 280.

52 Gill-Peterson, 'Haunting the Queer Spaces of AIDS', 281; Derrida, *Specters of Marx*, 54–5, 64–5, 101.

53 Gill-Peterson, 'Haunting the Queer Spaces of AIDS', 280.

54 The Visual AIDS Artist+ Registry is the largest database of works by artists with HIV/AIDS, and is open to all HIV+ artists. https://visualaids.org/artists (accessed 10 March 2022).

Bibliography

Abbott, Alysia. *Fairyland: A Memoir of My Father*. New York and London: W.W. Norton, 2013.

Abraham, Amelia. 'Photographing Black, Female, HIV Positive Power'. *Refinery 29* (blog), 30 December 2016. https://www.refinery29.com/en-us/kia-labeija-on-photographing-black-queer-femme-power.

ACT UP New York. 'Drawing Attention to the Modern HIV Epidemic for ACT up Artist David Wojnarowicz'. n.d. https://actupny.com/drawing-attention-to-the-modern-hiv-epidemic-for-act-up-artist-david-wojnarowicz/.

ACT UP New York. 'The Whitney Actions and the Historicization of HIV/AIDS'. n.d. https://actupny.com/the-whitney-actions-and-the-historicization-of-hiv-aids/#comment-44.

Ahmed, Sara. *The Cultural Politics of Emotion*. Edinburgh: Edinburgh University Press, 2014.

Aletti, Vince. 'Shot Through the Heart'. *Village Voice*, 8 February 2000.

Altman, Lawrence K. 'Rare Cancer Seen in 41 Homosexuals'. *The New York Times*, 3 July 1981.

Anzieu, Didier. *The Skin Ego*. Translated by Chris Turner. New Haven: Yale University Press, 1989.

Apter, Emily. 'Fantom Images: Hervé Guibert and the Writing of 'Sida' in France'. In *Writing AIDS: Gay Literature, Language, and Analysis*, edited by Timothy F. Murphy and Suzanne Poirier, 83–97. New York: Columbia University Press, 1993.

Archibald, Sasha. 'Robert Blanchon's Archive of Absence'. In *Robert Blanchon*, edited by Tania Duvergne and Amy Sadao, 23–31. New York: Visual AIDS, 2006.

Atkins, Robert. 'Stream of Conscience: Andres Serrano's "Piss Christ"'. *Village Voice*, 30 May 1989.

Ault, Julie, ed. *Felix Gonzalez-Torres*. New York and Gottingen: Steidl, 2006.

Ault, Julie, ed. *Show and Tell: A Chronicle of Group Material*. London: Four Corners Books, 2010.

Avgikos, Jan. 'This Is My Body: Felix Gonzalez-Torres'. *Artforum* 29, no. 6 (February 1991): 79–83.

Bachelard, Gaston. *The Poetics of Space*. New York: Penguin, 2014.

Baltz, Lewis. '(Sans Titre), Felix Gonzalez-Torres'. In *Felix Gonzalez-Torres*, edited by Julie Ault, 211–15. New York and Gottingen: Steidl, 2006.

Baraister, Lisa. *Enduring Time*. London and New York: Bloomsbury, 2017.

Baraister, Lisa, and William Brook. 'Watchful Waiting: Temporalities of Crisis and Care in the UK National Health Service'. In *Vulnerability and the Politics of Care*, edited by

Victoria Browne, Jason Danely, Tina Managhan, and Doerthe Rosenow, 235:230–47. Proceedings of the British Academy. Oxford: Oxford University Press, n.d.

Barthes, Roland. *Camera Lucida: Reflections on Photography*. Translated by Richard Howard. London: Vintage, 2000.

Barthes, Roland. *Roland Barthes by Roland Barthes*. Translated by Richard Howard. New York: Hill and Wang, 1977.

Barthes, Roland. 'The Death of the Author'. In *Image, Music, Text*, translated by Stephen Heath, 142–8. London: Fontana, 1977.

Bataille, Georges. *Erotism*. Translated by Mary Dalwood. London and New York: Marion Boyars, 1987.

Bataille, Georges. *Visions of Excess: Selected Writings, 1927–39*. Edited and translated by Allan Stoekl. Minneapolis: University of Minnesota Press, 1985.

Beaujour, Michel. *Poetics of the Literary Self-Portrait*. Translated by Yara Milos. New York and London: New York University Press, 1991.

Bellacasa, María Puig de la. *Matters of Care: Speculative Ethics in More than Human Worlds*. Minneapolis: University of Minnesota Press, 2017.

Ben-Levi, Jack, Craig Houser, Leslie C. Jones, and Simon Taylor. 'Introduction'. In *Abject Art: Repulsion and Desire in American Art*, 7–15. New York: Whitney Museum of American Art, 1993.

Berger, John. *Ways of Seeing*. London and Harmondsworth: BBC and Penguin, 1972.

Bersani, Leo. 'Foucault, Freud, Fantasy and Power'. *GLQ: A Journal of Lesbian and Gay Studies* 2, no. 1–2 (1995): 11–33.

Bersani, Leo. 'Is the Rectum a Grave?' *October* 43 (1987): 197–222.

Best, Susan. *Visualizing Feeling: Affect and the Feminine Avant-Garde*. London and New York: I.B. Tauris, 2011.

Blackshaw, Gemma. 'The Pathological Body: Modernist Strategising in Egon Schiele's Self-Portraiture'. *Oxford Art Journal* 30, no. 3 (2007): 379–401.

Blanchon, Robert. '[Never Realized]: 4 Opportunistic Infections for Public Viewing and Consumption'. In *Robert Blanchon*, edited by Tania Duvergne and Amy Sadao, 109–15. New York: Visual AIDS, 2006.

Bolaki, Stella. *Illness as Many Narratives: Arts, Medicine and Culture*. Edinburgh: Edinburgh University Press, 2016.

Bordowitz, Gregg. *General Idea: Imagevirus*. London: Afterall, 2010.

Bordowitz, Gregg. 'My Postmodernism'. In *The AIDS Crisis Is Ridiculous and Other Writings: 1986–2003, by Gregg Bordowitz*, edited by James Meyer, 221–39. Cambridge, MA: MIT Press, 2004.

Bordowitz, Gregg. *The AIDS Crisis Is Ridiculous and Other Writings, 1986–2003*. Edited by James Meyer. Cambridge, MA: MIT Press, 2004.

Bordowitz, Gregg and David Deitcher. 'Art, Activism, and Everyday Life'. *Documents* 11 (1998): 30–8.

Bourriaud, Nicolas. *Relational Aesthetics*. Translated by Simon Pleasance and Fronza Woods. Dijon: Presses du reel, 2002.

Brier, Jennifer. *Infectious Ideas: U.S. Political Responses to the AIDS Crisis*. North Carolina: University of North Carolina Press, 2009.

Brilliant, Richard. *Portraiture*. London: Reaktion Books, 1991.

Butler, Isaac, and Dan Kois. *The Worlkd Only Spins Forward: The Ascent of Angels in America*. New York and London: Bloomsbury, 2018.

Butler, Judith. *Bodies That Matter*. London and New York: Routledge, 1993.

Butler, Judith. *Gender Trouble*. London and New York: Routledge, 1990.

Butler, Judith. *Precarious Life: The Powers of Mourning and Violence*. London and New York: Verso, 2006.

Callen, Michael. 'Remarks of Michael Callen, American Public Health Association Annual Meeting, Las Vegas, Nevada, 1986'. *Surviving and Thriving with AIDS: Hints for the Newly Diagnosed*, March 1987.

Campbell, Alyson and Dirk Gindt, eds. *Viral Dramaturgies: HIV and AIDS in Performance in the Twenty-First Century*. London: Palgrave Macmillan, 2018.

Camper, Fred. 'Shooting Star'. *Chicago Reader*, 26 January 2001.

Camper, Fred. 'Writing on the Wall/Robert Blanchon: Gum, Waste, Indentations, Stains, and Envelopes'. *Chicago Reader*, 2 February 1996.

Capsuto, Steven. *Alternate Channels: The Uncensored Story of Gay and Lesbian Images on Radio and Television*. New York: Ballantine Books, 2000.

Carr, Cynthia. *Fire in the Belly: The Life and Times of David Wojnarowicz*. New York: Bloomsbury, 2012.

Cartwright, Lisa. *Screening the Body: Tracing Medicine's Visual Culture*. Minneapolis: University of Minnesota Press, 1995.

Centres for Disease Control and Prevention. 'HIV Surveillance Report, 2016; Vol. 28'. November 2017. https://www.cdc.gov/hiv/pdf/library/reports/surveillance/cdc-hiv-surveillance-report-2016-vol-28.pdf.

Chambers, Ross. *Facing It: AIDS Diaries and the Death of the Author*. Ann Arbor: University of Michigan Press, 1998.

Chambers, Ross. *Untimely Interventions: AIDS Writing, Testimonial, and the Rhetoric of Haunting*. Ann Arbor: University of Michigan Press, 2004.

Chapman, Roger. 'Andres Serrano'. In *Culture Wars: An Encyclopedia of Issues, Viewpoints, and Voices*, edited by Roger Chapman, 506–7. New York: M.E. Sharpe, 2010.

Charon, Rita. *Narrative Medicine: Honoring the Stories of Illness*. Oxford: Oxford University Press, 2006.

Chau, Lawrence. 'Mark Morrisroe'. *Flash Art*, October 1988.

Chave, Anna C. 'Minimalism and Biography'. *The Art Bulletin* 82, no. 1 (2000): 149–63.

Chave, Anna C.. 'Pollock and Krasner: Script and Postscript'. In *Pollock and After: The Critical Debate*, 2nd edition, edited by Francis Frascina, 329–47. London and New York: Routledge, 2000.

Cheng, Jih-Fei. 'How to Survive: AIDS and Its Afterlives in Popular Media'. *Women's Studies Quarterly* 44, no. 1/2 (2016): 73–92.

Cheng, Jih-Fei, Alexandra Juhasz, and Nishant Shahani. 'Foreword'. In *AIDS and the Distribution of Crises*, xvii–xxvi. Durham: Duke University Press, 2020.

Chevalier, Vincent and Ian Bradley-Perrin. 'Your Nostalgia Is Killing Me' Tumblr. *PosterVirus* (blog), 20 November 2013. https://postervirus.tumblr.com/post/67569099579/your-nostalgia-is-killing-me-vincent-chevalier.

Cifor, Maria and Cait McKinney. 'Reclaiming HIV/AIDS in Digital Media Studies'. *First Monday* 25, no. 10 (2020).

Cifor, Marika Louise. '"Your Nostalgia Is Killing Me": Activism, Affect and the Archives of HIV/AIDS'. Doctoral Thesis, University of California, 2017. https://escholarship.org/uc/item/2312c9bb.

Clark, Kenneth. *The Nude: A Study of Ideal Art*. London: John Murray, 1956.

Clark, T.J. *The Painting of Modern Life: Paris in the Art of Manet and His Followers*. London: Thames & Hudson, 1985.

Clements, Alexis. 'We Were Not Making Art, We Were at War'. 21 November 2012. http://hyperallergic.com/60650/gran-fury-in-2012/.

Cohen, Cathy J. *The Boundaries of Blackness: AIDS and the Breakdown of Black Politics*. Chicago and London: Chicago University Press, 1999.

Colucci, Emily. 'Touch Across Time: Familial Loss And Its Remains in Art During the Ongoing HIV/AIDS Pandemic'. Edited by Theodore (Ted) Kerr. *On Curating, What You Don't Know About AIDS Could Fill a Museum*, no. 42 (2019): 272–82.

Copier, Laura and Eliza Steinbock. 'On Not Really Being There: Trans* Presence/Absence in Dallas Buyers Club'. *Feminist Media Studies* 18, no. 5 (2018): 923–41.

Coulthard, E. and Nan Goldin. *I'll Be Your Mirror*. Blast! Films, 1995.

Crimp, Douglas. 'AIDS: Cultural Analysis/Cultural Activism'. *October* 43, no. Winter (1987): 3–16.

Crimp, Douglas. 'How to Have Promiscuity in an Epidemic'. *October* 43 (Winter 1987): 237–71.

Crimp, Douglas. Interview with Douglas Crimp: ACT UP Oral History Project. Interview by Sarah Schulman, 16 May 2007. www.actuporalhistory.org/interviews/images/Crimp.pdf.

Crimp, Douglas. 'Melancholia and Moralism: An Introduction'. In *Melancholia and Moralism: Essays on AIDS and Queer Politics*, 1–26. Cambridge, MA: MIT Press, 2002.

Crimp, Douglas. *Melancholia and Moralism: Essays on AIDS and Queer Politics*. Cambridge, MA: MIT Press, 2002.

Crimp, Douglas. 'Mourning and Militancy'. *October* 51 (1989): 3–18.

Crimp, Douglas. 'Mourning and Militancy'. In *Melancholia and Moralism: Essays on AIDS and Queer Politics*, edited by Douglas Crimp, 129–49. Cambridge, MA: MIT Press, 2002.

Crimp, Douglas. 'On the Museum's Ruins'. *October* 13 (1980): 41–57.

Crimp, Douglas. 'On the Museum's Ruins'. In *Postmodern Culture*, edited by Hal Foster, 43–56. London: Pluto Press, 1985.

Crimp, Douglas. 'Portraits of People with AIDS'. In *Melancholia and Moralism: Essays on AIDS and Queer Politics*, 83–107. Cambridge, MA: MIT Press, 2002.

Crimp, Douglas. 'The End of Painting'. *October* 16 (n.d.): 69–86.

Crimp, Douglas. 'The Spectacle of Mourning'. In *Melancholia and Moralism: Essays on AIDS and Queer Politics*, 195–202. Cambridge, MA: MIT Press, 2002.

Crimp, Douglas and Adam Rolston. *AIDS Demographics*. Seattle: Bay Press, 1990.

Croce, Arlene. 'Discussing the Undiscussable'. In *The Crisis of Criticism*, edited by Maurice Berger, 15–29. New York: The New Press, 1998.

Cruz, Amanda, Suzanne Ghez, and Ann Goldstein. 'Reflections on a Proposal for 1995'. In *Felix Gonzalez-Torres: America*, edited by Nancy Spector, 47–59. New York: Guggenheim Museum Publications, 2007.

Cullen, Deborah. 'Felix Gonzalez-Torres: The Jigsaw Puzzles'. In *Searching for Sebald: Photography as W.G. Sebald*, edited by Lise Patt and Christel Dillbohner, 350–9. Los Angeles: ICI Press, 2007.

Curiger, Bice. *Meret Oppenheim: Defiance in the Face of Freedom*. Cambridge, MA: MIT Press, 1989.

Dalrymple Henderson, Linda. 'X Rays and the Quest for Invisible Reality in the Art of Kupka, Duchamp, and the Cubists'. *Art Journal* 47 (Winter 1988): 323–40.

Deitcher, David. 'Death and the Marketplace'. *Frieze* 29 (1996): 40–5.

Deitcher, David. 'What Does Silence Equal Now?' In *Art Matters: How the Culture Wars Changed America*, edited by Brian Wallis, Marianne Weems, and Philip Yenawine, 92–125. New York and London: New York University Press, 1999.

Derrida, Jacques. *Specters of Marx: The State of Debt, the Work of Mourning, and the New International*. Translated by Peggy Kamuf. New York and London: Routledge, 1994.

Dick, Kirby. *Sick: The Life and Death of Bob Flanagan, Supermasochist*. Lexicon Home Entertainment, 1997.

diCorcia, Philip-Lorca. *Hustlers*. Gottingen: Steidl, 2013.

Diedrich, Lisa. *Indirect Action: Schizophrenia, Epilepsy, AIDS, and the Course of Health Activism*. Minneapolis: University of Minnesota Press, 2016.

Diedrich, Lisa. *Treatments: Language, Politics, and the Culture of Illness*. Minneapolis: University of Minnesota Press, 2007.

Dinshaw, Carolyn, Lee Edelman, Roderick A. Ferguson, and Carla Freccero. 'Theorizing Queer Temporalities: A Roundtable Discussion'. *GLQ: A Journal of Lesbian and Gay Studies* 13, no. 2–3 (2007): 177–95.

Doane, Mary Ann. 'Film and the Masquerade: Theorising the Female Spectator'. *Screen* 23, no. 3–4 (1982): 74–88.

Duve, Pascal de. *Cargo Vie*. Paris: J.C. Lattes, 1993.

Duvergne, Tania and Amy Sadao, eds. *Robert Blanchon*. New York: Visual AIDS, 2006.

Edelman, Lee. *Homographesis: Essays in Gay Literature and Cultural Theory*. New York and London: Routledge, 1994.

Edelman, Lee. *No Future: Queer Theory and the Death Drive*. Durham and London: Duke University Press, 2004.

Edelman, Lee. 'Tearooms and Sympathy; or, The Epistemology of the Water Closet'. In *Homographesis: Essays in Gay Literary and Cultural Theory*, 148–72. New York and London: Routledge, 1994.

Edwards, Steve. *Martha Rosler: The Bowery in Two Inadequate Descriptive Systems*. London: Afterall, 2012.

Egan, Susanna. *Mirror Talk: Genres of Crisis in Contemporary Autobiography*. Chapel Hill and London: University of North Carolina Press, 1999.

Elger, Dietmar, ed. *Felix Gonzalez-Torres: Catalogue Raisonné*. Stuttgart: Cantz Verlag, 1997.

Ellis, Havelock. *The Criminal*, 4th edition. London: The Walter Scott Publishing Company, 1910.

Engelmann, Lukas. *Mapping AIDS: Visual Histories of an Enduring Epidemic*. Cambridge: Cambridge University Press, 2018.

Engelmann, Lukas. 'Photographing AIDS: Capturing AIDS in Pictures of People with AIDS'. *Bulletin of the History of Medicine* 90, no. 2 (2016): 250–78.

Fanthome, Christine. 'The Influence and Treatment of Autobiography in Confessional Art: Observations on Tracey Emin's Feature Film Top Spot'. *Biography* 29, no. 1 (Winter 2006): 30–42.

Feldman, Melissa E. 'The Portrait: From Somebody to Nobody'. In *Face-Off: The Portrait in Recent Art*, edited by Melissa E. Feldman, 9–10. Philadelphia: Institute of Contemporary Art, University of Pennsylvania, 1994.

Finkelstein, Avram. *After Silence: A History of AIDS through Its Images*. Oakland: University of California Press, 2018.

Flood, Richard. 'The Law of Indirections'. In *Robert Gober: Sculpture and Drawing*, edited by by Richard Flood, Gary Garrels, and Ann Temkin, 9–31. Minneapolis: Walker Arts Center, 1999.

Ford, Akkadia. 'The Dallas Buyers Club: Who's Buying It?'. *TSQ: Transgender Studies Quarterly* 4, no. 1 (2017): 135–40.

Foster, Hal. 'Postmodernism: A Preface'. In *Postmodern Culture*, edited by Hal Foster, vii–xiv. London: Pluto Press, 1985.

Foster, Hal. 'The Crux of Minimalism'. In *The Return of the Real: Art and Theory at the End of the Century*, 35–70. Cambridge, MA: MIT Press, 1996.

Foucault, Michel. *Discipline and Punish: The Birth of the Prison*. Translated by Alan Sheridan. London: Penguin, 1991.

Foucault, Michel. *Society Must Be Defended: Lectures at the College de France, 1975–76*. Translated by David Macey. London and New York: Penguin, 2003.

Foucault, Michel. *The Birth of the Clinic*. Translated by A.M. Sheridan. London: Routledge, 1989.

Foucault, Michel. *The History of Sexuality, Volume 1*. Translated by Robert Hurley. London: Penguin, 1990.

Foucault, Michel. *The Order of Things*. Translated by Tavistock/ Routledge, 1970. London and New York: Routledge, 1989.

Foucault, Michel. 'What Is an Author?'. In *The Foucault Reader: An Introduction to Foucault's Thought*, edited by Paul Rabinow, 101–20. London and New York: Penguin, 1991.

Fournier, Lauren. *Autotheory as Feminist Practice in Art, Writing, and Criticism*. Cambridge, MA: MIT Press, 2021.

Fournier, Lauren. 'Sick Women, Sad Girls, and Selfie Theory: Autotheory as Contemporary Feminist Practice'. *Auto/Biography Studies* 33, no. 3 (2018): 643–62.

Frank, Arthur. *The Wounded Storyteller: Body, Illness, and Ethics*. Chicago and London: University of Chicago Press, 1995.

Freeman, Elizabeth. 'Introduction'. *GLQ: A Journal of Lesbian and Gay Studies* 13, no. 2–3 (2007): 159–76.

Freeman, Elizabeth. *Time Binds: Queer Temporalities, Queer Histories*. Durham and London: Duke University Press, 2010.

Freud, Sigmund. 'Beyond the Pleasure Principle (1920)'. In *Beyond the Pleasure Principle, Group Psychology and Other Works, Vol. XVIII (1920-1922)*, XVIII:7–64. The Standard Edition of the Complete Psychological Works of Sigmund Freud. London: Hogarth Press & The Institute of Psychoanalysis, 1955.

Freud, Sigmund. 'Fragment of an Analysis of a Case Study of Hysteria (1905 [1901])'. In *A Case of Hysteria: Three Essays on Sexuality and Other Works, Vol. VII (1901-1905)*, 1–122. The Standard Edition of the Complete Psychological Works of Sigmund Freud. London: Hogarth Press & The Institute of Psychoanalysis, 1953.

Freud, Sigmund. 'Mourning and Melancholia'. In *On the History of the Psycho-Analytic Movement, Volume XIV (1914–16)*, XIV (1914–16):243–58. The Standard Edition of the Complete Psychological Works of Sigmund Freud. London: Hogarth Press & The Institute of Psychoanalysis, 1993.

Freud, Sigmund. 'Remembering, Repeating and Working Through (Further Recommendations on the Technique of Psycho-Analysis) (1914)'. In *The Case of Schreber, Papers on Technique, and Other Works, Vol. XII (1911-1913)*, XII:145–56. The Standard Edition of the Complete Psychological Works of Sigmund Freud. London: The Hogarth Press and the Institute of Psychoanalysis, 1958.

Freud, Sigmund. *The Interpretation of Dreams*, 8th edition. Translated by James Strachey. Vol. 4. The Penguin Freud Library. London and New York: Penguin, 1976.

Freud, Sigmund. *Three Essays on the Theory of Sexuality*. Edited by James Strachey. London: Hogarth Press & The Institute of Psychoanalysis, 1962.

Fried, Michael. 'Art and Objecthood'. In *Art in Theory, 1900–2000*, edited by Charles Harrison and Paul Wood, 835–46. Oxford: Blackwell, 1992.

Galassi, Peter. 'Introduction'. In *Pictures of People*, edited by Nicholas Nixon, 9–28. New York: The Museum of Modern Art, New York, 1988.

Galton, Francis. 'Composite Portraits, Made by Combining Those of Many Different Persons Into a Single Figure'. *The Journal of the Anthropological Institute of Great Britain and Ireland* 8 (1879): 132–44.

Gangitano, Lia, ed. *Boston School: Mark Morrisroe (1969–89): A Survey from the Estate*. Boston: Institute of Contemporary Art, 1995.

Geary, Adam. *Antiblack Racism and the AIDS Epidemic: State Intimacies*. New York: Palgrave Macmillan, 2014.

Gever, Martha. 'Pictures of Sickness: Stuart Marshall's 'Bright Eyes''. *October* 43 (1987): 108–26.

Gill-Peterson, Julian. 'Haunting the Queer Spaces of AIDS: Remembering ACT UP/ New York and an Ethics for an Endemic'. *GLQ: A Journal of Lesbian and Gay Studies* 19, no. 3 (2013): 279–300.

Gilman, Sander. 'AIDS and Syphilis: The Iconography of Disease'. *October* 43 (1987): 87–107.

Gilman, Sander. *Disease and Representation: Images of Illness from Madness to AIDS*. Ithaca and London: Cornell University Press, 1988.

Gilman, Sander. *Health and Illness: Images of Difference*. London: Reaktion Books, 1995.

Giroux, Henry A. 'Consuming Social Change: The "United Colors of Benetton"'. *Cultural Critique* 26 (1993–94): 5–32.

Gober, Robert. 'Interview: Richard Flood and Robert Gober'. In *Robert Gober: Sculpture and Drawing*, edited by Richard Flood, Gary Garrels, and Ann Temkin, 121–43. Minneapolis: Walker Arts Center, 1999.

Gober, Robert. Robert Gober by Craig Gholson. Interview by Craig Gholson, Fall 1989. http://bombmagazine.org/article/1252/robert-gober.

Goldin, Nan. '20 Years: AIDS and Photography'. *The Digital Journalist* (blog), June 2001. http://digitaljournalist.org/issue0106/voices_goldin.htm.

Goldin, Nan. *Cookie Mueller: Photographs*. New York: Pace/MacGill, 1991.

Goldin, Nan. 'In the Valley of the Shadow'. In *Witnesses: Against Our Vanishing*, 4–5. New York: Artists Space, 1989.

Goldin, Nan. 'Nan Goldin on Cookie Mueller'. *The Digital Journalist. 20 Years: AIDS and Photography* (blog), 2001. http://digitaljournalist.org/issue0106/voices_goldin.htm.

Goldin, Nan. 'On Acceptance: A Conversation. Nan Goldin Talking with David Armstrong and Walter Keller'. In *Nan Goldin: I'll Be Your Mirror*, edited by Nan Goldin, David Armstrong and Hans Werner Holzworth, 447–54. New York: Whitney Museum of American Art, 1996.

Goldin, Nan. *The Ballad of Sexual Dependency*. Edited by Marvin Heiferman, Mark Holborn, and Suzanne Fletcher. New York and London: Aperture, 1986.

Goldstein, Ann. 'Bring in the World'. In *Barbara Kruger*, edited by Ann Goldstein, 24–36. Los Angeles: The Museum of Contemporary Art, Los Angeles, 1999.

Gould, Deborah. *Moving Politics: Emotion and ACT UP's Fight Against AIDS*. Chicago and London: University of Chicago Press, 2009.

Graham, Annabel. 'The Underside of Glamour: An Interview of Kia LaBeija'. *Autre.Love* (blog), 18 January 2018. https://autre.love/interviewsmain/2018/1/18/the-underside-of-glamour-an-interview-of-kia-labeija.

Gran Fury. 'Art and Politics of the 1980s: Language in the Public Sphere: Gran Fury (Tom Kalin and Members) and Helen Molesworth'. *Panel Discussion, Columbia University, NYC*, 12 November 2012.

Gran Fury. 'Good Luck . . . Miss You – Gran Fury'. In *AIDS RIOT: Artists Collectives Against AIDS, 1987-1994*, edited by 12th Session of the Ecole du Magasin (Caroline Engel, Nicholas Fenouillat, Aurélie Guitton, Benedetta di Loreto, Flora Loyau, Ivana Mestrov, Anna Olszewska), 301–6. Grenoble: Magasin, 2003.

Gran Fury. Gran Fury Talks to Douglas Crimp. Interview by Douglas Crimp, April 2003. http://www.artforum.com/inprint/id=4466.

Graves, Jen. 'Tacoma Art Museum's Art AIDS America Is a Messy Masterpeice That Reframes the Past 40 Years of American Art'. *The Stranger*, 7 October 2015. https://www.thestranger.com/visual-art/features/2015/10/07/22970740/viral.

Griffin, Gabriele. *Visibility Blue/s: Representations of HIV and AIDS*. Manchester: Manchester University Press, 2000.

Grosz, Elizabeth. *Space, Time, and Perversion*. New York and London: Routledge, 1995.

Grover, Jan Zita. 'Introduction'. In *AIDS: The Artists' Response*, 2–3. Columbus: Ohio State University, 1989.

Grover, Jan Zita. 'Visible Lesions: Images of the PWA'. In *Out in Culture: Gay, Lesbian and Queer Essays on Popular Culture*, edited by Corey K. Creekmur and Alexander Doty, 354–81. Durham and London: Duke University Press, 1995.

Gruber, Teresa. 'Biography'. In *Mark Morrisroe*, edited by Beatrix Ruf and Thomas Seelig, 442–7. Zurich: Ringier Collection, 2010.

Gruber, Teresa. *'There Was a Sense of Family . . .' The Friends of Mark Morrisroe*. Nurnberg: Verlag fur Moderne Kunst, 2012.

Grundberg, Andy. 'Nicholas Nixon Seeks a Path to the Heart'. *New York Times*, 11 September 1988.

Guibert, Herve. *Cytomegalovirus: A Hospitalization Diary*. Translated by Clara Orban and Elliot Weisenberg. Lanham and London: University Press of America, 1996.

Guibert, Herve. *Ghost Image*. Translated by Robert Bononno. Los Angeles: Sun & Moon Press, 1996.

Guibert, Herve. 'The Cancerous Image'. In *Ghost Image*, 154–8. Los Angeles: Sun & Moon Press, 1996.

Guibert, Herve. *The Compassionate Protocol*. Translated by James Kirkup. London: Quartet, 1993.

Guibert, Herve. *To The Friend Who Did Not Save My Life*. Translated by Linda Coverdale. London: Quartet, 1995.

Hagenmaier, Emily Boone. 'Untitled (Queer Mourning and the Art of Felix Gonzalez-Torres)'. In *Dying, Assisted Death and Mourning*, edited by Asa Kasher, 157–68. Amsterdam and New York: Editions Rodolphi BV, 2009.

Hagestad, Gunhild. 'On-Time, off-Time, out of Time? Reflections of Continuity and Discontinuity from an Illness Perspective'. In *Adulthood and Aging: Research on Continuities and Discontinuities*, edited by V.L. Bengston, 204–22. New York: Springer, 1996.

Halberstam, Judith. *In a Queer Time and Place: Transgender Bodies, Subcultural Lives.* New York and London: New York University Press, 2005.

Hall, Stuart. 'The Work of Representation'. In *Representation: Cultural Representations and Signifying Practices*, edited by Stuart Hall, 44–51. London: Sage and Open University Press, 1997.

Hallas, Roger. *Reframing Bodies: AIDS, Bearing Witness, and the Queer Moving Image.* Durham and London: Duke University Press, 2009.

Halperin, David. *Saint Foucault: Towards a Gay Hagiography.* New York and Oxford: Oxford University Press, 1995.

Hart, Kylo-Patrick R. *The AIDS Movie: Representing a Pandemic in Film and Television*, 2nd edition. London and New York: Routledge, 2013.

Hawkins, Anne Hunsaker. *Reconstructing Illness: Studies in Pathography*, 2nd edition. West Lafayette: Purdue University Press, 1998.

Hearn, Pat. 'Mark Morrisroe: A Survey from the Estate'. In *Boston School: Mark Morrisroe (1959–80), A Survey from the Estate*, edited by Lia Gangitano, 58–60. Boston: Institute of Contemporary Art, 1995.

Hebdige, Dick. 'Posing . . . Threats, Striking . . . Poses: Youth, Surveillance, and Display'. *SubStance* 37–38 (1983): 66–88.

Hedva, Johanna. 'Sick Woman Theory'. 2016. http://johannahedva.com/SickWomanTheory_Hedva_2020.pdf.

Heiferman, Marvin. 'Pictures of Life and Loss'. In *Nan Goldin: I'll Be Your Mirror*, edited by Nan Goldin, David Armstrong and Hans Werner Holzworth, 277–82. New York: Whitney Museum of American Art, 1996.

Hess, Elizabeth. 'Safe Combat in the Erogenous Zone'. *The Village Voice*, 10 January 1989.

hooks, bell. 'Is Paris Burning?' In *Black Looks: Race and Representation*, 145–56. London: South End Press, 1992.

Houser, Craig. 'I, Abject'. In *Abject Art: Repulsion and Desire in American Art*, edited by Jack Ben-Levi, Leslie C. Jones, Craig Houser, and Simon Taylor, 85–100. New York: Whitney Museum of American Art, 1993.

Howgate, Sarah and Sandy Nairne. *A Guide to Contemporary Portraits.* London: National Portrait Gallery, 2009.

Hudson, Jane. 'Comments on Mark Morrisroe: The Punk Years at the Museum School'. In *Boston School: Mark Morrisroe (1959–80), A Survey from the Estate*, edited by Lia Gangitano, 63–5. Boston: Institute of Contemporary Art, 1995.

Interview at the Bronx Museum of Art with Sur Rodney (Sur) and Kia LaBeija), 12 February 2016. https://youtu.be/AOLShR_Vq48.

Jay, Martin. 'The Uncanny Nineties'. In *Cultural Semantics: Keywords of Our Time*, 157–64. Cambridge, MA: University of Massachusetts Press, 1998.

Johnstone, Fiona. 'Mark Morrisroe's Self-Portraits and Jacques Derrida's "Ruin"'. *Third Text* 25, no. 6 (2011): 799–809.

Johnstone, Fiona and Kirstie Imber. 'Introducting the Anti-Portrait'. In *Anti-Portraiture: Challenging the Limits of the Portrait*, edited by Fiona Johnstone, 1–23. London and New York: Bloomsbury, 2020.

Jones, Amelia. *Self/Image: Technology, Representation, and the Contemporary Subject*. New York: Routledge, 2006.

Jones, Darren. 'Galleries Representing Felix Gonzalez-Torres Are Editing HIV/AIDS from His Legacy: It Needs To Stop'. *Artslant* (blog), May 2017. https://www.poz.com/article/galleries-representing-felix-gonzalez-torres-editing-hiv-aids-from-his-legacy.

Jordan-Zachery, Julia S. 'Safe, Soulful Sex: HIV/AIDS Talk'. In *AIDS and the Distribution of Crises*, edited by Jih-Fei Cheng, Alexandra Juhasz, and Nishant Shahani, 93–130. Durham: Duke University Press, 2020.

Jordan-Zachery, Julia S.. *Shadow Bodies: Black Women, Ideology, Representation, and Politics*. New Brunswick: Rutgers University Press, 2017.

Joselit, David. 'Mark Morrisroe's Photographic Masquerade'. In *Boston School: Mark Morrisroe (1959–80), A Survey from the Estate*, edited by Lia Gangitano, 66–80. Boston: Institute of Contemporary Art, 1995.

Joselit, David and Collier Schorr. 'Mark Morrisroe: Photographic Process and Psychic Structure'. *Panel Discussion, Artists Space, New York*, 16 April 2011.

Juhasz, Alexandra. *AIDS TV: Identity, Community, and Alternative Video*. Durham and London: Duke University Press, 1995.

Juhasz, Alexandra. 'The Contained Threat: Women in Mainstream AIDS Documentary'. *Journal of Sex Research* 21, no. 1 (1990): 25–46.

Juhasz, Alexandra and Theodore (Ted) Kerr. 'On Care, Activism, and HIV'. In *Health*, edited by Bárbara Rodríguez Muñoz, Whitechapel Documents of Contemporary Art, 37–42, London and Cambridge MA: Whitechapel Gallery and the MIT Press, 2020.

Juhasz, Alexandra and Theodore (Ted) Kerr. *We Are Having This Conversation Now: The Times of AIDS Cultural Production*. Durham: Duke University Press, 2022.

Juhasz, Alexandra and Theodore (Ted) Kerr. 'Who Are the Stewards of the AIDS Archive? Sharing the Political Weight of the Intimate'. In *The Unfinished Queer Agenda After Marraige Equality*, edited by Angela Jones, Joseph Nicholas DeFilippis, and Michael W. Yarbrough, 88–101. London: Routledge, 2018.

Juno, Andrea and V. Vale. *Bob Flanagan: Supermasochist*. San Francisco: Research Publications, 1993.

Kafer, Alison. *Feminist, Queer, Crip*. Bloomington and Indianapolis: Indiana University Press, 2013.

Kagan, Dion. *Positive Images: Gay Men and HIV/AIDS in the Culture of 'Post-Crisis'*. London and New York: IB Tauris, 2018.

Katz, Jonathan. 'Hide/Seek: Portraits by Felix Gonzalez-Torres and David Wojnarowicz'. Accessed 8 April 2014. https://www.youtube.com/watch?v=4iiLMJru7SY.

Katz, Jonathan. 'How AIDS Changed American Art'. In *Art AIDS America*, edited by Jonathan D. Katz and Rock Hushka, 24–45. Tacoma, Seattle and London: Tacoma Art Museum in association with University of Washington Press, 2015.

Katz, Jonathan. 'In/Different America and AIDS'. In *Art AIDS America Chicago*, edited by Staci Boris, 37–47. Chicago: Alphawood Foundation, 2018.

Kern, Stephen. *The Culture of Time and Space, 1880–1918*. Cambridge, MA: Harvard University Press, 1983.

Kerr, Theodore (Ted). 'A History of Erasing Black Artists and Bodies from the AIDS Conversation'. *Hyperallergic*, 31 December 2015. https://hyperallergic.com/264934/a-history-of-erasing-black-artists-and-bodies-from-the-aids-conversation/.

Kerr, Theodore (Ted). 'AIDS – Based on a True Story'. *Dandelion* 7, no. 1 (2016). https://dandelionjournal.org/article/doi/10.16995/ddl.341/.

Kerr, Theodore (Ted). 'AIDS 1969: HIV, History, and Race'. *Drain*, 2016. http://drainmag.com/aids-1969-hiv-history-and-race/.

Kerr, Theodore (Ted). 'As We Canonize Certain Producers of Culture We Are Closing Space for a Complication of Narratives'. *The Visual AIDS Blog* (blog), 10 December 2013. https://visualaids.org/blog/as-we-canonize-certain-producers-of-culture-we-are-closing-space-for-a-comp.

Kerr, Theodore (Ted). 'Time Is Not a Line: Conversations, Essays, and Images about HIV/AIDS Now'. *We Who Feel Differently*, Fall 2014. http://wewhofeeldifferently.info/journal.php.

Kerr, Theodore (Ted). 'What You Don't Know About AIDS Could Fill a Museum: Curatorial Ethics and the Ongoing Epidemic in the 21st Century'. *On Curating* 42 (2019): 5–17.

Kerr, Theodore (Ted), Amy Sadao, and Nelson Santos. 'Love Happended Here: Art, Archives, and a Living History'. In *Art AIDS America*, edited by Jonathan Katz and Rock Hushka, 62–73. Tacoma, Seattle and London: Tacoma Art Museum in association with University of Washington Press, 2016.

Kevles, Bettyann. *Naked to the Bone: Medical Imaging in the Twentieth Century*. New Brunswick: Rutgers University Press, 1997.

Kleinman, Arthur. *The Illness Narratives: Suffering, Healing, and the Human Condition*. New York: Basic Books, 1988.

Knezevich, Steve. 'Robert Blanchon at LACPS'. *LA Weekly*, 26 December 1996.

Kotz, Liz. 'Aesthetics of "Intimacy"'. In *The Passionate Camera: Photography and Bodies of Desire*, edited by Deborah Bright, 204–15. London and New York: Routledge, 1998.

Kramer, Larry. *The Normal Heart*. London: Methuen and the Royal Court Theatre, 1986.

Krauss, Rosalind. 'Notes on the Index: Part 1'. *October* 3 (Spring 1977): 68–81.

Krauss, Rosalind. 'The Crisis of the Easel Picture'. In *Jackson Pollock: New Approaches*, edited by Kirk Varnedoe and Pepe Karmel, 155–79. New York: The Museum of Modern Art & Harry Abrams, 1999.

Krauss, Rosalind. *The Optical Unconscious*. Cambridge, MA: MIT Press, 1993.

Kraynak, Janet. 'Nan Goldin's "Witnesses: Against Our Vanishing"'. In *Witness to Her Art: Art and Writings*, edited by Michael Brenson and Rhea Anastas, 34–41. New York: Bard College, 2006.

Kristeva, Julia. *Black Sun: Depression and Melancholia*. Translated by Leon S. Roudiez. New York: Columbia University Press, 1989.

Kristeva, Julia. *Powers of Horror: An Essay on Abjection*. Translated by Leon S. Roudiez. New York: Columbia University Press, 1982.

Kwon, Miwon. 'The Becoming of a Work of Art: FGT and a Possibility of Renewal, a Chance to Share, a Fragile Truce'. In *Felix Gonzalez-Torres*, edited by Julie Ault, 281–314. New York and Gottingen: Steidl, 2006.

LaBeija, Kia. 'Rebirth'. *TDR: The Drama Review* 60, no. 4 (2016): 2–3.

LaBeija, Kia and Alex Fialho. 'Living Free: Kia LaBeija, From Pathology to Wholeness'. *Lecture and Conversation, IDA Stanford*, 17 May 2017. https://www.youtube.com/watch?v=7jrbUspNXkE.

Lampert, Catherine. 'Family of Own Gender'. In *The Devil's Playground*, edited by Nan Goldin, 56–7. London: Phaidon, 2003.

Leader, Darian. *The New Black: Mourning, Melancholia and Depression*. London: Penguin, 2009.

Lebovici, Elisabeth. 'In the Darkroom'. In *Mark Morrisroe*, edited by Beatrix Ruf and Thomas Seelig, 228–39. Zurich: JPR Ringier, 2010.

L'Ecole, du Magasin, ed. *AIDS RIOT: Artist Collectives Against AIDS, New York, 1987–94*. 12e Session de l'Ecole Du Magasin. Grenoble: Magasin, 2003.

Leiris, Michel. *Scratches*. Translated by Lydia Davis. Vol. 1. The Rules of the Game. Baltimore and London: The John Hopkins University Press, 1991.

Levinas, Emmanuel. *Ethics and Infinity: Conversations with Philippe Nemo*. Translated by Richard A. Cohen. Pittsburgh: Duquesne University Press, 1985.

Levinas, Emmanuel and Richard Kearney. 'Dialogue with Emmanuel Levinas'. In *Face to Face with Levinas*, edited by Richard A. Cohen, 13–33. Albany: State University of New York Press, 1986.

Levine, Sherrie. 'Five Comments'. In *Blasted Allegories: An Anthology of Writing by Contemporary Artists*, edited by Brian Wallis, 92–3. New York: The New Museum, 1987.

Linfield, Susie. *The Cruel Radiance: Photography and Political Violence*. Chicago: Chicago University Press, 2011.

Lingis, Alphonso. *Libido*. Albany: SUNY Press, 1985.

Lippit, Akira Mizuta. *Atomic Light (Shadow Optics)*. Minneapolis: University of Minnesota Press, 2005.

Lippit, Akira Mizuta. 'Reflections on Spectral Life'. *Discourse* 30, no. 1–2 (2008): 242–54.

Livingston, Jane. 'Man Ray and Surrealist Photography'. In *L'Amour Fou: Photography & Surrealism*, edited by Rosalind Krauss and Jane Livingston, 115–47. New York: Abbeville Press, 1985.

Lombroso, Cesare. *Criminal Man*. Translated by Mary Gibson and Nicole Hahn Rafter. Durham: Duke University Press, 2006.

Lowery, Jack. *It Was Vulgar And It Was Beautiful: How AIDS Activists Used Art to Fight a Pandemic*. New York: Bold Type Books, 2022.

MacKinnon, Kenneth. 'After Mulvey: Male Erotic Objectification'. In *The Body's Perilous Pleasures: Dangerous Desires and Contemporary Culture*, edited by Michele Aaron, 13–29. Edinburgh: Edinburgh University Press, 1999.

Mann, Thomas. *The Magic Mountain*. Translated by H.T. Lowe-Porter. London: Secker and Warburg, 1946.

Marks, Laura U. *The Skin of the Film: Intercultural Cinema, Embodiment, and the Senses*. Durham and London: Duke University Press, 2000.

Marshall, Richard, ed. *Robert Mapplethorpe: Autoportrait*. Santa Fe: Arena Editions, 2001.

Mattison, Robert. *Robert Rauschenberg: Breaking Boundaries*. New Haven: Yale University Press, 2003.

McClelland, Alexander and Jessica Whitbread. 'PosterVirus: Claiming Sexual Autonomy for People with HIV through Collective Action'. In *Mobilizing Metaphor: Art, Culture, and Disability Activism in Canada*, edited by Christine Kelly and Michael Orsini, 76–97. Vancouver and Toronto: UBC Press, 2016.

McKay, Richard A. *Patient Zero and the Making of the AIDS Epidemic*. Chicago and London: University of Chicago Press, 2017.

McPhillips, Ramsey. 'Who Turned out the Limelight? The Tragi-Comedy of Mark Morrisroe'. In *Loss Within Loss: Artists in the Age of AIDS*, edited by Edmund White, 98–112. Madison: University of Wisconsin Press, 2001.

Meade, Fionn. 'At the Eleventh Hour'. In *Mark Morrisroe*, edited by Beatrix Ruf and Thomas Seelig, 130–7. Zurich: JRP Ringier, 2010.

Mercer, Kobena. 'Stuart Hall and the Visual Arts'. *Small Axe* 19, no. 1 (2015): 78–87.

Merleau-Ponty, Maurice. *The Phenomenology of Perception*. Translated by Colin Smith. London and New York: Routledge, 2002.

Meyer, Richard. 'Imagining Sadomasochism: Robert Mapplethorpe and the Masquerade of Photography'. *Qui Parle* 4, no. 1 (Fall 1990): 62–78.

Meyer, Richard. 'Rock Hudson's Body'. In *The Passionate Camera: Photography and Bodies of Desire*, edited by Deborah Bright, 341–60. London and New York: Routledge, 1998.

Molesworth, Helen. 'Stops and Starts'. *October* 92 (2000): 157–62.

Mulvey, Laura. 'A Phantasmagoria of the Female Body: The Work of Cindy Sherman'. *New Left Review* 1, no. 188 (August 1991): 137–51.

Mulvey, Laura. 'Visual Pleasure and Narrative Cinema'. *Screen* 16, no. 3 (1975): 6–18.

Muñoz, José Esteban. 'Morrisroe's Melodramatics'. presentation, Artists Space, New York, 23 April 2011. http://artistsspace.org/programs/mark-morrisroe-neo-romantic-iconography-and-the-performance-of-self/.

Nead, Lynda. *The Female Nude: Art, Obscenity and Sexuality*. London and New York: Routledge, 1992.
Nickas, Robert. 'Felix Gonzalez-Torres: All the Time in the World'. In *Felix Gonzalez-Torres*, edited by Julie Ault, 39–51. New York and Gottingen: Steidl, 2006.
Nixon, Nicholas and Bébé Nixon. *People with AIDS*. Boston: David R. Godine, 1991.
Ogden, Bethany. 'Through the Image: Nicholas Nixon's 'People With AIDS''. *Discourse* 23, no. 3 (2001): 75–105.
Olander, William. 'The Window on Broadway by ACT UP/On View at the New Museum, November 20, 1987, to January 24, 1988'. *New Museum Digital Archive*, 20 November 1987. http://archive.newmuseum.org/index.php/Detail/Object/Show/object_id/7910.
Omer-Sherman, Ranen. 'The Fate of the Other in Tony Kushner's "Angels in America"'. *Melus* 32, no. 2 (2007): 7–30.
Owens, Craig. 'Posing'. In *Beyond Recognition: Representation, Power, and Culture*, edited by Scott Bryson, Barbara Kruger, Lynne Tillman and Jane Weinstock, 201–17. Berkeley: University of California Press, 1992.
Owens, Craig. 'The Discourse of Others: Feminists and Postmodernism'. In *Postmodern Culture*, edited by Hal Foster, 57–82. London: Pluto Press, 1985.
Palmer, Tyrone. 'Under the Rainbow'. *The New Inquiry*, 28 July 2015. https://thenewinquiry.com/under-the-rainbow/.
Paster, Gail Kern. *The Body Embarrased: Drama and the Discipline of Shame in Early Modern England*. New York: Cornell University Press, 1993.
Patton, Cindy. *Last Served? Gendering the AIDS Pandemic*. London: Taylor and Francis, 1994.
Pearl, Monica. '"A Thousand Kindred Spirits" Reflections on AIDS Activism and Representations of AIDS in US Culture and Conversation'. *Radical History Review* 140 (2021): 217–25.
Pearl, Monica. *AIDS Literature and Gay Identity: The Literature of Loss*. New York and London: Routledge, 2013.
Phelan, Peggy. *Unmarked: The Politics of Performance*. London and New York: Routledge, 1993.
Piggford, George. '"In Time of Plague": AIDS and Its Significations in Hervé Guibert, Tony Kushner and Thom Gunn'. *Cultural Critique* 44 (2000): 169–96.
Pollock, Griselda. 'Artists, Mythologies and Media – Genius, Madness and Art History'. *Screen* 21, no. 3 (1980): 57–96.
PWA Coalition. 'PWA Coalition Portfolio'. *October* 43 (1987): 147–68.
Radley, Alan. *Works of Illness: Narrative, Picturing and the Social Response to Disease*. Ashby-de-la-Zouch: Inkerman Press, 2009.
Riese Hubert, Renée. 'From Déjeuner En Fourrure to Caroline: Meret Oppenheim's Chronicle of Surrealism'. In *Surrealism and Women*, edited by Mary Ann Caws, Rudolf Kuenzli, and Gwen Raaberg, 37–49. Cambridge, MA: MIT Press, 1991.

Riviere, Joan. 'Womanliness as Masquerade'. In *Psychoanalysis and Female Sexuality*, edited by Henrik M Ruitenbeck, 209–20. New Haven: College and University Press, 1966.

Roberts, John. 'The Museum and the Crisis of Critical Postmodernism'. *Third Text* 11, no. 41 (1997): 67–74.

Rodriguez, Bill. 'Biomedical Models of HIV and Women'. In *The Gender Politics of HIV/AIDS in Women*, edited by Nancy Goldstein and Jennifer L. Manlowe, 25–42. Perspectives on the Pandemic in the United States. New York and London: New York University Press, 1997.

Rollins, Tim. 'Felix Gonzalez-Torres: Interview'. In *Felix Gonzalez-Torres*, edited by William S. Bartman, 5–31. New York: ART Press, 1993.

Rosen, Andrea. '"Untitled" (The Neverending Portrait)'. In *Felix Gonzalez-Torres*, edited by Dietmar Elger, 44–59. Stuttgart: Cantz Verlag, 1997.

Rosenblum, Robert. 'Life Versus Death: The Art World in Crisis'. In *Art against AIDS*, edited by Rosenblum, 28–32. New York: American Foundation for AIDS Research, 1987.

Rosler, Martha. 'In, Around, and Afterthoughts (on Documentary Photography)'. In *3 Works*, 59–86. Halifax: The Press of Nova Scotia College of Art and Design, 1981.

Rounthwaite, Adair. 'Split Witness: Metaphorical Extensions of Life in the Art of Felix Gonzalez-Torres'. *Representations* 109 (Winter 2010): 35–56.

Russell, John. 'Images of Grief and Rage in Exhibition on AIDS'. *The New York Times*, 16 November 1989.

Sadao, Amy. 'Foreword'. In *Robert Blanchon*, edited by Tania Duvergne and Amy Sadao, 9–10. New York: Visual AIDS, 2006.

Saltzmann, Lisa. 'Reconsidering the Stain: On Gender, Identity, and the New York School Painting'. In *Reading Abstract Expressionism: Context and Critique*, edited by Ellen Landau, 560–80. New Haven: Yale University Press, 2005.

Sanchez, Rafael and Sur Rodney Sur. The Architecture of Loss: Mark Morrisroe, 1959–89, April 2011. http://www.thebody.com/visualaids/web_gallery/2011/sanchez/statement_full.html.

Sandahl, Carrie. 'Bob Flanagan: Taking It Like a Man'. *Journal of Dramatic Theory and Criticism* XV, no. 1 (2000): 97–104.

Sandell, Richard. *Museums, Moralities, and Human Rights*. London and New York: Routledge, 2017.

Sante, Luc. 'All Yesterday's Parties'. In *Nan Goldin: I'll Be Your Mirror*, edited by Nan Goldin, David Armstrong and Hans Werner Holzworth, 97–103. New York: Whitney Museum of American Art, 1996.

Schwabsky, Barry. 'Irresponsible Images: The Photographs of Mark Morrisroe'. *The Print Collector's Newsletter* 25, no. 2 (June 1994): 49–50.

Sekula, Allan. 'Dismantling Modernism, Reinventing Documentary (Notes on the Politics of Representation)'. *The Massachusetts Review* 19, no. 4 (1978): 859–83.

Sekula, Allan. *Photography Against the Grain: Essays and Photo Works, 1973–83*. Halifax: Press of the Nova Scotia College of Art and Design, 1984.

Sekula, Allan. 'The Body and the Archive'. *October* 39 (1986): 3–64.

Serres, Michel. *Rome: The Book of Foundations*. Stanford: Stanford University Press, 1991.

Shahani, Nishant. 'How to Survive the Whitewashing of AIDS: Global Pasts, Transnational Futures'. *QED: A Journal in GLBTQ Worldmaking* 3, no. 1 (2016): 1–33.

Sheehan, Carrie C. 'Securitizing the HIV/AIDS Pandemic in U.S. Foreign Policy'. Doctoral Thesis, American University, 2008.

Shilts, Randy. *And the Band Played On*. London and New York: Penguin, 1987.

Sikora, Tomasz. 'Queer Life-Worlds and the Art of David Wojnarowicz'. *Journal of Gender Studies* 29, no. 1 (2020): 76–87.

Singerman, Howard. 'In Theory and Practice: A History of the Whitney Independent Study Program'. *Artforum*, February 2004, 112–17 and 170–1.

Sirasi, Nancy. *Medieval and Early Renaissance Medicine*. Chicago: University of Chicago Press, 1990.

Smith, Giulia. 'Carolyn Lazard'. *Art Monthly*, 2019.

Smith, Giulia. 'Chronic Illness as Critique: Crip Aesthetics Across the Atlantic'. *Art History* 44, no. 2 (2021): 286–310.

Smith, Roberta. 'Felix Gonzalez-Torres, 38, A Sculptor of Love and Loss'. *The New York Times*, 11 January 1996.

Smith, Sidonie and Julia Watson. *Reading Autobiography: A Guide for Interpreting Life Narratives*. Minneapolis: University of Minnesota Press, 2001.

Smith, Sidonie and Julia Watson. 'The Rumpled Bed of Autobiography: Extravagant Lives, Extravagant Questions'. *Biography* 24, no. 1 (Winter 2001): 1–14.

Sokolowski, Thomas. 'Preface'. In *Portraits in the Time of AIDS*, edited by Rosalind Solomon. New York: Grey Art Gallery & Study Center, 1988.

Solomon, Rosalind. *Portraits in the Time of AIDS*. New York: Grey Art Gallery & Study Center, 1988.

Sontag, Susan. *On Photography*. Harmondsworth: Penguin, 1979.

Spector, Nancy. *Felix Gonzalez-Torres*. New York: Guggenheim Museum Publications, 1995.

Spender, Stephen. 'Confessions and Autobiography'. In *Autobiography: Essays Theoretical and Critical*, edited by James Olney, 115–21. Princeton: Princeton University Press, 1980.

Stacey, Jackie, and Mary Bryson. 'Queering the Temporality of Cancer Survivorship'. *Aporia* 4, no. 1 (January 2012): 5–17.

Stahl, Devan. 'Living into the Imagined Body: How the Diagnostic Image Confronts the Lived Body'. *Medical Humanities* 39, no. 1 (2013): 53–8.

Stallybrass, Peter and Allon White. 'The Sewer, the Gaze and the Contaminating Touch'. In *The Politics and Poetics of Transgression*, 125–48. London: Methuen, 1986.

Stoller, Nancy E. 'Foucault in the Streets: New York City Act(s) UP'. In *Lessons from the Damned: Queers, Whores, and Junkies Respond to AIDS*, edited by Nancy E. Stoller, 113–33. New York and London: Routledge, 1988.

Storr, Robert. 'Felix Gonzalez-Torres: Being a Spy'. *Art Press* 198 (January 1995): 24–32.

Storr, Robert. 'Felix Gonzalez-Torres: Être Un Espion'. In *Felix Gonzalez-Torres*, edited by Julie Ault, 229–39. New York and Gottingen: Steidl, 2006.

Storr, Robert. 'When This You See Remember Me'. In *Felix Gonzalez-Torres*, edited by Julie Ault, 5–37. New York and Gottingen: Steidl, 2006.

Sturken, Marita. *Tangled Memories: The Vietnam War, the AIDS Epidemic, and the Politics of Remembering*. Berkeley and London: University of California Press, 1997.

Sullivan, Andrew. 'When Plagues End'. *New York Times Magazine*, 10 November 1996.

Sussman, Elisabeth. *Nan Goldin: I'll Be Your Mirror*. New York: Whitney Museum of American Art, 1996.

Sussman, Elisabeth. 'Robert Gober: Installation and Sculpture'. In *Robert Gober: Sculptures and Installations, 1979–2007*, edited by Theodora Vischer, 16–31. Basel: Schaulager Basel, 2007.

Tacoma Action Collective. 'Press Release, Die In Protest 12/7 at Tacoma Art Museum'. Tumblr, 24 December 2015. https://stoperasingblackpeoplenow.tumblr.com.

Taylor, Simon. 'The Phobic Object: Abjection in Contemporary Art'. In *Abject Art: Repulsion and Desire in American Art*, 59–83. New York: Whitney Museum of American Art, 1993.

Teigrob, Robert. 'Robert Mapplethorpe'. In *Culture Wars: An Encyclopedia of Issues, Viewpoints, and Voices*, edited by Roger Chapman, 336–7. New York: M.E. Sharpe, 2010.

Tembeck, Tamar, ed. *Auto/Pathographies*. Alma: Sagamie édition d'art, 2014.

Tembeck, Tamar. 'Selfies of Ill Health: Online Autopathographic Photography and the Dramaturgy of the Everyday'. *Social Media + Society* 2, no. 1 (2016). https://doi.org/10.1177/2056305116641343.

Townsend, Chris. *Art and Death*. London and New York: I.B. Tauris, 2008.

Treichler, Paula. 'AIDS, Homophobia and Biomedical Discourse: An Epidemic of Signification'. *October* 43 (1987): 31–70.

Treichler, Paula. *How to Have Theory in an Epidemic: Cultural Chronicles of AIDS*. Durham and London: Duke University Press, 1999.

Tronto, Joan. *Moral Boundaries: A Political Arguement for an Ethics of Care*. London: Routledge, 1993.

Vance, Carol S. 'The Pleasures of Looking: The Attorney General's Commission on Pornography versus Visual Images'. In *The Critical Image: Essays on Contemporary Photography*, edited by Carol Squiers, 38–58. Seattle: Bay Press, 1990.

'Visual AIDS' Panel, The Personal and the Political: Losing Parents to AIDS, with Alysia Abbott, Kia Benbow, Mathew Rodrigues, and Sarah Shulman, Hosted by the New York Public Library'. April 2014. https://www.youtube.com/watch?v=BnZsMDEZV98.

Waldman, Diane. 'The Language of Signs'. In *Jenny Holzer*, 17–27. New York: Guggenheim Museum Publications, 1989.

Wallis, Brian, Marianne Weems, and Philip Yenawine, eds. *Art Matters: How the Culture Wars Changed America*. New York: New York University Press, 1999.

Watney, Simon. 'In Purgatory: The Work of Felix Gonzalez-Torres'. *Parkett* 39 (1994): 38–44.

Watney, Simon. *Policing Desire: Pornography, AIDS and The Media*, 3rd edition. London: Cassell, 1997.

Watney, Simon. 'The Spectacle of AIDS'. *October* 43 (Winter 1987): 71–86.

Weinberg, Jonathan. *Fantastic Tales: The Photography of Nan Goldin*. London: Tate Publishing/The Pennsylvania State University Press, 2005.

Whitehead, Anne and Angela Woods. 'Introduction'. In *The Edinburgh Companion to the Critical Medical Humanities*, edited by Anne Whitehead and Angela Woods, 1–49. Edinburgh: Edinburgh University Press, 2016.

Wojnarowicz, David. 'Postcards from America: X-Rays from Hell'. In *Witnesses: Against Our Vanishing*, edited by Nan Goldin, 6–11. New York: Artists Space, 1989.

Wollen, Audrey. 'Tell Me about Sad Girl Theory'. Instagram photo. *@tragicqueen* (blog), 22 June 2014.

Woods, Angela. 'Beyond the Wounded Storyteller: Rethinking Narrativity, Illness and Embodied Self-Experience'. In *Health, Illness and Disease: Philosophical Essays*, edited by Havi Carel and Rachel Cooper. Newcastle: Acumen, 2013.

Woods, Angela. 'The Limits of Narrative: Provocations for the Medical Humanities'. *Med Humanities* 37 (2011): 73–8.

Yablonsky, Linda. 'Mark Morrisroe in New York'. In *Mark Morrisroe*, edited by Beatrix Ruf and Thomas Seelig, 296–303. Zurich: JRP Ringier, 2010.

Yingling, Thomas E. *AIDS and the National Body*. Durham and London: Duke University Press, 1997.

Index